Published by Placedo Publishing

ISBN-13 978-1-51934-585-1

Also available as a Kindle ebook
ISBN-13 978-1-84396-263-2

A CIP catalogue record for this
book is available from the British Library

Pre-press production
eBook Versions
127 Old Gloucester Street
London WC1N 3AX
www.ebookversions.com

Real Secrets of Alternative Medicine

An Exposé

Dr Richard Rawlins
MB BS MBA FRCS MMC

Honorary Consultant Orthopaedic and Trauma Surgeon, Bedford Hospital
Fellow of the British Orthopaedic Association
Member of the Representative Body, British Medical Association
Liveryman of the Worshipful Society of Apothecaries
Freeman of the City of London

Member of The Magic Circle

Formerly:
Lecturer in Anatomy, King's College, London
Recognised Clinical Teacher, Cambridge University

Chairman:
Hospital Doctors Association
UK Consultants Conference
BMA Clinical Audit Committee
Advisory Council, Health Quality Service

Member:
Management Board, National Centre for Clinical Audit
Board of Science, BMA
Associate Member:
General Medical Council

Member of the Editorial Boards of:
Hospital Doctor
Journal of the Association for Quality in Healthcare
Journal of Evaluation in Clinical Practice
Forum for Alternative and Complementary Therapies

Surgeon Lieutenant Commander, Royal Naval Reserve

Mentalist of the Year, Riviera Circle of Magicians

Placebo Publishing
Dartmouth, Devon, UK

Contents

Copyright & Credits

For further information about styles and titles used in
orthodox medicine, bibliography, further guidance and frequently
asked questions, please refer to:

www.placedo.co.uk

A Conversation with Mrs. Smith

'Now Mrs. Smith, let us see where we've got to. Your family doctor sent you to see me because of pain around your hips, which he was no longer able to treat with straightforward painkillers. I agree that you will now have to consider having reconstructive surgery – a total hip joint replacement. I am going to give you information sheets explaining this proposal in detail and will be seeing you again to answer any questions.'

I could tell Mrs. Smith had already considered the possibility of a hip replacement. I knew she had discussed the issues with her family doctor, but she remained undecided.

'I thought that is what you would be saying doctor, but I've been doing a bit of reading on the Internet and I wondered if I might try any alternative medicine before I have to have an operation.'

One or two patients a week raised this issue, and I reiterated my standard reply:

'I have absolutely no objection to you trying any supplementary, complementary, or alternative medicine you fancy. Some patients say they benefit, but interesting anecdotes of personal experience are no substitute for critical analysis of plausible evidence and I know of no evidence to suggest that you will have any significant benefit. I appreciate some patients are dissatisfied with conventional treatment and tell me they do feel better after seeing an alternative medicine practitioner, so by all means go ahead and try.'

'But do you know which is most likely to help me? Can there be side effects? It seems a lot of patients are trying complementary approaches and alternative medicine nowadays. Is it a waste of time and money? Are they being fooled? Or are they just fooling themselves?'

'Very interesting questions but I can make no recommendations. I cannot see that any modality claimed to be 'complementary' is needed to complete any conventional treatment. The term 'alternative medicine' describes systems requiring an alternative mindset and belief system to that of rational science. 'Integrative medicine' is used by those who are in denial as to the nature of reality and those who intend misleading patients by using novel terms for marketing purposes. Although I have read a little about these alternative medical systems, I have not studied them in any detail.'

'Perhaps you should doctor. And then write a book...'

1

Part One:
In the beginning

Chapter 1

Beyond the Syringe

There cannot be two kinds of medicine – conventional and alternative. There is only medicine that has been adequately tested and medicine that has not, medicine that works and medicine that may or may not work.
Marcy Angell, Jerome Kassirer[1]

Either it is true that a medicine works or it isn't.
It cannot be false in the ordinary sense but true in some "alternative" sense.
Richard Dawkins[2]

The history of medicine is largely the history of placebo effects.
Arthur Shapiro[3]

When science is abused, hijacked or distorted in order to serve political or ideological belief systems, ethical standards will inevitably slip. The resulting pseudoscience is a deceit perpetrated on the weak and vulnerable. We owe it to ourselves and to those who come after us, to stand up for the truth, no matter how much trouble this might bring.
Edzard Ernst[4]

There's no such thing as alternative medicine. If an alternative medicine works, then it's medicine, and if an alternative medicine doesn't work, then it's not an alternative.
Paul Offit[5]

Medicine: 'The science or practice of the diagnosis, treatment, and prevention of disease.' Disease: 'A disorder of structure or function in a human, animal, or plant, especially one that produces specific symptoms or that affects a specific location.'
Oxford Dictionaries

Patient care and 'medicine' has evolved. In addition to conventional orthodox medicine, a group of systems known as Supplementary, Complementary and Alternative Medicine has become more clearly delineated. The 'S' is usually set aside and these alternative systems are now commonly referred to as 'CAM'. Direct out of pocket expenditure on eight of the more established alternative therapies in the UK has been estimated at between £580M and £1.6B per year and the NHS funds nearly ten per cent of this. Each year, Americans spend more than $34 billion on Complementary and Alternative Medicine; the French, €279M for homeopathic remedies; Australians, $A164M on 'natural therapies'. Is this wise? Are resources being wasted? Could they be better spent? Wikipedia advises:

> Alternative medicine is any practice that is presented as having the healing effects of medicine, but is not based on evidence gathered using the scientific method. The treatments are those that are not part of the conventional, science-based healthcare system. Complementary medicine is alternative medicine used together with conventional medical treatment in a belief, not proven by using scientific methods, that it 'complements' the treatment.

By the definitions applied in this book, there is no plausible evidence these practices actually do have any 'healing effects of medicine'. There is no reproducible evidence that CAM pills, pin punctures, pushing, prodding, potions or paranormal preternatural powers have any effect on specific disease processes – though patients may 'feel better'. Revelation of this simple fact is tantamount to exposure of how magicians' tricks are done, and can meet with comparable antagonism from those who would prefer to have patients duped, politicians inveigled, the public misled and health care fraud committed. Inevitably, revealing these secrets causes opposition from the deluded – and denigration from the greedy who prey on the needy.

The term *alternative medicine* entered common use during the 1970s with the alternative lifestyle movement. Later, stimulated by the requirements of marketing and branding and in an attempt to have alternative systems included in conventional medicine, *complementary* became fashionable. I coin *camistry* as a synonym to describe the field of practices and philosophies which are represented by CAM and which provide treatment, remedies and care metaphorically 'beyond the syringe' of scientific evidence-based conventional medicine. I term those who practice camistry, *camists*. In 2005 the Health Survey for England found 44% of respondents had used camistry at some time. I style these patients *camees,* as in 'trainees' or 'interviewees'.

In recent trends, the terms 'alternative' and even 'complementary' are avoided and *integrated* or *integrative* substituted. The US is now seeing the term 'complementary and integrative health disciplines' (CIH) used. This may be simple denial on the part of proponents as to the true nature of their practices, but may also be a deliberate attempt to mislead. You must be the judge as to whether there are attempts at an insurgency of fundamentalist and irrational beliefs, driven by the commercial interests of manufacturers and academic institutions who provide courses and seek funds for 'research'. Camees may find camistry pleasing, but tax-payers and insurance company clients should not be expected to pay for placebos which have no therapeutic effects on specific diseases. Making funds available for camistry represents a moral hazard by encouraging the consumption of unnecessary services. Those funds would be better spent on counselling, physiotherapy and support services. Fooling vulnerable and gullible patients on the grounds that 'it makes them feel better' and 'it's what they want' is patronising and unethical.

In this book, the term 'medicine' is applied widely – to the practice of registered medical practitioners, doctors, dentists, nurses, midwives and all colleagues in pharmacy and the fifteen other healthcare professions regulated by the UK Health Professions Council as of 1st January 2011, namely: arts therapists, biomedical scientists, chiropodists/podiatrists, clinical scientists, dieticians, hearing aid dispensers, occupational therapists, operating department practitioners, orthoptists, paramedics, physiotherapists, prosthetists/orthotists, clinical psychologists, radiographers, speech and language therapists. The HPC was renamed Health and Care Professions Council in 2012 when social workers were added.

Real Secrets deals with how 'healing practices' are perceived to provide benefit and to make patients 'feel better'. Any disease or illness may deteriorate. Beneficial outcomes patients perceive might be as a result of the specific treatment, but also as a result of non-specific factors such as spontaneous improvement, remission, fluctuation of symptoms, regression to the mean (a statistical phenomenon which will be considered later), and effects resulting from the consolation, hope and care provided by an empathetic practitioner in a constructive therapeutic relationship. The latter can be described as placebo or contextual effects.

Directed to patients, users of CAM, health practitioners, politicians, funders and members of the public more generally, *Real Secrets of Alternative Medicine* reveals how these placebo effects contribute to conventional holistic care and wellbeing. Care that provides opportunities for compassion, listening, explaining, encouraging. Care which offers consolation for present suffering, hope for the future and love at all times. *Real Secrets* considers how health professionals should answer Mrs. Smith's question – 'Will any alternative medicine help me?'

The origin of words is important in understanding their meaning and judging whether they are being used with integrity or with the intention of misleading the reader. In brackets I offer the origin of selected words – from Ancient Greek unless otherwise stated.

Part One considers the origins and development of scientific evidence based healthcare practices. Important considerations of happiness, a sense of wellbeing, contentment, emotional satisfaction and stress reduction are regarded as 'part of life' and are not considered here as being within the domain of 'medicine'. Part Two reviews Camistry – the remedies and practices which are used as alternatives to conventional, mainstream practices for treating disease, illness and injury, and/ or which require an alternative mind-set and way of thinking to the scientific.' Part

Three reveals how Camistry works, that is, by enabling patients to respond to their own expectations – effects described as *placebo* (Latin: I will please). Offit again: 'I think the placebo effect is often dismissed as "just in my head" and that's seen as dismissive. But the mind can be a powerful healing tool. The mind can regulate endorphins and cortisol, influencing one's immune system, blood pressure, and level of stress. So I think there is a physiology to placebo medicine.'[6]

Some people are attracted to the esoteric, and I coin *placedo,* with a *d,* to reflect those interests. Derived from *placere* – the Latin for 'to please' and *dō,* Japanese: 'the way' as in *judo,* the way of gentleness and *shinto,* the way of the gods. *Placedo* considers the 'way' or path to better understanding and use of placebo effects in the realm beyond the metaphorical syringe of convention. Placedo is practised by *placebists.*

Camistry works – but most camists would prefer you did not know the mechanism. Most practitioners and proponents of camistry prefer to keep secret the simple fact that camistry works through the power of placebo. That is the biggest of many secrets. Secrets which are hidden by camists' deliberate failure to publish plausible evidence, their pretence of being 'science-based practitioners', their attempts to mislead by using flowery and meaningless language, by disregarding critics and ignoring the conventions of modern medicine. This book might well have been titled *What Camists Don't Tell You.*

Camists claim their methods have direct effects on specific diseases. Many homeopaths and other camists even deride attempts to obtain evidence for the effects of their remedies, claiming evidence obtained by scientific methods is not necessary in order to endorse their beliefs. That is why their views represent faiths and are 'alternative'.

Throughout this book, the term 'belief' is taken to mean a firmly held opinion or conviction – 'an acceptance that something exists or is true, especially one without proof.' 'Knowledge' is taken to mean 'justified true belief' – with justification provided by scientific methods. 'Faith' is 'a strongly held belief' (Oxford Dictionaries). Absolute truth is like absolute zero temperature – it can never quite be reached. Most evidence relied on by camists is anecdotal and historical, not scientific and rational.

The difficulty of assessing whether a particular CAM 'works' was acknowledged by the Prince of Wales' Initiative on Integrated Medicine in 1997: 'To answer questions on the effectiveness of a therapy such as "Does it work?" requires clarity about the change that is expected as a result of an intervention and by whom; patient, therapist, relative, policy maker, etc. This can be particularly problematic in CAM if the desired outcome is not to "cure" or "fix" a problem but is to enable a condition to be better managed or coped with by a patient and carers, or for the patient to "heal" in a "deeper" sense and "come to terms" with their circumstances.' This is a coy way of explaining that CAMs provide no evidence of affecting diseases or illness any more than would be achieved by the powerful placebo effects from spending time in a constructive therapeutic relationship with an empathic practitioner.

In this book, I refer to some practitioners, some therapies and treatments, and some systems of medicine, not all. There is no absolute proof CAMs do not work as their proponents claim, but the probabilities are considered and opinions given are based on what is plausible, likely, reasonable and reproducible. Respect is given to people with different opinions, they are invited to reciprocate.

Some patients desire to follow the path of nothingness. Camistry may enhance a sense of wellbeing but there is no plausible evidence for therapeutically active forces or energies which can be manipulated or transmitted by ultra-dilutions, needles, hand movements, manipulation, crystals, talismans, symbols, or the stars. There is no plausible evidence that any of these dimensions exist in the real, substantive, immanent world − they are nonexistent nothingness. I term the path to wellbeing followed by their committed adherents *Wudo.* (Chinese: *wú,* nothing, nothingness, also 'spirit medium, shaman, magician, witch doctor'; Japanese: *dō,* way or path). Those who study and use placebo effects transparently and who seek a deeper understanding of the cultural, physiological, psychological, emotional and spiritual determinants which underline these effects I refer to as *placebists.*

The holism and attention to the spiritual domain which camists expound is not exclusive to them. As David Colquhoun and Steve Novella have emphasised: 'All good doctors are empathetic and patient-centered. The idea that empathy is restricted to those who practice unscientific medicine seems both condescending to doctors and it verges on an admission that empathy is all that alternative treatments have to offer.'

Most conventional practitioners now have special interests in one domain of practice. Many sub-specialise further, concentrating on one joint, organ, system or disease. The intellectual and professional landscape of modern practice is simply too large to do otherwise. But we all work in teams and together should be providing care for 'the whole person'. 'Holism' is not the exclusive preserve of camistry. All health care systems give consideration to diet, nutrition, exercise, massage, counselling, stress reduction, social determinants of health, the natural and built environment, employment, education, architecture, arts, and agriculture. Most CAMs are anachronistic − time has passed them by, being antithetical and opposed to modern advances of regulated scientific medicine. The majority of camists are not qualified in an orthodox profession. Those who are conventionally qualified may be practising unethically if they do not properly inform their patients as to the principles of their camist practices.

The Prince of Wales's Foundation for Integrated Health issued a report on the consumer perspective of CAM in 2001. In its forward, David Peters suggested the findings 'are of particular interest to anyone concerned with developing integrated health care.' He did not mean the integration of medical, social, mental and environmental health care but rather an insurgency so that CAM becomes incorporated with conventional medicine. Pseudo-science with science. He started from the premise that such integration *is* 'a good thing' rather than setting out to discover *whether* it is. This report failed to distinguish between the therapist and the therapy, practitioner and practice, style and substance. Camistry works. That is because of the time, care and attention paid by the therapist – not the specifics of the therapy. Conflating these two dimensions harms any critical analysis that can be given to each. By degrading this analysis, the advances made by scientific evidence-based health care are contaminated and impaired. That may be the intention of those associated with the 'College of Medicine' and similar lobby groups who endorse the insurgency of irrationality and camist 'integration'.

The World Health Organization (WHO) defines complementary or alternative medicine as 'a broad set of health care practices that are not part of that country's own tradition and are not integrated into the dominant health care system.' This could be why many CAM practitioners and supporters are currently keen to use the term 'integrated'. If CAMs were to be integrated, by definition, they would cease to be complementary or alternative. This may satisfy the ambitions of *wudoka* following the path of mysticism and *wu*, but patients would then be misled and denied their choice of preferred systems. Dr Mark Crislip puts it more bluntly: 'If you integrate fantasy with reality, you do not instantiate reality. If you mix cow pie with apple pie, it does not make the cow pie taste better; it makes the apple pie worse.'

'Integration' is opposed by some camists themselves as they fear the unique qualities and benefits of their practices would become subservient to the demands and dictates of modern health systems. Their systems would have to comply with the standards of scientific evidence and practice demanded by commissioners of regular health services and camists would no longer be able to offer patients the alternatives they desire. 'Integration' arises from Latin: *integrare*: 'to make whole'. 'Integrity' has the same origin, reflecting a 'sense of wholeness, perfect condition and hence 'the quality of being honest and having strong moral principles.' Whether those trying to turn the clock back and integrate anachronistic treatment methods with modern medicine are acting with integrity is for us all to judge.

In 2000, the House of Lords Select Committee on Science and Technology reported on Supplementary, Complementary, and Alternative Medicine, CAM.[7] The Lords' report identified three groups of different autonomous systems of medicine, based on novel theories of health and wellbeing, and which offer alternatives to evidence-based scientific, Conventional Orthodox Medicine, COM:

Group One: Systems regarded by the committee as being 'professionally organised': Osteopathy, chiropractic, homeopathy, acupuncture, and herbal medicine.

Group Two: Complementary Therapies which seem 'better established', but do not purport to embrace diagnostic skills: Alexander technique, bodywork therapies (including massage), counselling, stress therapy, hypnotherapy, reflexology, meditation, healing and shiatsu.

Group Three: Alternative Disciplines: (a) Long established and traditional systems of healthcare such as Indian Ayurvedic and Traditional Chinese. Often based on local flora, massage of different sorts and elaborate ceremonies and rituals. A wide variation of practices are seen, even within each tradition. (b) Other disciplines which lack any credible evidence base and comprise a wide variety of theatrical systems of 'medicine' and belief systems: Crystal therapy, iridology, radionics, dousing, applied kinesiology, energy therapies, spirit reading and 'other disciplines'.

The Lords' Committee did not consider every therapy, discipline or practice regarded as 'alternative'. The Prince's Foundation added aromatherapy, Bowen technique, cranial therapy, naturopathy, nutritional therapy, Reiki, and Yoga therapy. The British Complementary Medicine Association adds, amongst others: Angelic Reiki, Angel Therapy, Breathwork, Chakra Balancing, Colour Breathing, Buteyko Breathing, Bio-energy treatment, Colonic Hydrotherapy and irrigation, Completeness, Dianetics, Emotional Freedom Technique, Feng Shui, Flower Remedies, Gerson Therapy, Grounding, Holistic Massage, Holistic Podiatry, Holographic Re-patterning, Hopi Ear Candles, Indian Head Massage, Integrated Kabbalistic Healing, Iridology, Life Alignment, Lightening Process, Magno-Therapy, Magitherapy, Metamorphic Technique, Moxibustion, Multidimensional Healing, New German Medicine, Polarity Therapy, Shamballa, Tarot Reading, Therapeutic Magic, Theta Healing, Time Line Therapy, Thought Field Therapy, Transformative Mindfulness, Unani Tibb, Universal White Time Healing, Vibrational Energy Release.

All these practices are alternatives to evidence-based scientific medicine, each system and practice is individually autonomous, and being founded on incompatible principles, they are alternatives to each other. Some practitioners declare they are 'primary health-care professionals' (and are appropriate as the first to be consulted with a healthcare problem), but if they diagnose and treat diseases they are practicing medicine without being licensed. Unless prohibited by regulations, many camists claim they are able to diagnose and treat cancer. Restrictive laws and the regulation of conventional practitioners have been established over the years precisely to prevent advantage being taken of patients, especially the vulnerable. Who would wish otherwise?

Many alternative disciplines are based on concepts of 'energy', 'vital force', or 'spirits' which operate 'beyond' and have no basis in proper scientific understanding. That is why this book briefly reviews the origin of the universe and of human evolution. Camists and even some otherwise conventional health professionals generally favour metaphysical approaches, utilising physiological principles quite unknown to biological science and being indifferent to the scientific principles of conventional medicine.

The word 'complementary' refers to completion (Latin: *complere*, to fill up, complete). *Complementary medicine* is not in fact complementary as it is not necessary for the completion of conventional treatments. 'Complementary' is a term introduced for branding and marketing purposes. 'Complimentary' spelt with an 'i' refers to an act of respect and civility. Taken from the same Latin origin but implying 'completing the obligations of politeness', today implies 'free'. Spelling has differentiated the meanings from the mid seventeenth century. CAMs underline the same elements of lifestyle, diets, weight loss, stress reduction, and exercise that are emphasised by conventional medicine but CAMs are alternative by virtue of their unsubstantiated claims to provide medical treatment of specific conditions. Do camists intend to mislead when they use the term 'complementary'? You must be the judge.

Camists conduct research to prove that CAM methods do work, rather than to discover whether they do. Medical science hypothesises that a treatment, drug, or remedy does not work unless and until proved otherwise – it is null. Research is then carried out to find enough evidence to reject the initial 'null hypothesis' – to establish with plausible reproducible evidence that the null hypothesis is wrong and that the treatment studied does indeed have an effect. This scientific method cannot rely on anecdotes provided by individuals – they are too liable to subjective bias. Medical research rarely shows a zero result but may simply show that any effect is so small as to be undetectable by current methods – the probability of any genuine beneficial effect is very close indeed to zero. It is through this narrow chink of scientific integrity that camists squeeze the rationale for their practices. Camists dogmatically claim camistry has specific effects on illness, and then selectively present evidence to support those beliefs. As Professor Steve Novella points out:

> The burden of proof lies with demonstrating adequate evidence to reject the null hypothesis...Clinical research may not be able to detect the difference between zero effect and a tiny effect, but at some point it becomes irrelevant. Acupuncture is a case in point: Acupuncture does not work – for anything. This has profound clinical, ethical, scientific and practical implications. In my opinion, humanity should not waste another penny, another moment, another patient, any further resources on this dead end. We should consider this a lesson learned, cut our losses, and move on.[8]

Real Secrets of Alternative Medicine is recommended to all patients who are giving consideration to CAM and who wish to ensure they are not taken advantage of or defrauded. Camees may have largely given up on conventional treatments, may feel they need something extra, may be desperate and are attracted to alternatives. They may simply prefer non-conventional treatments and be prepared to run the risk of turning down the advantages of modern evidence-based medicine.

Those who want an alternative should not be denied. If a patient feels they derive benefit, we can be delighted for them, but it is important patients can trust their practitioner to provide all relevant information so that they can give fully informed consent to whatever it is the proposed intervention comprises. That is, patients are told all the facts necessary to make an intelligent choice, including the risks of wasting money, time and trouble on ineffective interventions and risks of being given false hope. These principles are particularly important in the care of children and those adults who lack the capacity to make wise decisions.

The UK General Medical Council requires doctors to 'Share with patients the information they want or need in order to make decisions...The doctor uses specialist knowledge and experience and clinical judgement to identify which treatments are likely to result in overall benefit for the patient...You should not make assumptions about the information a patient might want or need; the clinical or other factors a patient might consider significant, or a patient's level of knowledge or understanding of what is proposed...You should check whether patients have understood the information they have been given.' The Nursing and Midwifery Council requires that nurses 'Must ensure that the use of complementary or alternative therapies is safe and in the interests of patients and clients. This must be discussed with the team as part of the therapeutic process and the patient or client must consent to their use.' The General Pharmaceutical Council requires registered pharmacists to 'Make sure the services you provide are safe and of acceptable quality...You must explain the options available to patients and the public, including the risks and benefits, to help them make informed decisions. Make sure the information you give is impartial, relevant and up to date.' Pharmacists must explain that homeopathic remedies have no benefits. The General Dental Council requires dentists and members of their teams to act with integrity at all times. Whether recommendations by some dentists for the use of homeopathic remedies demonstrates that integrity has yet to be decided.

In order for any healthcare practitioner to comply with their professional obligations, the efficacy and effectiveness of any medicine, service, remedy, preparation or treatment offered must have been determined. The only effects of CAM which have been shown to be beneficial are due to their placebo effects. Unless this is explained, the practitioner cannot obtain fully informed consent. Simply saying 'some patients like them' is not adequate and is the first step to quackery.

Irrespective of their motive or intention, all readers should make decisions about healthcare and wellbeing for sound and sensible reasons. They should avoid being attracted to practitioners who take advantage of gullible and vulnerable patients, avoid expenditure on products or practices which have no therapeutic value and avoid being defrauded.

The UK General Medical Council requires that 'doctors must be aware that many patients are interested in and choose to use a range of alternative and complementary therapies. Graduates must be aware of the existence and ranges of such therapies, why some patients use them, and how these might affect other types of treatment that patients are receiving.'[9] Some medical schools now include modules on camistry to serve this requirement, but they are usually presented by proponents and enthusiasts who start from a viewpoint that CAMs do have specific effects on diseases, rather than considering whether they do. Concern has been expressed that pseudo-scientific medicine might be endorsed by universities, that there is an insurgency of irrationality and that critical reasoning is not adequately encouraged. *Real Secrets* is a resource which assists doctors and medical students meet GMC requirements and places CAM in a context which will assist nurses, therapists and other health professionals make up their own minds about the values, intellectual integrity, professional probity and ethics of camists.

To avoid quackery, fraud and harm, healthcare decisions and recommendations should be based on evidence which is rational, plausible, credible, reproducible and likely to meet with approbation from a significant consensus of professionals – not merely result from apocalyptic intuition as to how things might 'seem' (*apocalypse, revelation*). Doctors, nurses and other conventional professionals are all too aware that patients have minds, thoughts, emotions, feelings, which collectively represent a transcendent quality we can refer to as 'the human spirit.' (Latin: *transcendere:* to climb beyond, hence: 'a state of being which surpasses physical existence and is independent of it'). Mystics and the more religious might use terms such as 'soul'.

Scientific fact-based practice is often referred to as being 'clinical'. Originally referring to care carried out at the bedside, that term can now carry connotations of a dispassionate approach divorced from elements of caring about the mind and spirit at a human level (*klinos,* a bed). But good health professionals have always empathically incorporated these holistic, humanistic, psychological and emotional aspects into their regular practice as far as they have been able – without ascribing substance to metaphysical or supernatural entities or practices. Physicians are not fairymongers.

Many CAMs were founded in direct opposition to evolving scientific orthodox medicine, and their practitioners hold views on the nature of nature, reality, biology, chemistry, physics, pathology and physiology which are unconventional and not shared by the orthodox. Some orthodox practitioners nevertheless tolerate 'integration' for obscure reasons – possibly, self-interest. Rejection of the demands of science may be part of the attraction for those who seek the services of camists and why most camists have not joined one of the orthodox professions. Science is a hard task master. Obtaining knowledge requires attention to detail and intellectual imagination, a willingness to be shown to be wrong, significant modesty and preparedness to reject any theory or idea which does not stand up to testing by others. Scientists generally do not accept the authority of a particular teacher, master, or guru – but rather test any suggestions put forward. Camists are not as insistent upon evidence as obtained by the scientific method. They are more content to accept evidence based on anecdotes, 'experience,' 'intuition,' and the opinions of authoritative 'masters' who declare 'It seems to me…'

The concept of 'evidence' is taken very flexibly by camists, who too often set aside the generally accepted definition: 'the available body of facts or information indicating whether a belief or proposition is true or valid.' Science-based evidence is established by experiments and observations which have been repeated by other investigators. Other languages make distinctions more readily. Statements in Western Canadian Kwak'wala include an inflection on verbs indicating the strength and nature of the evidence for the assertion made: eye-witness, deduction, hearsay, anecdote, etc. Native speakers of Kwak'wala are especially clear-minded and precise about such matters, for instance when giving evidence in court.

Intuition is an excellent first step for scientific advance. Archimedes leapt from his bath crying 'Eureka!' when he realized the significance of density and how he could investigate adulteration of his king's gold crown with silver (*heurika*: I have discovered it). His experience is an early example of the rules of thumb, educated guesses and common sense which stimulate the solving of problems by observation and experimentation. Camists are often satisfied with evidence established by a heuristic approach alone. Scientific practitioners who are seeking higher levels of confirmation often start heuristically but then go on to subject their data to more thorough reviews, trials and statistical analyses. And it is expected that other scientists will be able to reproduce and confirm their results.

In this book I also address all those members of the general public, politicians and policy makers who are interested in public health strategy and policy, and are concerned about the impact of the demand for CAM on resources and investment in health services. This includes those journalists, editors and commentators who report on these issues in the public media, and who have ethical obligations to present the issues objectively and honestly.

Those responsible for allocating and rationing public resources have to consider that patients would 'benefit' were they able to choose from a vast number of various products and activities such as choosing a perfume, a stay in a spa, a new hairstyle, a fine wine, a ticket for a football match, or a visit to the gardens of Highgrove House. The list of products and experiences which might provide the benefit of 'feeling better' and 'feeling happier' is endless. The costs are infinite.

This is particularly relevant if consideration is to be given to the funding of unorthodox or non-conventional treatments, and if the taxpayer, insured population or charities are asked to support practices which lack a sound evidential base. The allocation of scarce healthcare resources is always controversial. Demand is infinite, but there are practical limits and decisions have to be made – rationally. 'The allocation of fixed amounts' is 'rationing' – but is a word which frightens dishonest politicians (Latin, *reri*, to think and reason).[10] We are all concerned that large commercial pharmaceutical companies may develop products with significant side effects. The impact on both personal budgets and international economics is also an issue. The term *Big Pharma* is used to draw attention to these concerns. (PhRMA: Pharmaceutical Research and Manufacturers of America – which represents biopharmaceutical researchers and companies). Camists use and recommend practices and products which are also part of large and commercially significant manufacturing interests and which can be termed *Big Charma* – 'Complementary Health and Alternative Remedy Manufacturers.' Any reservations or scepticism about the commercial impact and ethics of Big Pharma should be applied equally to Big Charma. Check out and compare the company accounts and directors' emoluments of any of the complementary and alternative medicine manufacturers and note practitioners who are sponsored to organise or attend camist meetings.

Healthcare managers and medical and executive directors with responsibility for funding and establishing the ethical basis of practice and research carried out in their institutions also need to consider the implications of any involvement with non-scientific CAM systems. If non-scientific systems are funded and practised, it makes it hard to justify requiring professional healthcare staff to base their own practices on scientifically established evidence. There should be only one standard. Additionally they will have to consider that the 'energies' employed by some camists are claimed to be very powerful, in some cases being transmissible over a distance. Managers and executives will need to ensure their use is in full compliance with regulations for the introduction of novel technologies and health and safety legislation. If the 'energies' or 'forces' cannot be measured, they cannot be managed. Authorities will need to be assured that patients give fully informed consent to any proposed therapy, including information that the proposed treatments are 'alternative' and may involve forces which could get out of control. If these energies can have effects on tissue and disease, there might also be unwanted side effects and harm.

Origins

This book has evolved, and will continue to do so. It has its origins in my youthful interests in magic as an entertainment and medicine as a career. I first demonstrated my powers of 'clairvoyance' as a schoolboy and later was asked to write a briefing paper on non-conventional therapies for the then President of the Royal College of Surgeons. The modern magician sets out to create illusion, misdirection and deception – but few claim to have assistance from the supernatural. Eminent magicians such as Harry Houdini, J.N. Maskelyne, James Randi and Derren Brown have exposed fraudulent mediums, fairymongers, quacks and charlatans and helped the public avoid being defrauded, gulled and cheated. The Magic Circle itself has a committee to investigate claims of paranormal activity. To date, all claims investigated have been trickery. Doctors and other clinicians are expected to be honest, open and act with integrity. Nevertheless it was only with the ascent of science during the 19th and 20th centuries that the needs for magic and mystery in medical practice could be discarded.[11] Experiences that lie outside the range of normal undestanding or scientific explanation are now referred to as 'paranormal'.

This book offers no recommendation for specific treatments. Placedo, the way of the placebo, is an appealing approach and often provides benefit. By definition, a placebo itself has no specific therapeutic effect, but placebo effects can initiate identifiable physiological, physical, emotional and spiritual responses of the body, mind and spirit. Placedo offers encouragement for the further study of these placebo effects. Placedo helps distinguish style from substance.

The title *Real Secrets* suggests there are secrets to be exposed. That is just a marketing ploy – and exemplifies the sleight of tongue all too prevalent when dealing with alternative medicine. This is not an academic textbook but may stimulate further study. References are suggested but for ease of reading are limited. A bibliography is available at www.placedo.co.uk and lists some of the books which have been of value and which should be consulted for details.

Communications

Much medical practice, whether conventional orthodox medicine (COM) or CAM, has become highly commercialised. Words, numbers, statistics are all used to promote services and products – sometimes with the deliberate intention of misleading patients, practitioners and politicians. In this book I offer definitions of relevant terms and words and, taking my cue from entrepreneurial camists, I have coined some new words to show that the devil does not have all the best tunes!

Numbers are often the best way of expressing size, shape and quantity and their use has evolved. In the eighteenth century, the numbers that describe larger groups, particularly of people and populations, were the subject of 'political arithmetic.' Now we use the term 'statistics.' Further consideration are given in chapter 8. Numbers are particularly important when considering homeopathic dilutions that are beyond the comprehension of most.

Numbers are not the only concept which needs clarification. CAMs are often presented and discussed using imaginative language designed to invoke response at an emotional level. The terms used by some practitioners, producers and promoters of CAMs seem to be deliberately designed to dupe. Why else would they be used?

The Nightingale Collaboration challenges misleading health claims and has expressed concern that:

> One of the hallmarks of pseudo-science is its attempts to commandeer established words and phrases from science and misuse them for its own purposes, giving it a veneer of authority and respectability. The prime example of this is the word 'quantum'. It refers to small, discrete steps such as the energy levels of an electron. In everyday use, however, it has come to mean the exact opposite: a quantum leap generally refers to some *huge* step in something or other. But the word is certainly sounds scientific and is used by purveyors of pseudo-science, trying to give their product (there usually is one) some legitimacy. The term 'quantum flapdoodle' was coined by Murray Gell-Mann to describe such usage.[12]

Examples abound in magazines purporting to advise patients. Claims that energies can be conjured from nothing to perform beneficial 'healing work', whether in pillules, meridians, chakras or 'energy fields', represents violation of the Second Law of Thermodynamics – and that is not possible except in the imagination.

There are numerous controversies but to the greatest extent possible, scientific evidence substantiates the knowledge and opinions offered in this book. Present opinion will change. Modern medicine is based on evidence, but the methods of obtaining that evidence should not exclude the personal experience of individual people in the context of their communities, values, hopes, fears and worries about themselves and relatives. These can be recorded as observations and be part of a scientific inquiry. That is what social scientists do. So should medical scientists. Science is never perfect and is always open to challenge, change, and the demands of sceptical inquiry. The scientific method is simply the best method yet devised to acquire true knowledge – probably.

The realm 'beyond the syringe' of modern medicine is appealing but 'medicine' has evolved. Myths, mysticism and metaphysics have been superseded. We now have alternatives to ancient superstition and sympathetic magic – that is, science based conventional orthodox medicine. Modern medicine is the new alternative.

Endnotes to Chapter 1

1. Marcy Angell, Jerome Kassirer. 1998. *Alternative Medicine: the Risks of Untested and Unregulated Remedies.* New England Journal of Medicine, 339 (12).

2. Richard Dawkins in the foreword to *Snake Oil* by John Diamond. Vintage, London, 2001.

3. Arthur K. Shapiro: *The Placebo Response.* In Modern Perspectives in World Psychiatry. Ed. John Howells. Oliver & Boyd. Edinburgh and London. 1968.

4. Edzard Ernst. *Placebo and other non-specific effects.* In *Healing, Hype or Harm.* Ed. Edzard Ernst. Imprint Academic, Exeter, 2008.

5. Edzard Ernst. *A Scientist in Wonderland.* Imprint Academic, Exeter, 2015.

6. Paul Offit. http://www.newsworks.org/index.php/thepulse/item/82346-why-healing-crystals-might-make-some-people-feel-better.

7. HL paper, Session 1999-2000. 12, (2000). The Stationery Office, London. Parliamentary information licensed under the Open Parliament Licence v1.0. www.publications.parliament.uk/pa/ld199900/ldsctech123/12301.

8. http://www.sciencebasedmedicine.org/acupuncture-doesnt-work/#more-27131

9. *Tomorrow's Doctors,* General Medical Council, Manchester.

10. Use of the term 'rationing' frightens politicians who like to promise everything, and who develop policies attractive to voters, not patients.

11. Shapiro, A. K. 1960. *A Contribution to the History of the Placebo Effect.* Behavioural Sciences, 5. www.nightingale-collaboration.org. Newsletter Number 38: WDDTY #8.

12. Murray Gell-Mann. www.nightingale-collaboration.org/component/acymailing/archive/
view/listid-1-mailinglist/mailid-52-newsletter-number-38. The first known use of 'flapdoodle'
being by Captain Frederick Marryat RN in his novel *Peter Simple* (1833) as 'The stuff they
feed fools on.'

Chapter 2

Conventional Orthodox Medicine (COM)
The Real Alternative to
Complementary and Alternative Medicine (CAM)

Legitimate medicine has no secrets. Of all her vast acquirements, she withholds nothing from the public. All that she has collected, from all ages, and nations, and countries, is freely offered to all the world, and whenever required is bestowed upon suffering humanity, without money and without price. Quackery may dash its mercenary waves against her, and send its spray mountains high; but she will still pursue the even tenor of her way, unmoved by its fitful storms.
Dan King
Quackery Unmasked 1858

Scientific medicine is defined as the set of practices which submit themselves to the ordeal of being tested. Alternative medicine is a set of practices that cannot be tested, refuse to be tested, or consistently fail tests.
Richard Dawkins

The real purpose of the scientific method is to make sure nature hasn't misled you into thinking you know something you actually don't know.
Robert M. Pirsig
Zen and the Art of Motorcycle Maintenance

The origins of 'medicine' are shrouded in the myths and mists of time. As mankind started to live in ever larger social groups, so our relationships with other humans and the environment developed. Abstract thought became the hallmark of our species, which is why we are termed *Homo sapiens* (Latin: wise man). Earlier versions of 'man' included more than twenty-five species of hominids, including *Homo neanderthalensis*. Modern DNA studies suggest *sapiens* probably interbred with *neanthalensis* over thousands of years – we have 4% of our DNA in common.[1]

Anthropologist W.H.R. Rivers considered three particular dimensions of our life and culture in *Medicine, Magic and Religion*: 'Medicine, magic, and religion are abstract terms, each of which connotes a large group of social processes, processes by means of which mankind has come to regulate his behaviour in the world around him. One has now gone altogether into the background of our social life, while the other two form distinct social categories widely different from one another, and having few elements in common.'[2]

Down the centuries, as more knowledge was gained, so a range of practices, treatments, remedies and potions came to be accepted as conventional, 'straight' or orthodox (*orthos,* straight). It was only in the nineteenth century that health care practitioners who complied with appropriate standards became regulated by law. The term 'nursing' was not used formally until the Nursing Society of Philadelphia did so in 1736, and nursing was not distinguished as a profession until Nightingale's reforms of the 1850s. In 1858, medicine became the first profession to be statutorily regulated in the UK. Today, a practicing registered medical practitioner has to have a licence issued by the General Medical Council.

Whether complementary and alternative (CAM) or conventional orthodox medicine (COM), there is now only one 'medicine': a system based on scientifically established plausible evidence. Some patients wish for alternatives to such a system and find that camistry offers more meaningful and satisfactory interpretations than orthodox explanations. Their rights to have a choice must be respected. At the heart of all systems is concern for the health and well-being of individuals and populations – which begs the question as to what is meant by 'health and wellbeing' and whether there is any difference in meaning between those two words. The World Health Organisation (1992) defines 'Health' as 'A state of complete, physical, mental and social wellbeing, and not merely the absence of disease and infirmity'. 'Health' and 'wellbeing' seem to be synonyms.

In order to achieve 'health and wellbeing', different civilizations and cultures have developed different systems at different times. Discrete bodies of organised thought and practices directed to the care of sufferers can be identified for over seven thousand years. Some have been discarded, some have evolved. Some new initiatives have become standard, conventional, orthodox and mainstream. Some have had their day and are no longer practised. Some have not been able to fit in with modern advances in understanding – but remain to offer alternative approaches. For those who like that sort of thing, that is the sort of thing they will like.

'Medicine' is not one dimensional – a variety of models have been described. Deborah Ragin has identified four which explore physiological, psychological, sociological, and environmental factors.[3] The classic is the Biomedical model: 'Health' constitutes freedom from illness, disability or dysfunction of the body caused by pathology, biochemistry and physiology. 'Disease' is the underlying pathological process, 'illness' is how the patient feels – and that fluctuates. This is often regarded as a modernist approach, but out of date with the post-modern world.

Professor George L. Engel added psychological factors of stress, emotions, social support and personal traits, creating a holistic Biopsychosocial model in which health outcomes are explained by multiple factors. For example, there is good scientific evidence that depression and stress affects heart disease.[4] Doctors find time constraints and institutional bureaucracy inhibit their application of this model as much as they would like – leaving the door open to alternative practitioners who can be more attentive.

The Wellness model incorporates two further health dimensions – spirituality and psychological quality of life. 'Spirituality' referring to an individual's perspective on the meaning of life and the impact of their values on their overall wellbeing – no religious connotation is intended. Some may believe that spirituality enables them to experience peace and tranquillity and a sense of transcendence, but not necessarily as the result of any divine influence.[5]

Fourthly, the Social-ecological model expands further to include five major determinants of health: The individual (biology and behaviour), social environment (family, community, cultural practices), physical environment (sanitation, safety, pollutants), care delivery organizations and government level health strategy and policy.[6]

There is current public criticism of conventional medicine, nursing and other healthcare professions for not taking these wider dimensions into account and for not being sufficiently holistic, caring and compassionate. Camists are keen to suggest that camistry will provide these missing or underprovided elements. Their patients appreciate a caring therapist, but do their treatments and remedies have any more effect than inert placebos? There is no plausible evidence that they do – so why spend any available funds on CAM? Why not spend on getting practitioners of conventional orthodox medicine (COM) to change their practices and give them time to do so?

The British Medical Association has recently given financial backing to the Institute of Health Equity at University College London (UCH) to tackle health inequalities through action on social determinants of health. This reflects the interests of Sir Michael Marmot, BMA President in 2010, whose Whitehall Study of cardio-respiratory disease and other social determinants in male British civil servants is a landmark in this field. However, University College Hospital is also the site of the former Royal London Homeopathic Hospital, now re-named as the Royal London Hospital and specialising in 'integrated medicine'. The hospital has advertised to employ 'Third Degree Reiki

Masters', who can train others to transmit energy from their hands over considerable distances in 'distant healing'. One can only hope that the powerful energies created by the 'masters' have been fully tested under Health and Safety legislation and that side effects have been fully investigated.

The hospital also employs pharmacists to dispense remedies which contain no therapeutically active ingredients. The Royal London Hospital at UCH has as its logo a caduceus – the winged staff of Hermes with two snakes entwined. Hermes was the messenger of the gods and regarded as the patron of thieves and liars. The RLH for 'Integrated Medicine' has had a number of complaints against it investigated by the Advertising Standards Authority which adjudicated on some in 2013.[7] The hospital had to correct its advertising to avoid misleading statements.

'Health and wellbeing' is a multi-factorial complex concept. This makes it all the more important that opinions are informed by evidence; that the evidence is of good quality, based on scientific precepts of observation and experimentation and that any evidence is accepted as plausible by a reasonable body of responsible people, acting with intellectual and professional integrity. Opinions in medicine are not determined solely by scientific evidence – the personal experience of individual patients and the clinical judgement of clinicians have much to contribute. Controversy arises in deciding the value to place on any piece of evidence and the probability is of it being 'correct and true'.

Dr C.J. Ewell emphasised: 'The emotional and psychological impact of illness cannot be underestimated, and the impact of pre-existing emotional and psychological disturbance on new health problems should be respected. A robust emotional and psychological reserve will always benefit a patient, while individuals with poor coping skills and underlying depression will fare worse than their better adjusted counterparts, if only on measures of quality of life. In the end, quality of life is what we all strive for.'[8]

Dr Sarah Burnett, Professor of Psychology, Rice University, Houston has commented: 'The problem with the 'Wellness' model is that the role of spirituality and quality of life on health are over emphasised by those who have taken up the concept. There are strong data that show that those who have good social support and who have meaning and purpose in their lives live longer than those who do not. But some Wellness practitioners claim that spirituality is everything. The same is true with the concept of stress. It is important, but some would have you believe that stress causes everything, including cancer, and thinking happy thoughts will cure everything, including cancer. People have a hard time with the concept of multiple factors being causative – it is easier to think in terms of single factors.'[9]

Spirituality is certainly of importance but need not have a religious dimension. The Royal College of Psychiatrists has defined 'spirituality' as 'being identified with experiencing a deep-seated sense of meaning and purpose in life, together with a sense of belonging.' Some ascribe the experience of a transcendent quality in life to a divine influence, but internal imagination is able to generate comparable feelings and humanists also recognise the inherent qualities of caring, compassion, harmony, contentment, altruism, and love. The conscientious placebist will be neutral on the origin of such experiences. NHS Standards for Spiritual Care Services (2010) sates: 'Spiritual care is usually given in a one to one relationship, is completely person-centred and makes no assumptions about personal conviction or life orientation. Spiritual care is not necessarily religious.'

In the UK, the term 'wellness' is used less often than 'wellbeing'. Essentially, they are synonyms – both mean a healthy balance of mind, body and spirit which results in an overall feeling of being well. The Oxford English Dictionary identifies the first use of *wellness,* as the opposite of illness, in the 1650s. 'Wellness' became formalised by Dr Halbert Dunn who defined 'wellness' as 'an integrated method of functioning which is oriented towards maximising the potential of which the individual is capable' (*High-Level Wellness*, 1961).

Today, 'wellness' or 'wellbeing' is seen as a state combining both health and happiness. 'Wellness' is particularly used by those interested in CAM, as it implies recognition of spirituality, destiny and other more esoteric concepts. At one time wellness was regarded as being the province of flaky therapists and enthusiasts for *wudo* – the Way of Nothingness. It can be a term which has simply distended the language, particularly as used in America. 'Wellness' or 'wellbeing' has now entered the mainstream of medical marketing and is used by more secular promoters of balanced health, often now without its New Age spiritual implications.

The problem with 'Wellness' or 'Wellbeing'
Reading books or articles on CAM can make the reader feel as if they had stepped through Lewis Carroll's Looking Glass. Logical fallacies abound, critical thinking is set aside, and imagination holds sway. This is acceptable in a work of literature, but may be thought patronising if it is intended that any sensible meaning should be conveyed to patients.

The promoters of some remedies seem to be deliberately intent on deception. Advertisements using imaginative language and slippery semantics proliferate: 'We are exempt from regulations covering conventional medicines because they are concerned with treating disease whereas we use natural resources and elements to optimise health.' The Advertising Standards Authority thinks otherwise and demands such claims are withdrawn, but the prevalence of quackery and fraud is pervasive.

It is a matter of regret that words in the healthcare lexicon are frequently used without clarification of meaning. There can be no reason for perfectly straightforward English words to be used in vague, novel, and original styles that cannot be properly comprehended by regular readers – unless it is intended they will be misled or that patients will delude themselves as to the implications. Even the terms 'health', 'wellness', 'wellbeing', and 'happiness' are elastic, and can mean practically anything you want them to mean. Perhaps they mean nothing in particular. Discuss.

The question of delusion has been considered in a talk to the Royal Society of Arts by Dr Barbra Ehrenreich.[10] In her view, delusion is always a mistake, for there can be no safe delusion (OED: 'An idiosyncratic belief or impression maintained despite being contradicted by reality or rational argument'). Problems of delusion are not helped when scientific terms are used wrongly. 'Energy', 'effectiveness', 'meridians of force', 'vital spirits', 'quantum effects', 'auras', 'toxins', 'chakras', 'natural' and like terms are all used regularly by camists, but not with any definitions or comprehensible explanation of what they mean.

Ehrenreich is particularly concerned about current resurgent enthusiasm for 'positive thinking and optimism'. She suggests it is cruel to delude people and to do so is morally corrupt. No doubt an optimistic approach can make patients feel better and assist them deal with their conditions more effectively and appropriately, but it is delusional to suggest that thoughts can affect pathological processes or cellular physiology. She encourages people to be real and to figure out what is really happening in the world. There is but one 'world'; that is where we exist and we have to face it as it is.

Sociologist Aaron Antonovsky described three components of emotional health in *Salutogenesis*: Comprehensibility: a sense that life events are reasonably predictable and orderly; Meaningfulness: the sense that life is interesting and offers satisfaction with a 'purpose'; Manageability: the sense that life is manageable and under control. Deficit of any element may drive patients to camistry. Not only patients are stressed – doctors' and nurses' own sense of worth and ability to manage their personal and professional affairs have been under sustained attack by politicians and health service managers. Doctors and nurses are no longer professionals serving patients in a civil health service, but civil servants working at the behest of managers. And progressively, with the aim and ultimate objective of increasing the financial return of investors and shareholders in the private companies which employ them. Sir Michael Marmot's study on civil servants showed the major correlate of illness amongst professionals is lack of control over their fate and a sense of disempowerment.[11] Patients need to bear in mind that if they do not look after their doctors, nurses and other health professionals – they will not be able to look after them.

Another issue with the concept of 'wellbeing' has been exposed by Prof. David Colquhoun who points out: 'Wellbeing is big business. And if it is no more than a branch of the multi-billion-dollar positive-thinking industry, save your money and get on with your life.'[12]

How Medicine Works

In the context of this book the term 'medicine' includes the professions of dentistry, nursing, midwifery and those regulated by the Health Professions Council as of 2011.

The basic art of a doctor is that of diagnosis of the patient's condition – by taking a clinical history, (identifying symptoms), carrying out a physical examination (observing signs) and performing further investigations based on laboratory and imaging techniques. Only when a diagnosis has been established (to the greatest extent possible) can treatment be considered. Not all camists establish a diagnosis before treatment.

Doctors may be individualists, but they are expected to work well in interdisciplinary and interprofessional, teams. The key attributes of a good health practitioner, of whatever profession, all initiate with 'C': Core knowledge and wisdom; Competence and proficiency; Care and an inclination to have genuine concern for the patient (Old English: *caru*); Compassion (Latin: *cum*, with; *patior*, to suffer); Consolation (Latin: *cum*, with; *solari*, to comfort); Charisma (grace, favour and a good 'bedside manner'); Commitment; Communication (an ability to ensure patients and colleagues are properly informed).

Taking the term 'benefit' to mean that patients report an improved sense of wellbeing, patients do seem to benefit from CAM – even though the Really Big Problem is that nobody knows how to measure 'wellbeing'. For most people, the days of arcane, mystical, irrational rituals have passed. We now have alternatives to that style of ancient practice. Today's medical practitioners are expected to be sceptical about claims for efficaciousness of treatments or medicines; to subject claims to rational analysis; and to base their practice on credible evidence provided by plausible scientific methodologies. The alternatives, once used by priests and magicians as well as physicians, have been superseded and left behind. Philosophers use the term *sceptic* to refer to someone who denies that we have knowledge in a given area (*skeptic* in the US). More generally, the term refers to someone unwilling to accept claims of extraordinary events which do not withstand close critical and scientific scrutiny. Scepticism is the best protection patients can have against being cheated and defrauded.

That is the basis of modern medicine, which is not to say that qualities of caring and empathy are not important to today's doctors. Many medical schools have introduced modules teaching interpersonal and communication skills as part of a more holistic approach. That can be overdone and a balance must be achieved. Psychiatrist and journalist Max Pemberton observes that more medical schools now place emphasis on the 'caring' side of being a doctor, but wonders whether this might be to the detriment of basic medical science. He expresses his worry 'that medicine is being reduced from an academic discipline to a protocol-driven tick-box subject, where students have poor grasp of the science underlying what they observe on the wards. It should worry us all that we're churning out young doctors who can smile and make good eye contact, but who panic when you collapse in front of them.'[13] His concern is shared by many of his medical colleagues.

Nevertheless, patients may remain disillusioned at the failure of even the most sophisticated of modern orthodox medical practice to alleviate their problems and ask their doctors for advice about supplements and CAM. Some doctors have come to believe that these non-orthodox medicines or remedies do 'work' – and they are content to promote and prescribe non-orthodox remedies. Whether such endorsement, founded on no plausible evidence, is contrary to the GMC's injunction that a doctor should 'Never abuse the public's trust in the profession' is for you to judge.

What is meant in this context by '*work*'? Parliament's Select Committee on the Evidence for Homeopathy (2010) offers no definition. The natural course of any illness may be to recover, irrespective or even in spite of any treatment offered.[14] From the patient's perspective, 'medicine', whether COM or CAM, 'works', that is – has an effect better than might be expected if left to nature, in one or both of two principal dimensions:

Type I effects: Firstly, therapies or remedies 'work' by making patients feel better – by affecting the 'ease' syllable of 'disease' (Middle English: *ese*; Anglo-French: *aise*, freedom from worry, agitation). In other words – by pleasing the patient. Type I effects result from constructive therapeutic relationships, conditioning and expectations and are seen in all healthcare practices to a greater or lesser extent. The Latin for 'I will please' is placebo – a term also applied to sham drugs which are used as controls in clinical trials and which have no significant effect on disease. Practitioners are always sensitive to the needs of patients for courtesy, care, compassion and consolation. The effects are seen when three year old Jimmy falls and grazes his knee and Mummy kisses it better, or when condolences are offered to the bereaved, perhaps with a hand on the arm or around shoulders. To the best of knowledge and understanding, Mummy does not pass energy to Jimmy to make it better, but Jimmy is placated. These effects are non-specific but, together with consolation, hope and love, provide meaningful interpretations which satisfy the patient.

Type II effects: Found when the medicine, surgery, remedy or treatment, whether physical or psychological, has a discernible effect on the physiological and pathological processes of a dis-ease or injury at an organic, cellular and molecular level. An effect on the 'dis' syllable (*dys*, bad, abnormal, faulty function). These are specific effects of the treatment. If there are effects which withstand scientific scrutiny, the practice will be accepted and cease to be 'alternative'. Orthodox medicine and health care practitioners will adopt the medicine or treatment. What do you call alternative medicine that works? Conventional Orthodox Medicine.

These two 'dimensions of work' should be distinguished and assessed separately for each treatment under consideration – the practitioner distinct from the practice, therapist from therapy, style from substance. Conflation of the two senses of 'work' leads to confusion. Clarity is all if intellectual integrity is to be maintained and fraud avoided.

Additionally, apparent effectiveness of treatments may be accounted for by regression towards the mean (outliers tend to move to the mean value); the natural history of the patient's condition (most conditions get better even without treatment); social desirability (patients tend to say they are better to please their friendly clinician); and concomitant treatments (patients often use treatments other than the prescribed one without telling their clinician). Real effectiveness may be an illusion.

Doctors and nurses want to help patients. Although doctors are trained to use the scientific method, their actual clinical job is not to be pure and unadulterated scientists but rather to help their patients by curing where possible and caring always. Deception and deceit is abhorrent, yet we all know that to a greater or lesser extent, doctors and health professionals do use placebos. At one time placebos such as 'the pink medicine' could even be bought from chemists and druggists specifically for the purpose. Such practice has been thought a 'pious fraud to placate ignorant, disappointed and incurable cases...an innocent deception on our hypochondriacal and fanciful patients.'[15]

Doctors have for long been aware that giving placebos may 'place the patient in circumstances as favourable as possible to the sanitive operations of nature' and that nature will then take its course. [15] The ethical issue is not so much the giving of a placebo but the deception when patients are not told of the 'pious fraud.' In a study of seventy one articles describing placebo use between 1840 and 1899, disclosure was reported in only one.[16]

In February 2010, the UK House of Commons Science and Technology Committee examined how the Government uses evidence to formulate and review its policies. Its Second Evidence Report considered Homeopathy, one of the more controversial alternatives to conventional medicine. *Evidence Check 2: Homeopathy* concluded:

> We were disappointed that, in light of its view on evidence for homeopathy, The Government has no appetite to review its policies in favour of an evidence-based approach. The Government was reluctant to address the issues of informed patient choice or the appropriateness and ethics of prescribing placebos to patients. By providing homeopathy on the NHS and allowing the Medicines and Healthcare Products Regulatory Agency (MHRA) licensing of products which subsequently appear on pharmacy shelves, the Government runs the risk of endorsing homeopathy as an efficacious system of medicine. To maintain patient trust, choice and safety, the Government should not endorse the use of placebo treatments including homeopathy. Homeopathy should not be funded on the NHS and the MHRA should stop licensing homoeopathic products.[17]

Reporting in March 2015 on more than 1800 papers on homeopathy, with 225 controlled studies, the Australian National Health and Medical Research Council concluded that 'homeopathy is not an effective treatment for any health condition.'

If a GP refers a patient for an alternative 'energy treatment', they must know just what powerful forces their patient will be subjected to, what the risks are of the patient suffering harm from these powerful energies and they will need to ensure the patient gives fully informed consent to be exposed to these forces. Patients need to trust their GP to ensure this. Through Clinical Commissioning Groups, GPs are also responsible for the commissioning and financing of these treatments, for establishing and ensuring the efficacy of the treatment, the cost effectiveness of the investment made and for ensuring that the chosen camist is not a quack, crook or defrauding the NHS.

The British Medical Association is mindful of its obligations to support rational evidence-based medical practice. In 2008, the BMA called on the National Institute for Health and Clinical Excellence (NICE) 'to review and report on the cost-effectiveness of homoeopathic remedies and to recommend whether they should continue to be funded by the NHS.' NICE has yet to report – its chairman indicated that such an inquiry would not be welcomed by some persons of influence.[18] At its annual meeting in 2009, the BMA urged the government 'to require by legislation that gullible or vulnerable patients who may wish to consider the purchase of 'complementary' or 'alternative' healthcare products or treatments have their interests protected by the requirement that terms such as 'toxins'; 'detox'; 'natural aid'; 'energy'; etc. be banned from marketing material unless and until they are defined and proven on a rational evidence basis.'

In 2010 the BMA expressed its belief that 'in the absence of valid scientific evidence of benefit, there should be no further commissioning of, nor funding for, homeopathic remedies or homeopathic hospitals in the NHS. Pharmacists and chemists should remove homeopathic remedies from shelves indicating they are 'medicines' of any description and place them on shelves clearly labelled 'placebos'.' Note the emphasis is on the 'remedies', not on homeopaths as practitioners or homeopathy as a philosophy.[19]

Not all doctors endorse these policies – a few actually practice homeopathy. Others do not prescribe homeopathy themselves, but like to be able to refer their patients to homeopaths. That is what some patients want. Some colleagues think this is simply shifting the responsibility for good patient care and passing the proverbial buck. Some doctors have patients who claim they have benefited from homeopathy or other CAMs and feel it might be in the patient's best interest for them to have at least some tender loving care and attention, even if there is no scientific evidence of actual therapeutic effectiveness. Such a need for solace deserves attention but the ethical issues raised by healthcare practitioners using, recommending, or allocating public finances to fund placebos also needs review, particularly if fully informed consent has not been obtained. Deception is always to be deprecated.

Nearly two hundred years after Dr Samuel Hahnemann published his *Organon of the Rational Art of Healing* as an alternative to conventional medicine, The Prince of Wales created the Prince's Foundation for Integrated Health to promote the use of CAM and to have it 'integrated' with conventional orthodox medicine. His Foundation was closed by its trustees in April 2010 after a police investigation into alleged fraudulent transactions. The Foundation's conference due to be held in July 2010 was cancelled.[20]

A private company and charity, the 'College of Medicine' has emerged since, with a number of its trustees and council members having previously been closely involved with the Prince's Foundation, although the College does not make that clear. Its inaugural annual conference was sponsored by a major manufacturer of homeopathic remedies and the venue was made available through a 'craniosacral therapist'. Its second conference was sponsored by Capita, a healthcare firm with interests in providing services including CAM to the NHS, and which employs the College's

President, Sir Graeme Catto. Concerns have been raised that the 'College' is a front for those who wish to see CAM integrated with conventional medicine, and is a College of Quackery.[21] Its constitution states the College's objectives include 'establishing an evidence base for integrated health and for individual complementary modalities; promoting, fostering and advancing an integrated approach to health care; raising public, professional and political awareness and cultivating a sentiment in favour of an integrated approach to health and care by publishing and distributing material on any media.' So, the old problem resurfaces – the College intends demonstrating that 'complementary modalities' have an effect, rather than discovering whether they do so. How this squares with its intention to be 'evidence-based' remains a mystery. It is unclear how its trustees can show they are not behind an insurgency of irrationality, seeking to promote quackery and harm the principles of NHS scientific-based medicine. The premise of conventional science – the 'null hypothesis' – is that a given treatment does not work. The 'College' starts from the premise that it does.

Edzard Ernst, Emeritus Professor of Complementary Medicine at the Peninsular Medical School has suggested 'These concepts are used for a classical "bait and switch": First you are baited by the seemingly good offers of patient-centred care and so on, only to be switched later to ineffective treatments like homeopathy. The College seems to be a smokescreen behind which unproven or disproven treatments are being promoted with a view to smuggling them into the NHS. This would not render the NHS more patient-centred. It would just make it less effective.'[22]

The same methods have been used by quacks, charlatans and fraudsters down the centuries. The Gold Brick is a classic swindle, with the mark/gullible victim believing he has invested in a valuable gold brick, only to find on getting it home that it was made of base metal painted gold. Authorities worldwide warn tourists that unscrupulous street hawkers and scam artists try similar tricks. Modern magicians offer demonstrations of the switching techniques used, and expose how the mark is taken in by their own vanity, credulity, and naivety.

In the US, the Institute of Medicine describes *integrative medicine* as 'orienting the healthcare process to engage patients and caregivers in the full range of physical, psychological, social, preventive, and therapeutic factors known to be effective and necessary for the achievement of optimal health.' 'Known to be effective and necessary' is part of this definition – but CAMs do not meet this criterion.[23] Why proponents of CAM are involved with the College of Medicine has not been explained. The tendency of camists and their supporters to turn platitudes into profundities should be recognised for what is – misleading metaphysics.

In 2010 the British Chiropractic Association sued physicist and science journalist Dr Simon Singh for libel. Reporting in the Guardian that the BCA website claimed chiropractic could be used for treating children with ear infections, asthma and colic, Singh had suggested that the BCA were happily promoting treatments for children and babies for which there was 'not a jot of evidence.'[24] This is an example of a SLAPP – a strategic lawsuit against public participation – a lawsuit intended to intimidate, and silence critics by burdening them with the cost of a legal defence until they abandon their criticism or opposition.[25] Many camists use this technique to avoid having their secrets exposed to scrutiny – particularly that their systems result in no type II effects on any specific condition.[26]

The BCA claimed there was a 'plethora of evidence' in respect of the use of chiropractic for these childhood problems and offered eighteen references. When the British Medical Journal published an exchange between the BCA and Professor Edzard Ernst, its editor Dr Fiona Godlee said: 'Ernst's demolition of the eighteen references is, to my mind, complete.'[27] The libel case was dropped. In order that scientists can publish honestly held opinions without the chilling fear of being sued, Singh remains actively involved in initiatives to see a change in libel law. Richard Brown, the President of the BCA continues to promote their beliefs – at the College of Medicine's annual conference 2012, he spoke on 'Active Aging in Europe'. He is 'Co-Chair, College of Medicine Neuro-musculoskeletal Faculty'- but chiropractic is based on non-scientific precepts and metaphysical approaches to healthcare which are incompatible with the advances in modern medicine and scientific advances in the understanding of anatomical, emotional and psychological components. Ernst has expressed concern that treatments such as chiropractic manipulation, acupuncture and herbal remedies often fail to record incidents when patients suffered adverse effects and that chiropractic manipulation could even be lethal.[28]

For a time, the BCA website included a video of what a patient might expect when visiting a chiropractor. The receptionist was seen describing to the patient what 'the doctor' would be doing. In the United Kingdom the title 'doctor' is customarily reserved for those with appropriate academic qualifications or who practise as registered medical practitioners. There is no law to prevent anyone using any title they wish – providing they do not seek to defraud by doing so. It might be thought that the use of such a title by a chiropractor in the United Kingdom is likely to mislead a patient as to the professional status of the practitioner and thereby defraud them. For what other reason would chiropractors wish to use the title 'doctor'? That video has now been removed from the BCA website but inexplicably the title of 'Dr' continues to be used by some chiropractors.

In response to the Singh case, Peter Dixon, president of the General Chiropractic Council, which regulates chiropractors, said the National Institute of Health and Clinical Excellence 'had recommended chiropractic manipulation for the treatment of lower back pain. If NICE had not thought it safe they would not have recommended it.'[29] In fact NICE made no such recommendation, and Mr Dixon's statement was wrong and misleading. NICE guidelines recommended 'one of the following treatment options, taking patient preference into account: consider offering structured exercise programme; manual therapy (including spinal manipulation); acupuncture. Manual therapy is a collective term that includes manipulation, spinal mobilisation and massage....The manual therapies reviewed were spinal manipulation, spinal mobilisation, and massage. Collectively these are all manual therapy. Mobilisation and massage are performed by a wide variety of practitioners. Manipulation can be performed by chiropractors and osteopaths, as well as by doctors and physiotherapists who have undergone specialist postgraduate training in manipulation.' There simply was no 'recommendation for chiropractic' in any specific sense.

The British Chiropractic Association itself claims 'Chiropractic is a primary health-care profession that specialises in the diagnosis, treatment and overall management of conditions that are due to problems with the joints, ligaments, tendons, and nerves, especially related to the spine.' In conventional medicine, making a diagnosis entails firstly determining what a problem is due to – it does not start from the assumption a condition is due to musculoskeletal problems. Who makes a primary diagnosis before referral to a chiropractor? As psychologist Abraham Maslow said: 'If all you've got is a hammer, everything looks like a nail.' The BCA web site offers no explanation of the fundamental principles of chiropractic, other than to say that its founder D. D. Palmer had been the first to adjust a 'subluxation' – to treat deafness. Palmer himself clearly stated: 'Chiropractic is founded on different principles than those of medicine.' Quite so.

Chiropractic is not simply a matter of spinal manipulation or mobilisation. If that is all it is, it could not usefully be distinguished from osteopathy, physiotherapy, or any other form of spinal manipulation. Chiropractic is more than that. It is a system of medicine predicated on a faith that 'innate intelligence', a 'vital spark' or 'soul' can be affected by adjusting 'subluxations' of the vertebrae. Anybody wanting to consider manipulation for low back problems needs to be fully informed about the therapeutic faiths of the practitioners they are considering and bear in mind that manipulation can also be offered by orthodox practitioners. If a patient wishes to have their 'innate intelligence' manipulated – then chiropractic could be considered. The GMC forbids doctors from proselytising their faith to patients. The General Chiropractic Council imposes no such ethical inhibition.

But change continues. Patient or person centred medicine/healthcare is becoming better established as a valuable more humanistic approach and conventional doctors and nurses are becoming ever more holistic. Nevertheless, patients do have to give informed consent to any treatment, and will need to better understand and appreciate why it is that so many doctors and other healthcare professionals are sceptical about CAM, are disinclined to recommend or support the use of CAM, and have called for the use of CAM within the NHS to be restricted or denied.

Duties of a Healthcare Professional
The duties, standards, and ethics of those responsible for the care for patients are set out in common law and in the codes of practice and guidance of regulatory authorities and professional associations. In the UK, some are established by statute – such as those regulating medical doctors, dentists, nurses, pharmacists and those regulated by the Health & Care Professions Council. Others rely on the strength of moral persuasion without resort to law. Each profession has developed its own

individual ethical requirements and recommendations and these continue to adapt and evolve. All have much in common but the exemplar of the medical profession, the first to be organised in any modern sense, serves a basis for them all.

From the Middle Ages, European workers banded together in 'fraternities' to share knowledge of techniques, set standards and establish the integrity of their crafts (Latin: *frater,* brother). These groups also became known as 'mysteries', as they possessed skills appearing to be secret by virtue of the long time needed to master them (Latin: *misterium,* an indentured trade or profession). Craft guilds developed in most major cities and can still be recognised. Members had to pay to join the guild, which acted much as do today's trade unions (Saxon: *gildan,* to pay). The guilds also protected customers by checking the standards of their members' work and fining them for selling substandard goods. In extreme cases a member could be expelled and so lose their livelihood.

In London the Guild of Pepperers was formed in 1180, and was joined by the Spicers in 1316. Some of these spicers dealt with herbs and other compounds which were used for healthcare treatments. They became known as Spicer-apothecaries (*apotheka,* storehouse, particularly of drugs and herbs – the same root produced the French, *boutique*). Other herb and spice merchants traded in dry goods *en gros* and established the Worshipful Company of Grocers in 1428. In 1617 the apothecaries who specialised in dealing with medicinal herbs and spices separated from the grocers and founded the Worshipful Society of Apothecaries of London. James VI granted them a Royal Charter commenting 'Grocers are but merchants, the business of an apothecary is a mystery.'[30]

Since 1511, the profession of medicine had been regulated by the College of Physicians, which was keen to limit the scope of practice of apothecaries. In the fullness of time, apothecaries who studied medicine became entitled to prescribe medicines as well as dispense them. Those apothecaries are now regarded as being forerunners of today's general medical practitioners. In 1841 the apothecaries helped chemists and druggists establish the Pharmaceutical Society which gained its Royal Charter in 1843. The Society of Apothecaries itself was the sole regulator of the profession of general medical practitioner until the General Medical Council was set up in 1858. Since 1998 all UK registered medical practitioners have been fully under the regulation of the General Medical Council.

Hospitals as distinct institutions had been established in the United Kingdom during the fifteenth century, but most were closed in 1536 when Henry VIII dissolved the monasteries. Thereafter patient care and healing was generally carried out in the home by women with varying degrees of wisdom. Qualifications as a physician became established in various universities, but these qualified doctors could only be afforded by the aristocracy.

In London, a Company of Barbers was established in 1308. Some barbers extended their scope of practice, and having experience of razors and scalpels, were particularly adept at caring for wounded soldiers on the battlefields. Those who treated their clients with more extensive manual techniques became known *chirurgeons* (*chiron*, a hand; Latin, *manus*). Hence: *surgeons*. In Scotland, the Royal College of Surgeons of Edinburgh was founded by James IV in 1505. In England the Company of Barber Surgeons was formed in 1540, eventually splitting in 1745 and creating the new Company of Surgeons. Royal Charters were granted in 1800 with the title of The Royal College of Surgeons of London, and in 1843, of England. The Barbers retained ownership of Barber-Surgeons Hall!

The three principal regulated professions of apothecary, physician and surgeon (including dentists) faced competition from a wide variety of other healers, corn cutters, bone setters, and teeth pullers. Some genuinely had a desire to care but were simply not qualified or officially recognised. Some set out to take advantage of the gullible, ignorant, and foolish, and were regarded as charlatans or quacks. That is not to say some qualified physicians, surgeons and apothecaries did not also act like charlatans, but as the principal professions became more extensively regulated, so it became possible to establish professional standards of entry, training, practice and ethics – and to exclude miscreants. Even surgeons are expected to think rationally. When teaching surgical trainees I emphasise that 'decisions are more important than incisions.'

Currently, those wishing to join any of the health professions have to comply with basic educational standards and professional training – in most cases, to graduate level. All require adherence to professional ethics setting out the principles and values on which each professional practice is founded. Each profession has its own guidelines, but those developed over the years by the General Medical Council serve as a basis for all: 'Make the care of your patient your first concern; Respect a patient's right to reach decisions with you about treatment and care; Be honest and open and act with integrity; Never abuse your patient's trust in you or the public's trust in the profession; You are personally accountable for your professional practice and must always be prepared to justify your decisions and actions.'

Healthcare professionals have a duty to act with integrity, probity and intellectual honesty. They can no longer hide behind the veils of mystery and superstition. They must ensure the patient has information they need in order to make their own choices and to give informed consent. Doctors must ensure that patients are aware of the 'alternative' nature of any practice or remedy proposed – and of the fact that there is no credible scientifically established evidence to suggest the proposed treatment will have any significant effects, over and above the placebo effects. That is, camistry works through the mechanism of placebo effects, not metaphysical vital spirits. Whether patients can trust their doctors on this point is for them to judge.

Providing patients are properly informed, conventional practitioners can use camistry. The question of how to tell the difference between a regulated healthcare professional using camistry sincerely and a quack seeking to take advantage of the gullibility of poorly informed and vulnerable patients has yet to be resolved. A professor of complementary medicine, concerned at the general lack of understanding of these issues exhibited by a past president of the BMA, has even described him as being 'a snake-oil salesman'. [31]

Times have moved on. Modern professional health care is demanding. Standards are high. The scientific method is not perfect and does not provide absolute truth, but it does get as close as possible and by rejecting false gods, ancient ways and pseudo-science, is prepared to change and develop where necessary. Alternatives are available for those who wish otherwise. Modern conventional, orthodox, medicine constantly challenges its own claims and seeks improvement. It provides a powerful alternative to the irrational, superstitious, misleading, and dishonest treatments of the past. Today, it is modern medicine which is the alternative, but in order to understand why complementary and alternative medicine persists, we need to start at the beginning...

Endnotes to Chapter 2

1. 'Man' is a term which is non-gender specific, as it is in 'chairman' and 'ombudsman'.

2. Paul Kegan. *Medicine, Magic and Religion.* Trench, Trubner & Co. Ltd. 1924.

3. Deborah F Ragin. *Psychology: an Interdisciplinary Approach to Health.* Prentice Hall 2011. pp. 12-17.

4. KD Mullen, RS McDermott, RJ Gold and PA Belcastro, 1996. *Connections for Health.* Fourth edition. Madison, WI: Brown & Benchmark.

5. GL Engel, 1977. *The need for a new medical model: a challenge for biomedicine.* Science 196.

6. Evolved from the work of: Urie Bronfenbrenner (1979); Kenneth McLeroy (1988); Daniel Stokol (1992, 2003).

7. Newsletters 33 and 44: http://www.nightingale-collaboration.org.

8. C.J. Ewell. Personal communication, 2011.

9. Sarah Burnett. Personal communication, 11.8.11.

10. www.dcscience.net/?p=4940. 2010.

11. Marmot M.G.; Rose, G.; Shipley, M.; Hamilton, P. *Emploment grade and coronary heart disease in British civil servants.* Journal of Epidemiology and Community Health. 32 (4): 244-249. 1978.

12. www.dcscience.net/?p=4308.

13. Max Pemberton, Daily Telegraph, December 19, 2011.

14. Glasser BG, Strauss A. *The discovery of grounded theory.* Transaction Publishers 1967.

15. West RU. *On the propriety of dispensing medicines.* BMJ.1849.

16. Jacqueline E. Raicek, Bradley H. Stone, Ted Kaptchuck. *Placebos in nineteenth century medicine.* BMJ. 2012;345:e8326. 22 December 2012.

Franklin Miller and Ted Kaptchuck. *The power of context: reconceptualising the placebo effect.* Journal of the Royal Society of Medicine May 1, 2008 vol 101 no. 5 222-115.

17. HC 45, the Stationery Office, 22 February 2010.

18. Personal Communication. In September 2012, David Cameron appointed Jeremy Hunt Secretary of State for Health. Hunt thinks homeopathy is effective. He has no evidence to support that assertion, yet expects doctors to base their practices on rational evidence-based concepts.

19. Declaration of interest: In order to establish BMA policy on a rational basis and give further guidance, those last proposals had been put forward by myself, as Honorary Secretary of the BMA's South Devon Division, where many of our patients have an interest in camistry. South Hams' chief town Totnes has had the sign on its approach road annotated advising the town is 'Twinned with Narnia' and with 'Area 51, Nevada'

20. www.homeopathyhome.com/reference/organon.

21. Prof. David Colquhoun. BMJ 16th July 2011, vol. 343. www.bmj.com/content/343/bmj.d4368.

22. Prof. Edzard Ernst. www.guardian.co.uk/science/blog/2012/jan/10/college-medicine.

23. www.medicalnewstoday.com/articles/139304.

24. Dr Simon Singh. *Beware the Spinal Trap*, Guardian, 19 April 2008.

25. https://en.wikipedia.org/wiki/Strategic_lawsuit_against_public_participation.

26. http://debunkingdenialism.com

27. Editorial. *'What next for the British Chiropractic Association?'* BMJ. & www.quackometer.net/blog. Both: July 10, 2009.

28. Prof. Edzard Ernst, Journal of New Zealand Medical Association. May 2012.

29. Stephen Adams, *Daily Telegraph*, May 14 2012.

30. At its dinners, the Master's Toast is to 'The Worshipful Society of the Art and Mystery of

Apothecaries of the City of London, may it flourish root and branch, bringing help to all, till time ceases.'

31. Prof. Edzard Ernst.www.guardian.co.uk/science/2011/jul/25/prince-charles.

Chapter 3

And then...

There was neither non-existence nor existence then.
There was neither the realm of space nor the sky which is beyond.
Darkness was swathed in darkness.
Creation Hymn of the Rig Veda, circa 1700 BC

The nameless is the beginning of heaven and earth...
darkness within darkness, the gate to all mystery.
Lao Tzu
Tao Te Ching, circa 600 BC

The Second Law of Thermodynamics is the only physical theory of universal
content which I am convinced will never be overthrown.
Albert Einstein

Once upon a time, there wasn't.
There wasn't any time. There wasn't any thing.
Nothing.
No up. No down, No left, No right. No Front, No Back. No past, No Future.
And then there was...

Energy

Camists and camees interested in CAM, use terms such as 'energy'; 'aura'; 'vital force'; 'work', 'ion', 'radical', 'quantum' but without the precision expected of scientists. That is why it is necessary to consider how these terms are used by those who apply rational and scientific thinking to their understanding of nature. It is a matter of regret that enthusiasts for camistry use terminology devised and defined by scientists, yet in different senses and with different meanings. Whether they do so deliberately in order to mislead and confuse has to be considered as a possibility and is for them to explain. If a camist ever suggests to you they can engage 'energies', just ask them to clarify what energies they mean.

This account considers the broad consensus of the majority of those who study these issues seriously. Other individuals or groups are of course quite entitled to use their own definitions – but to avoid misunderstanding and confusion they should offer clear explanations and definitions.

'Energy' has many forms. All are equivalent. If energy in one form disappears – it will reappear in another. 'Energy' is the quantity that can describe every particle, object, or system of objects. Changing energy from one form to another requires *work* – energy has to be transferred by a force acting over a distance. A *force* is any influence that causes a free body to accelerate – that is, speed up, slow down, or change direction. Even more basic are the fundamental forces: strong nuclear, electromagnetic, weak nuclear, and gravity. There may be other fundamental forces but so far only four have been discovered – so if a camist claims to have found another, get them to explain – and to apply for a Nobel Prize!

Although energy can be transferred from one system to another, the total amount of energy in an isolated system remains constant. The confidence we have in that statement being true is so high that it is the First Law of Thermodynamics or Law of Conservation of Energy.[1] The energy which was, at the beginning, had only length, as strings. No height or width. No up or down. No side to side. There was, if some modern physicists are to be believed, simply a 'quantum field'. That's the way it was.[2]

And then the little strings changed. They formed loops. They vibrated – and vibrate to this day. The dimension of that first change is called 'time' and in the next moment, the vibrating strands oscillated in eleven different ways, or dimensions. Three of these became large enough for us to perceive as those of height, width and length. So it is we can apply our own five senses to recognise four dimensions – three of space and one of time. The other dimensions are speculative and too small to have been detected to date. Their existence is inferred from mathematical analysis but physicists are currently seeking hard evidence of them.

The vibrating loops of energy are the most elementary particles there can be. More elementary particles are being discovered all the time but here mention is made of a few in order to give some sense of the extraordinary world of the subatomic particle. Except it is not extraordinary at all – indeed there is nothing more ordinary. It is just extraordinarily difficult for us to conceptualise and study.

Quarks are the only elementary particles to experience all four fundamental forces. The name 'quark' was coined by physicist Murray Gell-Mann in an attempt to simplify the terms used to describe the elementary particles. The word is attributed James Joyce's *Finnegan's Wake:* 'Three quarks for Muster Mark! Sure he has not got much of a bark.' Perhaps alluding to the cry of the gull – much as a duck 'quacks'. Gell-Mann's colleague Richard Feynman wanted to call these elementary particles 'partons' as they were part of the hadron group. Recognising Feynman's extra-curricular interests, Bill Bryson suggests Feynman's proposal referred to Dolly, but quark it is, though even the pronunciation varies – some preferring to rhyme the word with pork.[3] Bryson also reflects that the imaginative metaphorical terms 'flavours' and 'colours' used to describe them arose in California during the psychedelic 1960s!

The ancient Greeks had known that amber (*electron)* attracted light objects when rubbed. The English physician William Gilbert coined the term 'electricity' to describe these effects in his famous book *De Magnete.* Published in 1610, the year Gilbert was elected President of the College of Physicians, *De Magnete* is regarded as the first 'modern' scientific textbook based on experiments and observation.

The four fundamental forces of nature are carried by 'bosons'. Fifty years ago a fifth boson was described by English theoretical physicist Peter Higgs and others to explain how vector bosons can have mass. In July 2012 proof of its existence was confirmed using the Large Hadron Collider at Cern in Switzerland and at Fermilab in Illinois. The doors of perception into even more fundamental concepts of reality are slowly opening.

Writing in *Nature* Paul Davies commented: 'It is almost impossible for the non-scientist to discriminate between the legitimately weird and the outright crackpot.'[4] Things get weirder. In 1900 German physicist Max Planck had suggested that energy is not continuous like a flowing river but comes in little packets, later called quanta. (Latin: *quantus,* how much). Quanta are the dreams of stuff. Originally energy moved at the speed of dark but with the advent of photons – of light. Now all electromagnetic packets bear the name *photon.* They all move as a wave, but never faster than 3.10^8 meters, or 186,000 miles a second. The speed of light in empty space is designated c from *celeritas* (Latin: swiftness). It is because photons move both as packets and waves that quantum mechanics, which studies these small particles at the sub-atomic scale, is so often non-intuitive and barely comprehensible to the non-specialist.

The mind's eye picture of a little electron circling the nucleus of an atom should be replaced with one of 'fuzz' as electrons jump randomly in discrete steps from one shell like orbit to another. Not that we can ever know exactly where or when this happens. In 1925 Walter Heisenberg's *Indeterminacy Principle* stated it is impossible to determine both the position and velocity of a particle simultaneously. All that can be offered is the probability or likelihood of a particle behaving in a particular fashion. Currently this is termed *Heisenberg's Uncertainty Principle.*[5]

Camists will have you believe they can move these quanta by thought or hand waving and so achieve therapeutic benefit, but they must be questioned on just what they do believe. They have a tendency to use all these scientific words and terms in unique and imaginative ways but without defining them. Are they trying to deceive?

In the beginning there was no 'Big Bang.' It was not 'big' for there was nothing smaller to compare it against. There was no medium to transmit a bang – not even a little pop. In the beginning all the energy was in the smallest possible space and time. A place we now call a singularity, which was nothing more than a quantum field, and which some term 'God'. The field then fluctuated – as that is the nature of nothing. The term 'Big Bang' was coined by Sir Fred Hoyle in 1949 in order to distinguish between two rival hypotheses about the origin of the universe. In 1927 Georges Lemaître had suggested that a 'primeval atom' expanded to form the universe as we know it today. Intriguingly, not only was Lemaître professor of physics and astronomy at the Catholic University of Louvain, but a Roman Catholic priest. Conversely, Hoyle's preferred explanation was that the universe had always existed in a steady state. Currently the vast majority of physicists and other natural philosophers support Lemaître's hypothesis, but if suggestions that multiple universes can come into and out of existence are ever verified, perhaps Hoyle will be vindicated.

Other popular terms used by camists are 'ion', and 'radical'. If an atom or molecule has a positive or negative electric charge it is called an ion. That is how atoms and molecules function when they are in physical or chemical reactions. Michael Faraday applied the term *ion* to matter which went from one electrode to another (*ienai*, to go). Water, with two hydrogen and one oxygen atom is written as H_2O, but functions with a positive charge as hydroxonium: H_3O^+. An equal number of hydroxide ions, OH^- gives pure water its neutral pH, which expresses its hydrogen ion concentration. Marketing of CAM often makes much of ions and pH. The camee must assess whether such promoters are using the terms knowledgably or are seeking to deceive.

If an atom, molecule, or ion has an unpaired electron, the term used is *free radical* – much beloved by camists and CAM marketeers (Latin: *radix*, root. Surferspeak: *radical*, at the limits of control). *Free* because there is a spare electron which makes the atom, molecule, or ion available for reactions. It is in this configuration that critical biochemical reactions occur and without which, life would not.

Antioxidants are molecules which inhibit electrons becoming combined with molecules which can produce free radicals. Oxidation is necessary for life but can also cause damage. Cellular balance and harmony is needed lest disease is caused – the Ancients were right all along. The scientific jury is out as to whether the antioxidants used in dietary supplements provide benefit or do harm. If a claim of benefit is made, be sure the evidence to back it up is sound, or save your money.

These ideas and theories engage scientists who apply the most serious and advanced understanding. In the field of health, wellbeing and camistry, it is essential that anyone using terms such as 'quantum,' 'force,' 'radical', 'aura', 'spirits' or 'energy' must either use them in the proper scientific sense, or explain how they define the terms they use. Otherwise we have to accept that their musings are those of hyperactive imaginations, a deceit of deliberate quackery and merely marketing ploys designed to exploit the gullible. Camees have no more desire to be taken advantage of and defrauded than anyone else.

Life

This book is about humans – their hopes, fears, feelings. We have evolved as sentient beings capable of thought – thoughts which have themselves evolved. About 4.5 billion years ago enough debris and gas plasma had accreted under the force of gravity and inertia for our nebula to ignite as a star – the Sun. As it matured, the Sun and its nebula developed planets and asteroids. Our Earth became the third major rock out from the Sun about four billion years ago.

Over hundreds of millions years, chemical reactions occurred – binding groups of atoms as molecules. The larger aggregations and chains of atoms incorporated hydrogen, oxygen, nitrogen, phosphorus, and carbon in combinations we now recognize as phospholipids, nucleic acids and proteins. One particularly important biopolymer was deoxyribo-nucleic acid. DNA is the largest individual molecule yet discovered and is found in all life forms.

For the first billion years after self replicating molecules evolved, the only life on Earth is thought to have been simple single cells with no nucleus and a single strand of DNA. About 2.7 billion years ago bacteria emerged and at about 1.2 billion years ago, multi-cellular organisms. When DNA came to be exchanged between organisms, the fittest survived more readily, and reproduced more. We refer to this as sex (Latin: *secare*, to divide). Palaeontologist Nick Butterfield aptly named the earliest fossils found which show these features as *Bangiomorpha*.

Around 2.3 hundred million years ago, Archosaurs (ruling reptiles) including dinosaurs (terrible lizards) began their adventures on Earth. This lasted two hundred million years and ended with an extinction event about 6.5 million years ago.

Mammals had evolved during this period but whether any which had placentae ever lived at the same time as dinosaurs is highly debatable. Today we recognise eighteen orders of placental animals and we are in the in the 'first order', termed 'primates' (Latin: *primus,* first).[6]

Early hominids in Africa began walking on two legs around five million years ago and about one and a half million years ago there was a significant increase in brain size. Animal species are connected in genera (*genos,* race, kin). Our own genus, *Homo,* showed up in Africa between 3 and 1.4 million years ago but initially was not particularly wise. Current consensus suggests that our species, *sapiens* (Latin: wise), evolved about four hundred thousand years ago. Human evolution takes a very long time by our everyday scales, but is rapid when related to the time since the origin of the Earth. Evolution is not teleological – it does not describe a journey, nor have a purpose (*telos,* end, purpose). Evolution is what happens. It continues all the time under the pressures of the survival of the fittest in a process of natural selection. Not only the fittest life form, but also the fittest, or most selfish, gene.[7]

Civilisation

Currently it is suggested that modern humans separated from Neanderthals some three hundred and fifty thousand years ago and left Africa sixty thousand years ago. A *Science* report has suggested that 4% of some humans' DNA was from neanderthals, demonstrating past cross-breeding which probably strengthened our species' immune system.[8]

About twelve thousand years ago these peoples began settling in defined groups, organised under powerful leaders, influenced by those who felt a spiritual affinity with nature around them and with the supernatural. As human beings organised their tribes and grouped together to live in cities with shared practices of agriculture, philosophy and religion, so they are today identified as being distinct 'civilisations' (Latin, *civitas,* city). Philosophy and religion were of particular importance and developed layers of sophistication and knowledge as the 'culture' of these civilizations. Writing developed to record their administration and give accounts of the spirits and supernatural forces that influenced their lives. Some civilisations were more successful than others. Advances in agriculture, urbanization, the organisation of religion and development of arts and sciences varied significantly. Military conquest and enslavement was the order of the day.

The first clearly identifiable civilizations arose about six thousand years ago in Mesopotamia – between the Tigris and Euphrates. Today this area is Iraq and parts of Syria, Turkey, and Iran. Here the Akkadian, Babylonian, Sumerian and Assyrian Empires flourished. Other centres of civilisation developed in Egypt (about 3000 BC, when the Sahara was more fertile), in China, (notably the Valley of the Yellow River from 2000 BC), India, (particularly the Indus Valley from 1500 BC), the central Andes and middle Americas.

Ancient Egyptian civilisation developed writing in the hieratic cursive form and also as hieroglyphs. Hieratic pen and ink was used for one of the oldest papyri to have been discovered on medical subjects. The Edwin Smith Papyrus was written in about 1600 BC. Other papyri setting out systems of medicine were based in magic with emphasis on supernatural and occult forces. Smith's papyrus offered a more rational and 'scientific' system, particularly for treating trauma and injuries, though eight magic spells are also suggested. Smith bought the papyrus in Luxor in 1862 and it has now been donated to the New York Academy of Medicine. Eber's Papyrus of 1550 BC is regarded as the oldest book to set out details of medical, as opposed to surgical, treatments. Surgeons at the time of the first Babylonian dynasty (1792-1750 BC) had to take care. The code set down by Emperor Hammurabi included the penalty of amputation of a hand if a surgeon's patient died.

Other Egyptian texts, such as those associated with the priest Imhotep, established a pharmacopoeia which was used for 3000 years (*pharmako*, drug; *poi*, make). His recommendations for incantations and the conjuring of magic spirits to ward off demons were slowly set aside as the ancient Egyptians became more aware of the importance of moderation in all things, a balanced a diet and avoidance of too much beer.

Egyptian physicians were widely respected by other civilizations, and frequently acted as consultants. They recognised the connection between pulse and heartbeat, but not between arterial and venous blood. Influenced by their observations of the River Nile, and noticing how crops became unhealthy if its branches were blocked, they developed the concept that in humans, 'channels' were important for air, blood and food. Emetics, laxatives and bloodletting were therefore a logical method of treatment for ill patients.

Most illnesses were put down to the malign influence of evil gods, spirits, demons (*daimona*, spirits), jinns (Arabic: hidden) and other supernatural entities. As religions developed, so priests acted as both physicians and magicians. The powerful charisma exerted by priests' incantations and their dramatic demeanour enhanced placebo effects. As diseases regressed, so many patients recovered and were suitably grateful to their priest/physician/magician. Gradually some priests specialised in relationships with the supernatural, whilst others concentrated on specific practices for treating injuries and diseases and became physicians. The ancient Egyptians even had a *neru phuyt* – a 'shepherd of the anus'.

The Babylonian *Enuma Elis*, written around 1700 BC, described four cosmic elements: sea, wind, earth and sky. In common with virtually every other developing civilisation, the ancient Greeks also understood the world to be formed of four elements – in their case: water, air, earth and fire – related to the four phases of matter: fluid, gas, solid and fire. As the various elements were mixed, so four qualities emerged: fire and air gave hot; air and water gave wet; water and earth gave cold; and earth and fire gave dry. The Greeks then added a fifth element, the quintessence of 'aether'- spirit. Later still, the alchemists of medieval Europe added sulphur, mercury and salt.

Developing European thought took a strong steer from the ancient Greeks and knowledge of health and welfare was intimately bound with philosophical considerations of religion and metaphysics (*meta*, beyond; *physis*, nature). The term metaphysics was used in several Greek philosophical texts, particularly those of Aristotle. Initially 'beyond' may have simply meant chapters in the books after those on physics but the term came to mean the science of the immaterial, of reality, of the meaning of God and the nature of existence – beyond the physical world. That is the starting point for the next chapter's review of some of the traditional systems of healthcare and medicine which developed in ancient civilisations.

Endnotes to Chapter 3

1. The First Law of Thermodynamics states that energy can neither be created nor destroyed. The Second Law states that in a closed system, energy is spread randomly. If no energy enters or leaves a system, its potential energy will always be less than its initial state. 'Entropy', that is, disorder, increases (*en*, inside; *trope*, transformation). Healing energy simply cannot be conjured from nothing – not by diluting active compounds beyond the point of existence, waving hands, sticking needles in the skin, or releasing innate intelligence.
Prof. Jim Al-Khalili points out: '*Everything wears out, cools down, gets old and decays... the Second Law of Thermodynamics is statistical in nature...it is overwhelmingly more likely that states of low entropy will evolve into ones of high entropy than the reverse.*' (*Paradox.* Bantham Press, London, 2013).
If you consult a camist who claims they can conjure and move energies with their bare hands, you need to be sure they know of what they speak.

2. Lawrence M. Krauss. *A Universe from Nothing. Why there is Something rather than Nothing.* New York. Free Press. 2012.

3. Bill Bryson. *A Short history of Nearly Everything.* Black Swan 20044. Nature: 27 September 2001 p. 354.

5. It is said Heisenberg's Uncertainty Principle can be expressed as $\sigma_x \sigma_p \geq h/2$. But I cannot be certain.

6. My wife returned from her first visit to the antenatal clinic and claimed she had been told she was a 'elderly primate'. Being non-medical, she had misheard. At thirty five, she had been told she was an 'elderly primip', referring to her primiparous state (first time pregnant).

7. Michael J. Benton.*The History of Life.* Oxford University Press. 2008, and Richard Dawkins. *The Selfish Gene.* Oxford University Press. 1976.

8. *Science*, 25th August 2011.

Chapter 4

Traditional Medical Systems:
Shamanic, Indian, Chinese, Magnetic.

*When religion was strong and medicine weak, men mistook magic for medicine;
now when science is strong and religion weak, men mistake medicine for magic.*
Thomas Szasz

Ancient physicians, whose vocation and profession it was to help the sick, were often at the forefront of developing knowledge – but advances were slow from antiquity, through the middle ages, until the intellectual flowering of the Renaissance. The second half of the seventeenth and the eighteenth century then saw the blossoming of knowledge referred to today as the Enlightenment or Age of Reason. Ancient precepts and superstitions were largely set aside, outmoded ideas were recognised as having had their day and much traditional medicine slowly evolved to become grounded in evidence-based science. Some did not and remained antiquated.

There is no entirely coherent story to tell of the development of medicine, nursing and the other healthcare professions. There were false starts, some new ideas aroused misplaced enthusiasm and then faded as scrutiny exposed inconsistencies. Some old ideas became entrenched in spite of being irrational. Conventional medicine and healthcare continues to change and evolve under the relentless drive of scientific inquiry, the demands of patients and the need to provide healthcare on an acceptable economic and political basis. Most camists want more approbation from the public and more funding, yet have been slow to change and adapt to modern demands.

There are countless traditional systems of medicine – in this chapter, four are considered: Shamanic, Indian, Chinese and Magnetic. Our own systems of Traditional Western Medicine are considered in the next chapter.

Traditional Shamanic Medicine (TSM)

Different cultures developed different 'ancient wisdom' to help them relate to the 'spirit world'. There has been no single common belief. Shamanism is not a religion and has no single dogma, but a number of themes emerged and have been described by Mircea Eliade: Spirits exist and are important in the lives of individuals and society; imbalance of the spirits may cause harm, dysfunction, and disease; certain priests or magicians can communicate with the spirit world and treat sickness; these priests may use techniques of trance and may use plants and herbs such as 'magic' mushrooms, cannabis and tobacco which are known to have an effect on diseases or to have mind altering effects.[1] Stone Age peoples probably had the these ideas before cultures developed organised 'religions'.[2]

Anthropologist Sir Edward Tylor in *Primitive Culture* (1871) used the term 'animism' to describe beliefs prevalent in indigenous cultures that non-human entities such as animals, plants, rocks, rivers, and even thunder possess spirits – and that there is no difference between the immaterial spiritual world and the material physical world. Today some healthcare commentators and practitioners still refer to there being 'two worlds'. Controversy continues as to whether animism should be regarded as a religion or as component of some, if not all, religions.

As beliefs about the supernatural became organised, so society authorised certain knowledgeable and vocationally driven members to perform sacred rites and intercede between the human world and that of the gods. Ancient peoples regarded much they did not understand about the natural world as being due to 'magic'. Anyone who claimed to be able to assist in controlling these natural forces was a 'magician'. If the root cause was believed to be the gods, the magician who interceded was a priest. Organised religions turn to such priests to act vicariously in their dealings with their deities. (Latin: *vicarius,* substitute, deputy. From *vicis,* turn, change, substitute). At Apollo's Temple at Delphi, The Oracle was consulted for advice for a thousand years, not withstanding her invariably ambiguous prognostications (Latin: *orare,* to pray, plead). The Oracle herself was probably affected by the volcanic fumes issuing from the rocky cleft over which she sat, and which contained ethylene. Glue sniffing underpinned her ancient wisdom.

Modern magicians make no claim of divine or supernatural abilities – they simply intend to entertain by conjuring the illusion that they possess such expertise. The techniques of the modern magician are however adopted from those of their ancient brethren: misdirection; deception; false witness; lying; exaggeration; an ability to spot a weakness in an observer in order to take advantage; and use of sleights of hand, tongue and mind.

Before religions became organised, priests generally acted on their own authority, driven by a vivid imagination. Some shamans had suffered from an illness which caused psychological collapse – perhaps epilepsy. After recovery, a strong sense of vocation led to these individuals taking up shamanic practices as magicians, mystics, ritualists and healers. Indeed it might be considered that Abram (in a vision), Moses (at the burning bush), Saul of Tarsus (later called Paul – on the road to Damascus), Muhammad ibn Abdullah (during meditations on Mount Hira near Mecca) and Joseph Smith (in a grove in Manchester, New York) had intense emotional experiences which impinged on their fertile imaginations to such an extent that they reported they had been directly addressed by angels or their gods. Siddhartha Gautama Budda, (Sanskrit: *budda,* enlightened one) had similar experiences whilst meditating but did not ascribe them to any particular deity. Whether a god or gods were involved is a matter for theological interpretation.

Ancient priests claimed they could confront malign spirits directly, ensure rebalance of a patient's 'energy' and mend the soul. A wide variety of rituals and practices grew up to assist these processes. In addition to herbal medicines, rituals, chanting and trance inducing dance all helped restore balance. Some anthropologists have termed these ancient practices as shamanism, and those who practiced them, shamans. In the 1690s shamans were described as being priests of the Ural-Altaic peoples, many of whom eventually became absorbed into the Han Chinese culture. (Turkic: šamán, priest). Today, the term has come to be applied to all those who practice in the way described.

Philosopher Karl Jaspers described the middle of the first millennium BC as the Axial or Pivotal Age during which the rise of organised religions saw a decline in shamanism, though shamanic practices of ritual, chanting, singing and praying to spirits still play a part in modern Abrahamic religions. In Japan, shamanic elements were absorbed into Shinto, which is associated with Buddhism. The Jewish god Yaweh told Ezekiel: 'I am against your magic charms with which you in ensnare people like birds and I will tear them from your arms. I will set free the people that you ensnare like birds.' [3]

In Britain, Wales, Ireland and Gaul, shamanistic practices were found amongst the Ancient Druids from the late Iron Age of 100 BC to 200 AD. (Old Irish, *drui*, sorcerer; Welsh, *dryw*, seer). Theirs was an oral tradition, probably to preserve the secrecy of their inner working. [4] Our knowledge of their practice is limited, based on myths and a few writings by Roman authors, notably Julius Caesar who recorded the Druid belief that 'souls do not perish, but after death pass from one to another.' [5] In the Roman Empire, the mystery religion of Mithraism had comparable features of salvation through secret rituals.

In the early twentieth century, the Canadian Indian shaman Quesalid wrote an auto-biography in his Kwak'wala language which was studied by anthropologist Claude Lévi-Strauss. It transpired that Quesalid had always used tricks to produce the bloody 'tuft of illness' and knew full well that his success resulted from the powerful faith and placebo effects he engendered. More recently still, interest in 'New Age' philosophies and religions has stimulated an renewed awareness of shamanic practice, particularly as applied to 'spiritual and energy healing'. Shamanism remains a useful term to describe a range of traditional practices based on association with the spirit world, particularly in the field of healthcare and well-being. Recent work at the Kaiser Permanente Centre for Health Research in Portland, Oregon, suggests some patients with temporomandibular joint disorder have concomitant emotional and psychosocial difficulties and may benefit from shamanic healing.[6]

Camees will have to consider the extent to which their own preferred camist is using shamanic magic medical techniques to underpin the health care approach used, whether they are fairymongers and whether they consider that is appropriate.

Traditional Indian Medicine (TIM)

During the second millennium BC, various civilisations set down accounts of the universe, the Earth, humankind, and how all were interconnected in harmony and balance. Different tribes, races and cultures developed different traditions, based on their religions and practices of practical 'magic'. The oldest scriptures of the peoples who developed civilisations in the Indus valley of the second millennium BC were written in Sanskrit and are the Vedas. The Brahmins, hereditary priests, had originally passed down these extensive hymns and rituals from memory (Sanskrit: *veda,* knowledge; *brahmana,* priest). Europe at the time was in the Late Bronze and Iron ages.

The Indian sub-continent saw many religions evolve. Orthodox Hindus hold that their Vedas record the direct revelation of deities, specifically Brahma, the god of creation – who himself arose from the navel of the supreme god or cosmic spirit,

Vishnu. There was no unique founder or guru to whom these Vedic revelations were made but other distinct religions were founded under the stimulus of the *gurus* Mahavira (c.599-527 BC: Jainism), Siddhartha Gautama (c.560-485 BC: Buddhism) and Nanak Dev Ji (1469-1539 AD: Sikhism. Sanskrit: *sisya,* disciple; *siksa,* instruction. *Guru:* elder, teacher). All have their own medical traditions.[7] In this book, TIM is used as an umbrella term for them all.

Vedic philosophy is said to have originated from the Upanishads of the sixth century BC and which were still being added to in medieval times (Sanskrit: *upa,* near; *ni,* down; *sad,* sit -that is: 'lessons learned sitting near the teacher'). Originally the narratives were passed down by oral tradition, but then formed one of the basic scriptures for Hinduism.

A key concept of Hindu and Buddhist texts is that of *chakra* (Sanskrit: wheel). It is claimed there are a number of wheels, whorls, or vortices in the human body which act as a focus for *prana* (Sanskrit: breath, vital spirit. Comparable to Japanese, *kana;* Chinese, *ch'i* or *qi;* modern camist, *biophysical energy*). [8]

There is no consensus in TIM as to how many chakras there might be – together with their spokes, different texts set down anywhere between three and 365, the number of days in the year. All are said to be joined by 'meridians' along the spinal column, head and limbs. None have been identified by anatomists, physiologists or pathologists but the 'energy' in these chakras has to be balanced in order to achieve health and well-being. Usually 'balance' can only be achieved by employing the professional assistance of a healthcare practitioner or a donation to a temple. No surprise there.

The term *Hindu* was first used in Arabic to refer to the tribes which had migrated across the River Indus about ten thousand years ago. By the nineteenth century AD the term was applied to all the religious and philosophical traditions of Hindustan, now, India. Other texts of the traditional Indian philosophies, religions, magic and medicine include the Purana, Mahabharata, the Bhagavad Gita, the philosophies of Yoga and the final Vedic texts, the Vedanta.

Ayurveda
The Vedic texts that dealt with life and healthy living were termed *Ayurvedic* (Sanskrit: *ayus,* longevity; *veda,* knowledge, wisdom). There has been no coherent 'Vedic medicine,' rather a variety of precepts which later gave rise to more discrete forms of different systems. Numerous forms and expressions of ayurvedic medicine can be identified as they evolved over the centuries, but a fundamental principle is based on the 'five elements' of earth, water, fire, air and sky. In different combinations, these form the human body and the entire universe. The three most important humours (*doshas*) for health and well-being are: *Vita* (air and sky) for wind, nervous control and rheumatism; *Pitta* (fire and water) for bile and metabolism in the venous system; *Kapha* (water and earth) for phlegm and nutrients of the arterial system. Balance is essential if harmony is to be established

50

and wellbeing maintained. Good digestion, effective excretion and physical exercise is essential. The importance of moderation is strongly emphasised.

Panchakarma describes the five processes which Ayurveda uses to purify the body of toxins and balance the doshas (Sanskrit: *pancha,* five; *karma,* action). Different regions and practitioners offer a variety of methods – nasal washes, emesis, purging, enemas, and bloodletting (nowadays by leeches) often with douches, massage, yoga, meditation and vedic astrology, *Jyotish* (Sanskrit: *jyotis,* light/heavenly body). Hindu astrology is based on a sidereal system and fixed stars. The system familiar to Western astrologers today is tropical and based on the orientation of the Earth relative to the Sun and its planets. The two systems drift apart by about 1.4 arc degrees per century.

The original Vedic texts emphasised prevention as well as cure; public health as well as individual treatment. The Veda set down the use of various herbs, chemicals and medicines, and there is much in common with Ayurveda as it later came to be practised. There is much reliance on the personal experience of the practitioner but not on scientific observation and experimentation. Ayurveda is based on the Veda but with influence from aesthetic traditions of Buddhists, Jains and others which have more in common with shamanistic and spiritual dimensions. Ayurveda today holds that everything in the universe is made up of five great elements, with a human being having the addition of an 'immaterial self'. This idea parallels that of philosophies of vitalism in Europe. If you do not share these beliefs, you can set ayurvedic medicine aside. Conversely, if you are involved in ayurvedic medicine, it must be presumed you believe in the five elements of the cosmos and in the five processes of care – otherwise there would be no point to your practice.[9]

Ayurvedic theory and the practice of *rasa shastra* attributes importance to mercury and lead but few herbal medicines have been analysed to determine the effects of their constituents. There is concern at the heavy metal content of many 'traditional' medicines, which are not prepared to standards currently required in Western countries and may be at toxic levels. *Caveat emptor.*[10, 11]

Yoga
The Yogic system of healthcare has evolved from ancient Hindu philosophies and is now often a term applied to exercise, meditation, breathing and relaxation therapies (Sanskrit: *yoga,* union, join, yoke – implying 'union with the divine'). Many techniques have become orthodox – the original spiritual dimensions which raised non-scientific concepts of vital forces, chakras, and humoral balance have been left behind. There is good evidence that patients genuinely gain benefit from feeling more relaxed, calm, less stressed and gently exercised.

Traditional yoga developed under the stimulus of different masters and gurus and has been used by all the TIM systems. A wide variety of styles, concepts and practices have evolved since the rise of inter-religious movements in fifth century India. *Hatha Yoga* began as a branch of practices described as Tantric, whose devotees sought to fuse the male and female aspects of the universe into a state of mystical bliss, sometimes by decidedly intimate means (Sanskrit: *tantra*; principle, doctrine). Hatha Yoga, practised by Lord Shiva himself, seeks balance of positive and negative influences by contemplation, meditation, breathing control and positioning of the body (Sanskrit: *ha,* sun, the mind; *tha,* moon, 'vital energy' – also termed *prana*). *Raja Yoga*, the yoga sutras of Patanjali, combined the practice of meditation and exercise with mystical Samkhya philosophy arising from the early days of civilisation in the Indus Valley. Hindu, Buddhist and Jain Scriptures distinguished between *Jnana Yoga* based on knowledge, *Karma Yoga* based on action and *Bhakti Yoga* which emphasises a loving devotion to a personal god.

The objective of all styles of yoga is to improve health and well-being by inducing a release from suffering and the repeated cycle of death and reincarnation. In the Buddhist and Jain traditions, such liberation is aimed at achieving *nirvana* – the 'highest happiness', achieved by deep meditation, even reaching the level of cessation of thought. Such deep states are enhanced by relaxing the body into various yogic postures and achieving 'Kundalini arousal'. Kundalini is the serpent goddess in the base of the spine, who can be induced to travel upwards activating the patient's *prana* and clearing their *chakras* so that psychic healing powers are released. Hatha Yoga extended the original sitting postures to the 'full body poses' which are seen today in Western interpretations. Kundalini herself has never been identified, being more elusive than a Higg's boson.

The West of the 1960s saw an extraordinary release of philosophical, psychological and political inhibition with developing interest in Eastern esoteric spiritual practices. A number of gurus actively promoted yoga, which became part of the growing interest in health and well-being. The principles have also become adapted by twentieth century systems such as that of Joseph Pilates. Swami Satchidananda influenced cardiologist Dean Ornish who has developed a particular interest in the affects of lifestyle on coronary heart disease. His recommendations for yoga, meditation, low-fat diet, smoking cessation and regular exercise are now orthodox and the benefits of this approach for managing coronary disease have been demonstrated in randomised controlled trials.[12]

Controversies continue as to the value of a strict vegetarian diet and fish oil supplements recommended by gurus, but claims for benefit are now becoming subject to proper scientific scrutiny. Consensus will gradually emerge but until it does, yoga for disease management is classified as a CAM. Yoga seems likely to enter the orthodox canon as postural yoga (*asana*) and breath control (*pranayama)*. Stripped of the more spiritual, occult and esoteric elements of the original oriental philosophies and practices, yoga continues as a component of exercise programmes developing strength, mobility and stability through the *asanas*. Those interested should bear in mind that pushing body positions to the limit may cause injuries, and that traditional yogic practices were for supple young people training over years to reach nirvana, not middle aged westerners wanting to get fit.[13]

Unani Tibb

In the second century AD, Claudius Galenus wrote on many disciplines including philosophy, logic, anatomy, and pathology. He was a Roman physician and surgeon of Greek extraction whose theories influenced the development of medicine for over sixteen hundred years. In 1025, the Persian physician Abu ibn Sina (known in Europe as Avicenna) had written his *Canon of Medicine.* Although he emphasised the importance of observation and evidence-based opinion, his system was built on that of Galen and evidence was not of the highest standard – he still proposed that health was a matter of balancing the four Hippocratic humours of phlegm, blood, yellow bile and black bile. These influences entered South Asia and India with the Muslim conquests of the thirteenth century and evolved as 'Unani Tibb'. (Arabic: *Unani,* Ionian; *tibb,* medicine). Galen's opinions about human anatomy were wrong but not corrected until the work of Andreas Vesalius in 1543. His theory of the physiology of the circulation remained current until William Harvey's *De Motu Cordis* of 1628.

Unani physicians, *hakim* (Arabic: wise one), make diagnoses as do conventional doctors, but treatment is based on similar principles to Ayurveda – balancing the elements or humours. In 1997 the Indian government constituted an Act to standardise education in Unani medicine but such systems are still regarded by the World Health Organisation as alternative. The medicines and herbs used are simply not manufactured to the same standards as those in Western pharmacopoeias and the fundamental principles are pseudo-scientific.

Siddha

The Siddha tradition developed two thousand years ago, particularly amongst the Tamil people of southern India and Northern Sri Lanka. Basing their system on meditation, herbs, plants and trees, minerals and animal parts, there were eighteen important siddhar gurus and eight supernatural powers. (Tamil: *sidda,* from its root *chit,* heavenly bliss. Sanskrit: an accomplished, perfect one). A combination of priest, physician and magician, Guru Agathiyar received his wisdom from the son of Lord Shiva himself. The intention, as with most medical systems in India, is to achieve a 'heavenly bliss' with the body being in balance with the spirit. In this system there are five basic elements, corresponding with the five senses. The influence of the humours vata (air) in childhood, pitta (fire) in adults and kapha (earth and water) in old age is the reverse of beliefs of the Ayurveda system. Deep within the body are *varmam*, akin to chakras, which act to encourage free flow of prana. A hundred or so of these vital points are recognised, but not by conventional science.

Jains believe siddha are the souls of those who have meditated enough to loosen the bonds of *karma* – the deeds and actions of cause and effect in our lives. By meditation we can be truly liberated and achieve salvation.

In 2003 the Indian Government changed the term 'Indian System of Medicine and Homeopathy' and renamed it as AYUSH – Astang Ayurveda, Yog and Naturopathy,

Unani Tibb, Sidda and Homeopathy. There is now an Ayush Medical Association for practitioners of the 'Ayush System.' The AMA intends having the Ayush system 'removed from the complementary and alternative medical system and try to recognise it like other scientific medical system and national medical system as modern medical system' (Constitution of the AMA, *sic*). However the standards of scientific evidence-base are not those recognised by conventional systems and the various practices of Ayush remain faith based – some might think each practice is mutually contradictory. Toxic heavy metals are components in many remedies, and extreme care has to be taken in their use. In 2008, the Indian Government's Ministry of Health and Family Welfare made clear it 'has not recognised an Integrated System of Medicine. Moreover, currently there is no proposal to introduce or to develop Integrated System of Medicine by the Government of India. So the question of budget allocation does not arise.'[14]

Traditional Chinese Medicine (TCM)

As practised today, not traditional but rather developed during the 1950s by committees of the Peoples' Republic within their political ideology; not historically Chinese but rather Indian; not medicine in any modern sense but rather an alternative to scientific evidence-based systems – TCM is undoubtedly popular throughout the Far East and is now regularly seen in western shopping centres and high streets. China benefits from considerable exports of TCM products and marketeers are not likely to drop the term 'Traditional' any time soon.

TCM is based on ancient Chinese concepts and philosophies of diet and disease originating in India, with a variety of other techniques added – principally massage of numerous types, such as *Tui Na*, acupuncture, moxibustion and herbal medicine. Myths identify Shennong, the 'divine farmer' who devised a formulary of medicinal plants in the twenty fifth century BC. Accounts suggest he was a friend of Huang Di, the Yellow Emperor (after the Yellow River), and together they were party to secrets of medicine, alchemy and making gold. The same mythology suggests Shennong devised acupuncture, which is described extensively in the the Yellow Emperor's *Huangdi Neijing* and which became formalised by the third century BC.

The *Neijing* is regarded as the oldest organised medical textbook and the basis of the original TCM. Its ideas spread throughout China, Japan, Southeast Asia, and Korea but TCM as we know it today is a more recent development. Neijing is usually translated as 'Inner Canon of Medicine' (Chinese: *nei,* internal; *jing,* medicine). 'Canon' means 'law', and implies the authoritarian nature of the Emperor, which would not be appropriate in medicine today. Kings can now expect to have their opinions challenged.

The oldest beliefs of the peoples developing as Chinese were shamanistic, with influences of demons and spirits on health and well-being paramount. The *Neijing* additionally considered the effects of diet, the environment, emotions, the five elements, *qi* and *yin* and *yang* (the basic balanced forces of nature, or poles of

54

existence). Various combinations of *yin* and *yang* give rise to water, fire, wood, metal, and earth – the five elements which form our world. The vital energy then passes through channels styled *meridians*, affecting all parts of the human body. This 'vital energy' is termed in Chinese: *qi, chi, ch'i*, pronounced 'chee' – in Japanese: *ki;* Vietnamese*: xi;* Korean: *gi.* Blockage to free flow leads to imbalance and thereby, disease and illness. There are a wide variety of methods for making diagnoses by taking a detailed medical history including that of lifestyle, and examination of the pulse, tongue and eyes.

Balance and harmony between yin and yang is a fundamental concept of much traditional Chinese philosophy, science and medicine. Yin and yang are regarded as complementary but opposites and are particularly expressed in Buddhist adaptations of Taoist philosophy. Arising from an initial and ultimate nothingness (*wuji*) and finding expression in the works of traditional Chinese philosophers who sought to explain the mechanism of the universe, yin and yang are represented in the Taoist *taijitu* – a circle divided by an S-shaped line separating black and white, each side with a dot of opposite colour.

Different traditions offer different variants of the meridians. There is little coherence between them, and quite how a contemporary practitioner decides which to choose and use is mysterious and has no rational justification. The number of acupuncture points varies between four and 365 according to which practitioner is consulted. There is no consensus. There is considerable disagreement amongst TCM practitioners about how to diagnose patients and what treatments go with which disease. Modern scientific analysis cannot be applied to such metaphysical considerations. Given there is no scientific evidence of yin, yang, chi, meridians, nor the wide variety of pulse qualities practitioners claim to be able to detect – any diagnosis offered is clearly unscientific and any treatment based upon it must be regarded as alternative and incompatible with modern medicine and healthcare.

The Chinese know this perfectly well and today their doctors are trained in conventional medicine just as those in the West. A false dichotomy is presented – as if there is a difference between 'Western' and 'Eastern' medicine. There is not. There is simply 'medicine' – medical and healthcare practice which works and has an effect on disease, illness or injury, on all peoples of the world – and that which does not. Other medical systems are alternatives. For traditional, metaphysical and often political reasons, some healthcare systems are more tolerant of alternative medicine systems than others. Economic necessity in the West tends to require evidence of effectiveness before public funding of medical systems. In the East, tradition may hold greater sway, even in the absence of scientific evidence of effectiveness. Funding of some traditional systems might assuage the concerns of the populace and keep them tolerably contented but that is politics, not science. Karl Marx regarded religion as 'the opium of the people' in much the same way.[15]

In the 1840s Emperor Mianning had acupuncture removed from the curriculum of the Imperial Medical Institute as being old-fashioned and not in tune with developing science-based medicine. China has always used Western precepts when they clearly have value and does not cling on to tradition without good reason. After the communist revolution of 1949, the People's Republic of China determined that healthcare of some sort should be made available to all its citizens. There were clearly not enough regularly educated and trained doctors, so Mao Tse-tung took a pragmatic view and established a system of traditional healers known as 'barefoot doctors'. At least they provided the populace with some healthcare, irrespective of whether their practices actually worked or not. The fact patients were receiving some attention was better than nothing and good for morale. Mao himself described these practitioners as snake-oil salesmen and said: 'Even though I believe we should promote Chinese medicine, I personally do not believe in it. I do not take Chinese medicine.'[16] The Communist government founded the State Administration of Traditional Chinese Medicine in 1954.

Other current concerns relate to the composition of traditional medicines themselves. Many contain herbs of indeterminate origin which would not pass the basic tests required to be classified as a 'medicine' by orthodox regulatory authorities. Many might still contain compounds derived from endangered species. Indeed, this is the principal attraction of TCM for many camees.

The demand for rhinoceros horn in Traditional Chinese Medicine is rising. TCM practitioners use pulverised horn for a range of problems from skin disease to cancer. The horn is essentially composed of keratin, a fibrous structural protein found in the outer layer of human skin, forming the basis of hair and nails, as well as feathers and claws of birds and shells of animals such as tortoises. Rhino horn is now the most valuable commodity in the world and with widespread poaching there has been a serious decline in the numbers of rhinos. As a result, rhino farms are being developed in China to allow harvesting of horns, which are cut down and then allowed to re-grow.[17] The Duke of Cambridge's recent expression of concern over these traditional practices has been welcomed by those seeking to protect the rhinoceros.[18]

Bones of tigers have been regularly used in TCM, particularly in making medicines for arthritis. Some authorities suggest that enthusiasm for these medicines was behind the tiger conservation crisis in the 1990s. *Panthera tigris* is now an endangered species. TCM also has a need for the bile of the black bear, and bear farms have developed in China since the 1980s. Conservationists also express disquiet at the demands of TCM for musk deer and seahorses. In Korean medicine the endangered pangolin is slaughtered for its scales which are made simply of keratin, just like human nails. Given there is little or no scientific evidence of the efficaciousness of remedies prepared using these ingredients, conservationists' concerns are well founded. They should be borne in mind by camees interested in these systems of medicine, and by those minded to support them. Toe nail clippings are just as efficacious.

Moxibustion provides effects similar to acupuncture, stimulating 'meridians of chi' by burning dried mugwort herb, as a moxa stick, and applying it to the relevant point. Originally this process produced blistering, and whilst some practitioners still follow the traditional method, indirect moxibustion which stops short of scarring is now attracting adherents.

The origins of the methods used to make diagnoses and develop treatments may be from the West or East, but modern doctors and healthcare professionals of all traditions share a commonality of understanding which has become orthodox. Which is not to say it is unchanging or that there are not at times a very considerable disagreements amongst orthodox practitioners. Indeed – that is the nature of science. There will always be change and development. It is because traditional practitioners have been reluctant or unable to give up their beliefs and practices that they have been obliged to develop 'alternative medicine' and promote their practices as offering 'complementary approaches.' Many patients appreciate traditional approaches and gain benefit from them, in the sense they 'feel better'. It is essential however, that camees understand what it is they are exposing themselves to, the risks they are taking and that they are able to give fully informed consent. We are now some five thousand years from Shennong's time. There is some way to go.

Traditional Magnetic Medicine (TMM)

Animal Magnetism, Mesmerism, Hysteria, and Hypnosis.
From time immemorial various forces of nature were recognised, though their interconnectivity has taken until the latter part of the twentieth century to describe in detail and a 'Theory of Everything' still seems a long way off. One of the most mysterious forces, magnetism, has long been used by priests, magicians and medicine men. Six centuries before Christ, Thales of Miletus had written about magnetic properties of the lodestone he found in Magnesia.

Paracelsus
By the early sixteenth century Swiss physician Phillipus von Hohenheim was using magnetite for therapeutic purposes in his medical practice, attributing occult and magical powers to magnets. His adopted professional name of 'Paracelsus' meant 'equal to Celsus.' Perhaps not unsurprisingly, colleagues regarded him as arrogant. He wrote about the 'unconscious' in *Von den Krankeiten* (1567). 'The cause of the disease chorea lasciva is a mere opinion and idea, assumed by imagination, affecting those who believe in such a thing. In children their sight and hearing are so strong that unconsciously they have fantasies about what they have seen or heard.'

Chorea was a strange hysteric dancing sickness, also called *St. Vitus' dance* after the saint at whose shrine cures were sometimes prompted. Whole populations could be affected, wildly dancing and entering trances. In the sixteenth century, magnetic forces were held to have been at work in the unconscious minds of the afflicted. The Ancient Greeks had a word for such problems, *hysteria*, from *hysteron*: a womb – which was thought to move and trouble the female patient. Men did not have hysterics.

William Gilbert (1544-1603)
Gilbert eventually proved the Earth itself is a magnet, and explained why compass needles point north and south. His experiments, observations and detailed data analysis on magnetism and static electricity were reported in *De Magnete* (1600), regarded by some as the first great scientific work in English. He became physician to the Court of Elizabeth I.

William Maxwell (1581-1641)
Maxwell was a keen Paracelsian, physician to Charles I and a magnetiser, but recognised the importance of the imagination in healthcare: 'If you wish to work prodigies, abstract from the materiality of beings – increase the sum of spirituality in bodies – rouse the spirit from its slumbers. Unless you do one or other of these things – unless you can bind the idea, you can never perform anything good or great.'

Sir Kenelm Digby (1603-1665)
Son of Sir Edward Digby who had been executed for his part in the Gunpowder Plot, Kenelm promoted the idea of the *weapon-salve* and the *powder of sympathy* based on astrology. Applied to the weapon itself, they healed wounds by utilising magnetic forces created within the weapon which had caused them. Today we would today regard such Sympathetic Magic as a hypnotic effect.

Sebastian Wirdig (1613-1687)
The Professor of Medicine in Mecklenburg presented *The New Medicine of the Spirits* to the Royal Society in 1673, explaining how the whole world was influenced by magnetism and how living things could thereby influence each other and even cause death. During the seventeenth century, Valentine Greatrickes in London, Francisco Bagnone in Italy, Balthazar Gracian in Spain and Johann van Helmont in Switzerland all promoted their magnetic healing practices as being effected by 'the spirits' and even directly by God.

Richard Mead (1673-1754)
Mead was born in London, to which he returned after qualifying in medicine in Padua in 1695. He became a physician at St Thomas's Hospital, an Apothecary, a Fellow of the Royal Society, lecturer in Anatomy at Surgeon's Hall, and physician to George II. Sea captain Thomas Coram established The Foundling Hospital as a home for the children of unmarried mothers. As a hospital governor, Mead's house became the original Hospital for Sick Children, Great Ormond Street. Today its charitable activities continue as the Thomas Coram Foundation for Children. It was Coram who persuaded philanthropist Thomas Guy to found a hospital to the south of London Bridge. Mead delivered the thirteenth prestigious Harveian Oration of the Royal College of Physicians in 1723, on the *Status of Greek and Roman Physicians.*

In his younger days Mead imagined that he was able to account mechanically for the effects of several poisons, by their mixture with the blood; but he was afterwards convinced, that there is in all living creatures a vehicle infinitely more subtle, an ethereal and invisible liquor, over which poisons have a real, though inexplicable, power. This retracting of an opinion, earlier espoused, which procured him great credit in the literary world, shows a candour and ingenuity becoming a great man.[19]

Mead's *Mechanical Account of Poisons* was published in 1702. His *Short Discourse concerning Pestilential Contagion* (1720) formed the basis of subsequent theories of transmissible diseases and kick started the speciality of preventative medicine. Sir Isaac Newton was both a patient and a friend and Mead incorporated Newton's ideas of gravity and forces in his own work: *On the Influence of the Sun and Moon upon Human Bodies and the Diseases Arising Therefrom* (1704):

My new reasoning was founded upon experiments of electricity and attraction applied to the nervous fluid, which at the time of my writing were not known. The instructive Queries and Suppositions of Sir Isaac Newton, and the surprising electrical operations of Mr Stephen Gray, improved by Monsieur Du Fay at Paris, had not then enlightened the learned world. My reasoning upon this abstruse subject are grounded upon principles of planetary attraction, lately discovered by Sir Isaac Newton.[20]

Mead went on to set out a rationale for the effects of changing atmospheric pressure on the body by the same mechanism that caused tides, winds and weather. Mead reasoned:

The Moon has a greater influence on the nervous fluid or animal spirits than on the blood, or any other fluid of the animal body. Wherefore the moon's action will chiefly regard those diseases which are occasioned by the vitiation of those spirits. The moon, says Galen, governs the periods of epileptic cases. Upon this force, they, who were thus affected, were by the Greeks and Latins afterwards, called Lunatici.

Richard Mead sets a good example of the proper behaviour of a scientist: Faced with newer and better evidence, old ideas are abandoned and the new are further explored – in this case by the emerging sciences of physics and chemistry. Mead's approach to psychological phenomena and illness continued to have influence and were developed by Franz Anton Mesmer, whose name became used eponymously for a distinct style of therapy.

Maximillian Hell (1720-1792)
Originally named Höll, Hell was a Jesuit priest, astronomer and director of the Vienna Observatory in 1756. There he developed the therapeutic use of magnets and taught the medical student Anton Mesmer.

Franz Anton Mesmer (1734-1815)
Mesmer studied Mead's theory of 'nervous fluid or animal spirits' and the dissertation for his doctorate from Vienna University, *On the Influence of Planets on the Human Body,* was published in 1766. Advancing Mead's concepts, Mesmer set out his own principles which were recorded as *Mesmer's Aphorisms and Instructions.*[21]

Essentially Mesmer was concerned to remove any obstacle or obstruction to the free flow of universal fluid through unseen channels – much as those of oriental mien hold that *ch'i* affects us. Mesmer later set aside his initial idea that this could be done by lodestone magnets and introduced the idea of 'animal magnetism' – using the French word *animale* (soul, the basic force within animals). Mesmer devised the term 'animal magnetism' to distinguish this force from mineral, planetary and cosmic magnetism. By its means, health could be restored in a natural manner:

> Everything in nature has a communication by a universal fluid, in which all bodies are plunged; There is a constant circulation of acting mediums; There are several ways to ascertain them, and make them subservient to mankind: the surest method is, to place yourself opposite the person you mean to touch... you must put your hand upon his shoulder, then come down gently to the fingers and ... repeat this operation two to three times and by that means you will establish a communication agency from head to foot... The cause of the disorder must be enquired into.
>
> You keep constantly touching the cause of the disorder, and by aiding by degrees, the symptomatic pain produces a kind of crisis ... and effects a radical cure; You touch with advantage by the means of an extraneous conductor. We generally make use of a little wand about 10 or 15 inches long of a conic form, ending in a blunt point. These wands may be made of iron, steel, gold, or silver. A basin is magnetised by plunging a cane or any other conductor into the water, to communicate to it a medium. The person opposite to it will feel the effect of it. Many persons may be placed around the basin and will feel the magnetic power; The apparatus of magnetism consists in a flat tub containing some water about a foot high, with a cover screwed to the tub.

Mesmer went on to describe in detail how groups of patients could be treated, sat around the tub of water containing magnetised iron filings, applying the magnetised wands to their afflicted parts. Mesmer advised:

> There is an incredible number of other means to effect Magnetism, such as sounds, music, light and looking glasses. The magnetic fluid retains some of its virtue even after being extracted from the body... the greater quantity of patients, the greater power in the magnetism, for thereby the mediums multiply and the fluids gained strength by the union and the contacts.

Mesmer's 'animal magnetism' was not 'an attractive force emanating from an animal' but rather 'a force derived from the soul'. This vitalist force was not one of the four fundamental forces of nature as they are now understood. Mesmer felt the free flow of life's vital force was essential for health and that his methods would remove obstructions, produce crises and restore wellbeing. We have come across these beliefs before, and since. An early commission for Mesmer was from the Munich Academy of Sciences – to consider the exorcisms carried out by charismatic priest Johann Gassner. Mesmer's approach was secular and suggested the exorcisms were due to Gassner's 'animal magnetism'. Gassner, who had ascribed his success to the intercession of the divine, retired hurt. Some have regarded Mesmer's approach as initiating dynamic psychiatry. Mesmer based his methods on scientific principles but the excitement, even hysteria, caused by the group therapy in his salons and the success of his treatments, particularly on psychosomatic problems, inevitably created jealousies with other members of the medical profession. He had to give up his practice in Vienna, moving to Paris in 1777. Whereupon history repeated itself.

Parisian monk Abbe Faria emphasized that 'nothing comes from the magnetizer; everything comes from the subject and takes place in his imagination i.e., autosuggestion generated from within the mind.' Further challenges from the medical community followed and in 1784 King Louis XVI set up a Commission of Inquiry to investigate Mesmer's work. Commissioners were specifically charged with differentiating between 'the instantaneous effects of the magnetic fluid and all the illusions which might mix with them.' Mesmer did not co-operate and instead the commission had to audit the practice of Dr Charles d'Eslon, who had studied with Mesmer, but who was held by him to be inferior. As a result of the lack of co-operation by mesmerists and perhaps due to their lack of insight about scientific methods, the Commission largely set aside considerations of the undoubted clinical benefits and concentrated instead on the mechanism.

Members of the Commission included the father of modern chemistry, Antoine Lavoisier, Dr Joseph-Ignace Guillotin (whose humanity extended to promoting an 'ethical' method of execution he had imported from Germany) and the noted polymath, physicist and American ambassador to France, Dr Benjamin Franklin. It is ironic that during the Reign of Terror Guillotin's machine was to despatch Lavoisier, despised by the National Assembly for being a tax collector. Lavoisier's outstanding scientific work was totally disregarded by the new authorities. This approach to science is reflected even today in the activities of fundamentalists.

After extensive experiments, which we can regard as clinical trials, the Commission found no evidence of any universal magnetic fluid or animal magnetism. The Commission concluded that the music, wand waggling and general ambience of the sessions imparted such an intense experience to patients that they became entranced, exhibited convulsions and were 'mesmerised'. The benefits of the experience were due to the imagination of the participants. Expectations rose when attending such fashionable treatment sessions and gave added depth to the experience of the susceptible. The Commissioners declared that Mesmer's methods affected the imagination but otherwise were medically useless and unsafe.

Mesmer had also emphasised the importance of patients achieving 'harmony' with each other and the wider world. He founded *La Société de l'Harmonie Universelle* on democratic lines, where people of different ranks met on terms of equality. Membership was by subscription, from which the good doctor benefitted handsomely. Harmony became a theme of the French revolution and in 1793 Louis XVI was executed for treason when he failed to harmonise. By then Mesmer had retired quietly to Austria where he died in 1815.

Despised as a quack and charlatan, Thomas Jefferson described Mesmer as a maniac and his methods 'a compound of fraud and folly.' Nevertheless, these fashionable

61

trends were welcomed in the new United States and attracted many 'magnetic practitioners'. Mesmer's use of a metal wand as a conductor was reflected by Dr Elisha Perkins and his 'Patent Metallic Tractors'.

Mesmer had been convinced of the physiological reality of 'animal magnetism' and he sought scientific credibility. Eventually he came to realise that a trance like state could be induced by eye to eye contact and speaking in soft tones – the magnetised wands and bathwater were unnecessary. Mesmerism steadily developed to the therapeutic hypnotism we recognise today.

Amand-Marie-Jaques de Chastenet (1751-1825)
The Marquis de Puységur studied Mesmer's works and developed his own system for inducing a state of 'artificial somnambulism'. Now known as 'hypnotic induction', Puységur triggered the trance like state by assisting the subject concentrate, ignore peripheral awareness and relax – aided by focusing on bright objects such as a gently swung watch on a chain. He did not suggest the practitioner was transferring some form of force or energy to the subject, but rather was influencing the subject to control their own conscious state. Force of personality of the practitioner and susceptibility of the subject all played a part.

Puységur claimed; 'I believe in the existence within myself of a power; I believe I have the power to set into action the vital principle of my fellow-men; I want to make use of it; this is all my science and all my means. Believe and want – and you will do as much as I.' Readers must judge in what way Reiki and today's other energy therapies are any different.[22]

Elisha Perkins (1741-1799)
Perkins practised as a doctor in Connecticut. In 1796 his 'Metallic Tractors' were the first medical devices to be patented in the United States. At six centimetres, they were smaller than Mesmer's wands and claimed to be made of secret exotic alloys. Applied directly to the affected part, they were then drawn away, so removing the harmful forces and 'noxious electric fluid that lay at the root of suffering.' Though they cost about five pence to manufacture, they sold in pairs for over a thousand times that – five guineas (£5000 at today's prices). They made Perkins and his son Benjamin very rich indeed. – even George Washington bought a pair.

In 1797 the Connecticut Medical Society condemned use of the tractors as 'delusive quackery' and Perkins a 'user of nostrums'. Perkins was expelled from its membership. Elisha and Benjamin went to England and were initially well-received – the Quaker Society of Friends even built the Perkinean Institution to arrange treatments for the poor on a charitable basis. Eminent people enthusiastically attended public dinners and events in support of Perkins' 'grand medical discovery of the age.' To promote their worth more widely, tractors were given to ministers of religion gratuitously. After Elisha's death in 1799, Benjamin continued in practice and published his father's work on *The Influence of Metallic Tractors on the Human*

Body.

Sir Joseph Banks, the naturalist on Capt James Cook's first great voyage, was noted to be having 'a good deal of laughing about the Tractors'. His scepticism was shared by many doctors, notably John Haygarth.[23] Mesmer had done what he could to establish his therapies on a scientific basis. Perkins did not, and in 1799 Dr John Haygarth of Bath exposed his methods as quackery and charlatanism. Haygarth conducted placebo controlled trials and proved that the use of 'fictitious wooden tractors' worked as well as Perkins' expensive alloys. Benjamin returned to the United States, £800,000 better off (today's value).

Charles Poyen

A French self-styled 'Professor of Animal Magnetism', Poyen promoted Puységur's methods in America in 1836, giving lecture-demonstrations as stage performances. Phineas Quimby (1802-1866) was impressed and found common ground with a range of new religious, metaphysical and psychical approaches which were attracting acolytes at that time such as Swendenborgism and Spiritualism. Quimby set aside his original career as a watchmaker, studied with Poyen for two years and became a mesmerist in Maine. He eventually opined that all illness was illusionary and set out his philosophies as *New Thought*, later expressed as *Quimbyism*. Rather than put patients into a trance, Quimby entered into intensive conversation with them on the basis that 'the mind was spiritual matter and could be changed.' Quimby's ideas influenced a number of other newly developing religious groups, including San Francisco's Church of Divine Science and Mrs. Mary Baker Eddy's Christian Science – though Eddy later expressed concern that subjects could be under the influence of unscrupulous mesmerists who were 'channels for Satan's electric currents.'

It became clear orthodox medicine relied much on placebo effects. The American physician and author Dr Oliver Wendell Holmes Snr. gave detailed consideration to the placebo effects of Haygarth's fictitious tractors in *Homeopathy and Its Kindred Delusions* (1842). In this he discussed the ability of a physician's charisma and bedside manner to arouse patients' imaginations and emotional responses. He also suggested use of the word 'anaesthesia' to describe a state of having sensations blocked.

James Braid (1795-1860)

Born in Scotland, Braid was educated at the Royal College of Surgeons of Edinburgh. After private practice in Dumfries, he moved to Manchester where he became a well-known surgeon, successfully operating on conditions as disparate as clubfoot and squint, both of which can have an origin in muscular imbalance.

Having seen demonstrations by Charles Lafontaine, a travelling mesmerist and publisher of *Le Magnéitiseur,* Braid claimed he had discovered a natural psycho-physiological mechanism which accounted for the trances demonstrated by susceptical subjects. Initially he felt these were due to 'nervous sleep' which he termed 'neuro-hypnotism' after Hypnos, the Greek god of sleep. He later shortened this to 'hypnotism'. After lecture demonstrations in Manchester in 1842, Braid was reproached by the clergy and responded with *Satanic Agency and Mesmerism Reviewed.* His paper *On the Curative Agency of Neuro-Hypnotism* was submitted to the British Association but was declined and had to be published privately.

In 1843, John Elliotson, Professor of Medicine at University College, London reported *Numerous Cases of Surgical Operations without Pain in the Mesmeric State.* At that time, there were no anaesthetics. They had to wait until dentist William Morton's work with ether in 1846. Elliottson was denounced as a fraud, though his friend Charles Dickens regularly used hypnotism as entertainment for family and friends.

James Braid's initial theory that hypnotism was purely a physiological phenomenon did not stand the test of more critical experiment and analysis. He abandoned that original idea, as a true scientist should, and incorporated a more psychological approach. This emphasised the importance of assisting the subject focus or concentrate on a single idea, much as Puységur had suggested. Braid referred to this as *monoideism.* He considered various theories to account for the phenomena, considering most responses were due to delusion of the subjects but possibly the phenomena were real and produced by the imagination. Braid regarded Mesmer's theories which suggested that some form of transmissible magnetic force caused the phenomena as belonging to the occult worlds of the supernatural. His own preferred theory was that there was 'a peculiar physiological state of the brain and the spinal cord induced by the hypnotist' and said:

> I adopted the term 'hypnotism' to prevent my being confounded with those who entertain that the mesmeriser's will has an irresistible power over his subjects, and that clairvoyance and other 'higher phenomena' are manifested by those in the mesmeric state. I was the first to give a public explanation of the trick by which a fraudulent subject had been able to deceive his mesmeriser. I have never been a supporter of the imagination theory – that the induction of hypnosis is merely the result of imagination. My belief is quite the contrary. I attribute it to the induction of a habit of intense abstraction or concentration of attention, and maintain that it is most readily induced by causing the patient to fix his thoughts and sight on an object, and suppress his respiration.[24]

Braid felt that the eye muscles, being strained by concentration and fixation, would tire and induce sleep. Being used to operating on eye muscles he understood their function well. He did not regard hypnotism as a panacea, but used it sparingly: 'In the majority of cases I do not use hypnotism at all, but depend entirely upon the efficacy of medical, moral, dietetic, and hygienic treatment, prescribing active medicines in such doses as are calculated to produce obvious effects.'

Mesmerism and Magnetic healing in the USA of the mid-1800s

Mesmer's system of magnetic healing was introduced to America by the Marquis de Lafayette at the time of the Revolution and subsequently promoted by Charles Poyen.

Benjamin Franklin's scientific commission of inquiry had discredited Mesmer's theories of animal magnetism; however, faced with a burgeoning population and the relative paucity of orthodox medical practitioners, some States licensed these magnetic healers to practice. Having some caring practitioners, even if not medically qualified, was better than having none. A plethora of magnetic practitioners emerged at the beginning of the nineteenth century. Dr Charles Caldwell developed a practice in 'magnetic medicine' in Louisville, Kentucky, advocated phrenology and opposed general medical opinion that yellow fever was contagious. Rev. John Dods cured two deaf and dumb girls by 'electro psychology' in 1849. Numerous other healers claimed success for magnetic techniques admixed with spiritualism and metaphysics.

Magnetic medicine provided the early training and stimulus for two other Midwest practitioners who went on to establish distinctive medical systems, developed further as legitimate medical therapeutic hypnosis, and is the basis of stage hypnotism as presented by modern entertainers. Some entertainers have developed their careers laterally and now provide elements of health care, particularly for psychological issues. Other magnetic practitioners left 'magnetism' and devised original healing methods involving hands on manipulation.

Paul Caster (1827-1881)
Born 'Custer', Caster developed a thriving 'magnetic practice' in Ottumwa, Iowa. He declared his ability was a gift from God and although he had no formal qualification, he styled himself as 'Doctor'. Amongst his students were Andrew Taylor Still and David Daniel Palmer who both started out as magnetic practitioners before going on to develop their own idiosyncratic medical systems.
Andrew Taylor Still founded Osteopathy in 1892 and D. D. Palmer, Chiropractic in 1895. Neither practitioner was a medical doctor. Their systems of medicine were novel and out with the norms of conventional orthodox mainstream medicine. Even today these systems do not comply with the requirements of evidence-based scientific disciplines. These practices, and other proprietary systems of medicine based on them, remain 'alternative'. That is, they are alternatives to evidence-based scientific medicine and require an alternative mind-set and way of thinking to normal. They are belief systems. A fact which appeals to patients who feel conventional medicine has not been able to help them deal adequately with underlying disease or unhappiness and to practitioners (medically qualified or not) who share the esoteric beliefs established by Custer, Still, Palmer and the other founders of unorthodox medical systems. But once upon a time in the West...

Endnotes to Chapter 4

1. Mirca Eliade. *Shamanism: Archaic Techniques of Ecstasy*. Bolingen series LXXVI, Pantheon Books, NYNY 1964.

2. Karl J. Narr. *Prehistoric Religion*. Britannia Encyclopaedia 2008. Retrieved 2008-9-12.

3. Ezekiel 13:20 and 2 Kings 21:6; Acts 19.

4. Alice Beck Kehoe, *Shamans and Religion: An Anthropological Exploration in Critical Thinking.* 2000: Waveland Press, Long Grove, Illinois.

5. Julius Caesar. *De Bello Gallico.* VI.13-18. 50 BC.

6. Vuckovic N. H. et al. *Feasibility and short-term outcomes of a shamanic treatment from temporomandibular joint disorders.* Altern. Ther. Health Med. 2007 Nov-Dec; 13(6).

7. Mishnaic Hebrew *rabbi,* and English *doctor,* from Latin *docere,* 'to teach,' both mean essentially the same as *guru.*

8. *Chi* is a traditional Chinese unit of length of about 33cms. 'Vital force' is more correctly written as *ch'i* or *qi,* but commonly as *chi,* and pronounced 'chee'. The term *chi* was also used to describe the setting of coding wheels solved during decryption by Colossus, the world's first programmable electronic computer developed during WWII at Bletchley Park, Berkshire. The use of *chi* for the settings may have reflected not only 'force' but also the Greek chi (X) as used in mathematics to denote a probability distribution. Given the upshot of Enigma and other codes on the outcome of the war, both senses seem apposite.

9. Dominic Wujastyk, *Indian Medicine.* www.ucl.ac.uk/~ucgadkw/papers/hm.pdf.

10. *Lead poisoning in pregnant women who used Ayurvedic medications from India*: New York City, 2011-2012. MMWR 61:641-646,2012.

11. Saper R. B. et al. *Heavy metal content of Ayurvedic herbal medicine products.* JAMA 292:2868-2873, 2004.

12. Dean Ornish. Lancet: 1990 July 21st 336 (8708).

13. For them, the personal fitness consultancy *Raw Impact* advises: 'Lay off the cake fatty, and go for a run.'

14. www.ayushmedicalassociation.org/pdf/constitution.pdf.

15. Karl Marx, from introduction to *Contribution to Critique of Hegel's Philosophy of Right,* 1843. In 1797 the Maquis de Sade had referred to *'This opium you feed your people'* in *L'Histoire de Juliette.*

16. Zhisui Li, *The Private life of Chairman Mao,* quoted by Simon Singh and Edzard Ernst, *Trick or Treatment.*

17. Jonathan Leake, *The Times*: 7th March 2010. Daniel Foggo & Simon Parry, *The Sunday Times*: 12th June 2011.

18. The rhinoceros is the emblem of the Worshipful Society of Apothecaries, reflecting the use formerly made of powdered horn in medicinal preparations. The Society has recognised the errors of its ways, moved on, and is now active in the 'Save the Rhino' campaign. Not all

TCM practitioners have been so progressive.

19. Thomas Ewing. Introduction, *The Medical Works of Richard Mead*, Dublin, 1767. Google Books 2011.

20. Quoted *ibidem.*

21. Caullet de Veaumore *Mesmer's Aphorisms and and Instructions.* Sold at the Glass Warehouse, London in 1785, now available from Google Books.

22. Henri Ellenberger, *Discovery of the Unconscious: The History and Evolution of Dynamic Psychiatry.* Basic Books.New York. 1970.

23. Tom Clarke in *A Journal of American Postal History,* Vol 28, no. 2. May 1997 p.16. La Posta Publications, Oregon, 1997.

24. James Braid, *Hypnotism,* Letter to the Editor, *The Lancet,* Vol.45, No. 1135 31 May 18 45.

Chapter 5

Traditional Western Medicine: TWM

There are, in fact, two things, science and opinion; the former begets knowledge, the latter ignorance.

It is more important to know what sort of person has a disease than to know what sort of disease a person has.
Hippocrates

The four groups of traditional medical practice described in the last chapter encompass numerous sub-varieties and there is wide diversity. Some sense of order has to be brought to bear, and a review of developing European and Western systems of medicine which have become universal over the past two millennia follows:

Our Western culture has developed and evolved from those established by the Greeks and then the Romans, starting some five hundred years before the time of Christ. Modern American medicine is based on European, and can be considered under the heading of Western, though the indigenous peoples of North and South America originally developed their own shamanic traditions. North American content has also been derived from the cultures of India, China, Arabia and the Far East, and more recently, with the culture of the Far West as represented by California! The account that follows outlines the traditions of where we have come from, how the Renaissance led us from the European dark ages, how the intellectual Enlightenment encouraged more focused attention to philosophical detail, how the scientific method developed and how we continue to evolve our medical systems to take advantage of modern technology and better understanding. The term 'TWM' is novel, but its use serves to emphasise that just as ancient Chinese medicine can be described as TCM, so we, from European backgrounds, can think of our philosophical and scientific developments as gradually emerging from our traditions. TCM has become something of a trendy marketing term. TWM is entitled to the same benefits of branding in the crowded healthcare market place. As with all the other new words coined in this book, if inventing novel words is good enough for camistry, it is good enough for us all.

In the modern world there is only one 'medicine' – based on evidence derived from rational use of the scientific method. It is global, coherent, progressive, developing, constantly being refined and founded on the purest principles of nature and science. Now we have only 'medicine' which probably works – and that which probably does not. Other systems are alternatives to medicine. But once upon a time in the West, there were only systems revealed by the gods:

Gods and Goddesses

Apollo was the senior ancient Greek god of medicine and healing. His son Asklepios (Aesculapius to the Romans) carried a wand, entwined with a single snake and no wings. Today this symbolises medicine throughout the world. Snakes had important connotations, for it was thought they could never fall ill. The caduceus, a staff with two snakes and a pair of wings, was carried by Hermes, the messenger of the gods (Mercury to the Romans). The caduceus remains a symbol of commerce, but its current use in American healthcare may have origins in printers' marks used by book publishers such as that of John Churchill of London. He used the emblem to signify 'messages and communications'. In ancient times Hermes, and the device, also had connotations of trickery. The caduceus was used on the uniforms of American army hospital stewards who acted as messengers for doctors, and was adopted by the Marine Hospital Service in 1871, possibly for purely aesthetic reasons.[1]

Consideration of these symbols might seem unimportant, but indicates how slippery meaning can be and how in healthcare, marketing can trump exactitude.[2] No doubt the gods will forgive transgressors who use the symbol wrongly – unless US medics mean to proclaim they are commercial cunning tricksters...

In ancient times, sufferers visited temples where singing, ritual purification, charismatic and thaumaturgic performance of the priests, together with soporific drugs heightened their fertile imaginations and even induced trances (*kharisma*, divine or spiritual gift; *thaumatourgos*, wonder-worker, conjurer). Not too far from hypnotic inductions as developed by Mesmer and Braid in the eighteenth and nineteenth century.

At these *Asklepieia*, heightened expectations and the suggestions of the priests enabled patients to experience Asklepios and his daughters, Hygieia, Iaso, Aceso, Aglæa and Panacea in dreams and visions. Patients could even be prepared to subject themselves to surgery. Non-venomous snakes were given free rein of the accommodation, and intensified the experience. Offerings to the gods were obviously essential, and faithfully collected by the priests. Since time immemorial it has been recognised that 'thar's gold in them thar ills.'

Philosophical and scientific scepticism

I don't believe in astrology. I am a Sagittarius and we're very sceptical.
Arthur C. Clarke

Ancient Greek philosophy and logic became established during the sixth century BC, with distinct schools of thought emerging such as those of Epicurus and Zeno. Traditionally, the opinions of high-ranking authorities were accepted as facts and taken as 'givens'. The Skeptikoi, followers of Pyrrho, questioned this dogmatic approach, recognised that absolute certainty of scientific truth is impossible and expected all propositions to be investigated and supported by evidence (*skeptesthai*, to think, consider; *dogmatos*, opinion, belief. Hence 'doctrines').[3]

Sceptics were supportive of empiricism, suggesting knowledge can only come from sensory experience gained from observation and experiments (*empeiria*, experience, from *peira*, trial, experiment). Developments of scepticism were to become known as the 'scientific method' and distinguished the empiricist approach from dogmatic opinion which relied on revelation or reason alone along the lines 'it seems to me ...'

Thales of Miletus. (c. 624-547 BC)
Thales is regarded as the first Greek to remove myths from traditional accounts of the natural world and establish an identifiable and rational form of natural philosophy. Thales developed a scientific method to answer the questions of life, albeit not with the precision of the eighteenth century Enlightenment. He studied with priests and astronomers of Crete and Egypt at a time when the gods were thought to account for everything.

Thales accepted the theory of matter based on four elements and phases: water/fluid; earth/solid; air/gas and fire/plasma. He also believed that matter was created from a principal element – water, which imbued everything. His ideas about spontaneous generation of life continued until Louis Pasteur in the nineteenth century. Thales noted that lodestone from Magnesia attracted iron and described the phenomenon of magnetism, ascribing the force to its 'soul'. He posed a question that has still not been answered twenty six centuries later: 'What is the basic material of the universe?'

Alcmaeon of Crotone (born c. 510 BC)
The ancient Babylonian concept was that man, being made of the four cosmic elements, depended for health and well-being on the equilibrium of those elements. Alcmaeon was a physician, natural philosopher and noted anatomist who advanced this concept adding ideas about the importance of lifestyle and the environment. Alcmaeon called this 'democracy' in distinction to 'monarchy' where one domain gains supremacy and makes people ill. He seems to have been the first to have realised the importance of the brain in controlling the whole person – an idea that was not widely accepted at the time.

Empedocles (c.490-430 BC)
Empedocles is credited with establishing the four elements theory as a basis for Greek philosophy and of 'knowledge' for two thousand years. Love and Strife were responsible for mixing the elements in the manner we see in the world around us and which were incorporated in a human's basic spirit or soul – to be reincarnated after death.

Empedocles was regarded as an outstanding orator and poet, a physician who could cure epidemics, and a magician who could control storms, wind and rain. He died when he threw himself into the crater of Mount Etna but failed to overcome its volcanic forces. At least he did the experiment.

Socrates (469-399 BC)
The archetypical Greek philosopher is recognised as a prime founder of Western philosophy. His constant questioning of any idea he could get his hands on not only led to his method being given his name but to the exasperation of civic authorities, the Tyrants, who ultimately demanded his suicide. The Tyrants were then overthrown. Socrates has left no writing of his own but we learn of his work through his pupils, notably Plato. The Socratic method of establishing a hypothesis by questioning is a basis of the scientific method.

Hippocrates (c.460-377 BC)
Regarded as the first philosopher to put the practice of traditional western medicine on a defined rational basis Hippocrates established a school on Kos and travelled widely through the Mediterranean. Although he regarded himself as a lineal descendant of Asklepios, he set aside ancient wisdom that health and disease was

mediated by divine intervention, supernatural spirits, demons or magic. Hippocrates' medicine was secular, and he described practitioners who related diseases to the gods as magicians and charlatans, and as being foolish. Even now, those ancient ideas linger in some contemporary cultures and systems of medicine.

> For the first time in our tradition there was complete separation between killing and curing. Throughout the primitive world, the doctor and the sorcerer tended to be the same person. He with the power to kill had the power to cure. He who had the power to cure would necessarily also be able to kill ... with the Greeks that distinction was made clear. One profession, the followers of Aesklepios and Hippocrates, were to be dedicated completely to life under all circumstances, regardless of rank, age or intellect.[4]

Hippocrates endorsed Alcmaeon's principle that illness and disease was caused by loss of balance or equilibrium between the four elements – *dyscrasia* (bad balance). He went further, proposing that four 'nervous juices', *chymoi,* or humours were the essential agents of the traditional four elements. The humours were thought of as fluids: blood was associated with air; phlegm with water; yellow bile with fire; black bile with earth. To achieve balance, the practice of bloodletting developed; expectorants assisted discharge of phlegm; emetics – yellow bile; purgatives – black bile. Human personality and temperament was associated likewise: sanguine, phlegmatic, choleric, melancholic.

The original Hippocratic School promoted gentle care, placing great reliance on the fact that most diseases had a natural history of recovery and that nature held the power of healing. (Latin: *vis medicatrix naturae*). In the centuries that followed, treatments based on bloodletting, purging and emetics were taken to excess and reached 'heroic' levels.

Hippocrates recognised the importance of a crisis during the course of illness, after which the patient either survived, relapsed or succumbed (*crisis,* turning point in a disease). He did not believe in superstition or spirits as a cause of illness – the necessary balance and harmony of the four humours could be achieved naturally. It was the job of a physician to care for the patient whilst nature took its course – to encourage rest, warmth, good hygiene and nutrition. Drugs were used sparingly. Hippocrates theory of *Humourism* held sway for two millennia.

Prior to Hippocrates it was hard to distinguish a priest from a magician from a physician. Ancient Egypt's Imhotep is regarded as having been a physician, as well as a priest. Hippocrates was the first to establish a distinct profession of natural philosophers who cared for the sick and injured and he is now thought of as the 'Father of Western Medicine'.

Hippocrates insisted on his students having discipline, being honest and serious – just like today's medical students. Along with taking a history from the patient, he stressed the importance of observation. Physicians should not only examine and make observations of a patient's appearance, pulse, temperature, pain and effluents, but also record them conscientiously. Much of his teaching was set down as his famous Aphorisms, the first of which counselled: 'Experience is deceitful and judgement difficult'. Physicians were taught to be cautious. He emphasised the importance of establishing a distinctive *diagnosis* and of clinical record keeping (*dia*, apart; *gnoskein*, to learn). Hippocrates should be regarded as the 'Father of Clinical Audit'.

Hippocrates clearly had a good bedside manner and was a true clinician (*klinos*, bed). Nevertheless, he counselled: 'Keep a watch also on the faults of patients, which often make them lie about the taking of things prescribed. For through not taking disagreeable drinks, purgative or other, they sometimes die. What they have done never results in a confession, but the blame is thrown upon the physician.'

As a result of observations and records he was able to identify and classify diseases and illnesses as well as their associated symptoms and recommendations for treatment. The underlying humoral theory of illness is nowadays set aside but many of the descriptions of disease and treatment are still valid. The principles of Hippocratic medicine were adopted throughout Europe and Arabia with Humourism only dying out after the Renaissance. Hippocrates' basic principles of clinical observation remain an influence on the development of medicine today.

The famous Hippocratic Oath may in fact have been set out after his death, but he gets the credit, and its tenets have remained the basis of medical ethics ever since (*ethike*, study of customs, morals). The original Greek has been translated by different authorities and with different interpretations. Some newly qualified doctors still take the oath or have it displayed during graduation ceremonies, for most, it is only of historical interest. By declaring this oath the physician entered a profession (Latin: *professionem*, public declaration). The tenets of the oath included:

> I will be loyal to my teachers, and in turn teach their children the art; I will do no harm to a patient (*primun non nocere*); I will keep myself far from all intentional ill doing; I will keep secret and never reveal all that may come to my knowledge in the exercise of my profession or in daily commerce, which ought not to be spread abroad; If I keep this oath faithfully, I will enjoy my life and practice, my art respected by all men and in all times; If I transgress and forswear this oath, may the reverse be my lot.

The medical profession remains top of the list of those that hold the public's trust. No comment on that which is at the bottom.[5]

Hippocrates' approach to medicine was an alternative to the previous systems which relied on the gods, spirits and superstition. Eventually, by custom and practice, Hippocrates' alternative medicine became orthodox. Patients were reassured and many recovered from what were often self-limiting diseases. Those with incurable

73

diseases were also well cared for by conscientious professionals. More importantly, Hippocrates encouraged the Socratic method of constantly questioning and he expected this questioning to lead to change and improvement. In the course of time Hippocrates' works inevitably became regarded as authoritative and formed the basis of medical care down the centuries, very often without challenge by subsequent practitioners – until time and circumstance again encouraged more questioning approaches. Indeed, from Hippocrates times patients were expected to trust their doctors without question. The principle that doctors should trust their patients to be closely involved in decision making and for patients to give informed consent, has only become established in the last quarter of the twentieth century.

Hippocrates' son Thessalus and son-in law Polybus founded a school of medicine based on Hippocrates' works which emphasised the importance of knowledge of hidden causes of diseases as well as the obvious signs. Observations and experiments might be necessary, but they felt the most important practice of a physician was to reason – and hence to be 'Dogmatic' and their system of medicine also came to be known as 'Rationalist'.

Plato (429-347 BC)
Sophocles' student, and teacher of Aristotle, founded a school in the Grove of Hecademus at Athens. The 'Academy' was closed by the Eastern Roman Emperor Justinian in 529 AD when its philosophical teachings seemed a threat to the Christianity which Justinian wished to promote.

The authorities had decided that Socrates had corrupted the minds of the youth of Athens by his constant questioning. He was found guilty of impiety and heresy and sentenced to take his own life by drinking hemlock, when he commented: 'I know you won't believe me, but the highest form of human excellence is to question oneself and others.' [6]

Plato's approach was to present arguments as 'discussions' with Socrates, questioning others about their beliefs, claims, premises and promises. He wrote extensively on medicine noting: 'Medicine is an art, and attends to the nature and constitution of the patient, and has principles of action and reason in each case.'

Aristotle (384-322 BC)
The son of a physician, Aristotle described Thales of Miletus (d.547 BC) as the first notable Greek philosopher (*philo,* loving; *sophia,* knowledge). Two hundred years later, Aristotle himself wrote about natural theology (the study of the gods and the universal science of first principles which underpinned all other sciences including mathematics and astronomy) and ontology (*ontos,* of being; what is meant by existence). None of which would have been possible if sound reasoning and opinions based on valid inference from physical facts had not been part and parcel of the philosophers' approach. 'Logic' was applied in ancient philosophies, including those of India and China but Aristotle put the subject on a more formal basis, identifying two principal styles of reasoning – inductive and deductive. (*Logike,*

possessed of reason; *logos*, thought, idea, argument, or principle).

Any thought, idea or proposal which you wish to convey to somebody else has to be put forward as an 'argument'. That term simply describes a discussion about the reasons which you wish to advance in support of your opinion. Two or more reasons are stated as 'premises', from which a 'proposition', a rational conclusion, can be inferred. If enough other people agree with your conclusion, and a consensus can be reached, so your idea can be moved up the scale from hypothesis, to theory, to fact – even to a scientific 'law'.

In a deductive argument, if the premises in general are true, then the conclusion is guaranteed to be true. 'All men are mortal, Socrates is a man, and therefore Socrates is mortal'. But if a premise is false, the conclusion will be false, in spite of a valid argument. To establish 'truth' in any meaningful way, not only must the logical argument be applied validly, but also the premises themselves must be true. In Aristotle's time, much reliance was placed on the 'truth' of basic premises about life and the universe which were in fact nothing more than the opinions of religious and political authorities who grandly proclaimed 'it seems to me...'

Additionally Aristotle taught the 'inductive' method of reasoning and argument. This encouraged better testing of initial premises from which inferences can be drawn more reliably. The premises of inductive arguments, as used by the scientific method, are established empirically, by observation, though can still be shown to be wrong when further and better particulars come to hand after more comprehensive observations and experiments.

Aristotle set out his system for conducting arguments in three steps which he called a 'syllogism' (*syllogismos*, conclusion). Aristotle's style of reasoning, by using categorical syllogisms enabled facts to be inferred by making logical links between the premises. This approach was fundamental to critical thinking and reasoning for the next two thousand years and formed the basis of science and medicine, only beginning to decline with the fifteenth century Renaissance. Aristotle's book *On the Soul,* in which he refers to the human mind starting out as an 'unscribed tablet' or 'blank slate' is regarded as the first Western book on psychology. The traditional collection of Aristotle's six books on logic were called the *Organon* (instrument, tool, organ). A word later adopted by Francis Bacon and then by Samuel Hahnemann for his works on homeopathy.

As more philosophers began applying themselves to what we may regard as 'medicine', most based their practices on the dogmatic opinions of authorities and not on experimental observations. After the Greek conquest of Egypt in 330 BC, some physicians in Alexandria based their practice on observation and experimentation and the Empiric School of Medicine emerged (*empeiria,* experience).

The Empirics were often seen as rivals to the Dogmatics. During the first century before Christ, various other competing schools of medicine were founded. In some, remedies were selected because they were known to cause symptoms comparable to those caused by disease – a principle described as *simila similibus:* 'like with like'.

Epicurus (c. 341-270 BC)

Epicurus and his colleagues, including women and slaves, developed a philosophy that was materialistic, pleasure-seeking and secular. He is regarded as the earliest liberal and scientific humanist, and influenced all later Hellenistic thought. He supported Democritus' revolutionary view that the universe consists of atoms and space and which found parallels in China, India and near East during the axial age of 800-200 BC. What was 'good' was defined by what was pleasurable, and that usually meant an absence of pain.

Asclepiades (c. 125-40 BC)

Placing emphasis on sympathy, pain relief and the humane treatment of the mentally ill, Asclepiades introduced Greek medicine and Epicureanism to Rome. He rejected Hippocrates' humoral theory and introduced the concept that disease resulted from irregular motion of corpuscles of the body – atoms. He promoted music therapy and used sugar pills for their placebo effect. His student, Themison of Laodicea continued his work, supporting elements of both the dogmatic and empiric systems of medicine, but held that medicine is no more than applied understanding of general factors manifest in a methodical way. Like was not necessarily cured by like, though an accurate diagnosis would suggest the best methods. Known as the Methodists, their followers certainly applied reason – not to find any occult, innate, indeterminate force, but facts which were confirmed by observation. Both Reason and Experience were of value, but the Methodists largely rejected the four humours theory and held that 'corpuscles' had to pass freely through pores in the body. Health was seen as a balance between obstruction and laxity. The cures that were offered by their methodological approach would therefore involve enlarging small pores, and closing large ones – 'cure by opposites'. Methodist physicians used gentle medicines with emphasis on convalescence, massage, exercise and cold baths.

Aulus Aurelius Celsus (c. 25 BC-c. 50 AD)

Celsus was not a physician but is famed for his great encyclopaedia *Artes* (the Sciences). Not only are the dates of his life uncertain, but even his exact name. *De Medicina* is regarded as a prime source of medical knowledge during the Roman period, a masterpiece of prose, and the origin of scientific Latin. Celsus appears to have been disenchanted with the various systems of medicine then current, regarding them as sects and cults: the Dogmatists basing their system on the opinion of dogmatic authority – in turn based on reason, which so often meant 'imagination'. The Empirics emphasised the importance of the experience of observations, often of poor quality, and the Methodists concentrated on the practicalities of treating everyday conditions. Celsus suggested both reason and experience should be integrated. He emphasised the four classic signs of inflammation – *calor, rubor, dolor, tumor*: heat, redness, pain, and swelling. Hippocrates had been first to describe malignant growths as having the appearance of a crab or crayfish – Celsus translated the Greek into Latin as *cancer.*

During the first century AD the Romans developed other systems. Methodists gave emphasis to the corpuscles, which were 'atoms', as they could not be cut (*a,* not; *tomos,* cutting).[7] The physicians of the Pneumatic school of medicine opined that the most important element involved in health and disease, over and above the humours, was immaterial spirit, *pneuma.* Notwithstanding Celsus' ambition that the different systems should be integrated, the Methodic, Dogmatic, Empiric and Pneumatic systems of medicine were all widely but independently used until synthesised by Galen.

Klaudios Galenos (129 AD-200AD)
Galen was a Greek physician and philosopher who made major contributions to virtually every known science. After extensive travel and studying different medical systems, he settled in Rome and became physician to a number of emperors. Subscribing to Hippocrates' Humourism, Galen's descriptions of human anatomy, based on non-human dissection, were accepted almost universally until Andreas Vesalius dissected humans in the middle of the sixteenth century. Galen barely distinguished between arteries and veins, though he recognised venous and arterial blood had different qualities. He taught that the body had two circulatory systems, based respectively on the heart and liver. He did not appreciate that blood circulated in one system and thought all the blood was freshly made in the liver each day. His 'two vascular systems' created a 'divine breath' or 'vital spirit' which maintained life, action and thought. His physiological opinions were regarded as authoritative until William Harvey's *De moto cordis,* in 1628.

As a philosopher, Galen wrote on logic and explained in *The Best Physician is also a Philosopher* that medicine should be closely aligned with philosophy. He is thought to have written more than six hundred books on virtually every subject.

The Western Roman Empire slowly collapsed over three centuries until the last emperor, Romulus Augustus, was deposed in 476 AD. Galen's works, along with most Greek philosophical and scientific works largely disappeared. Fortunately, even after Muslim Arab conquests in the seventh century they were still actively being used in Byzantium of the Eastern Roman Empire. Galen's rational and systematic system of medicine was an important influence on Islamic medicine, though experiments carried out by physicians such as Rhases raised doubts about the theory of Humourism.

Muhammad ibn Zakariya Razi (865-925 AD)
Rhases was a pre-eminent Persian physician from the city of Rey, whose influence was long felt throughout the Middle East and beyond. He studied Greek and Indian medicine and wrote more than two hundred books on medicine, alchemy, philosophy and music. Rhases based much of his own medical system on the original Hippocratic principles. He was particularly concerned about diseases of children, and was the first doctor to differentiate smallpox from measles. He described allergic rhinitis and

believed that fever represented the body's natural defence mechanism.

In a forerunner to the Internet, Rhases wrote a medical book for the public, so that they could have some guidance as to what diseases they might be suffering from and what remedies might be appropriate – even if they could not afford the services of a professional physician. He described how to make up the various drugs and in what proportions the components should be mixed in the appropriate 'recipe' (Latin: *recipe,* take).[8]

Rhases recognised that being a doctor required an education in all the then known sciences and philosophies, and he was highly critical of fakes and charlatans who sold their nostrums without having such an education. He did not claim the educated doctor had all the answers, but suggested they were at least more true to the basic ethic of being compassionate and acting with reason. He also expressed concern for doctors who cared for princes because their instructions, particularly for moderation, were not always obeyed!

Abu Ali al-Husayn ibn Abd Allah ibn Sina (c. 980-1037 AD)
Ibn Sina or Avicenna was a Persian who qualified as a physician at the age of eighteen. He found that 'medicine is no hard and thorny science, like mathematics and metaphysics, so I soon made great progress.' He was also a philosopher whose wrote extensively on many subjects. His *Canon of Medicine* was the standard medical text of the Middle Ages. Based on Hippocrates and Galen, incorporating the rational and logical approach of Aristotle, he shared with the Greeks the view that epidemics were caused by air pollution (*miasma*), but he also introduced the idea of contagion (*contact*). Infections could be communicated by physical contact or secretions from diseased patients.

Avicenna's approach to medical studies were rational and logical and in centuries to come his system became more popular than that of Rhases. He still based his approach on the four humours, to which he added emotional aspects, self-awareness, moral attitudes and influence of dreams. Importantly, Avicenna also wrote about the value of experimental medicine and clinical trials in a fore runner of what we now term 'evidence-based medicine'.

The Middle Ages: 500-1500 AD

During this period, doctors in Europe continued to care for their patients very much in line with Galen's teaching. Christianity flourished and was closely involved in civil governance. Disputes between church and state were common. Henry II appointed one of his best friends, Thomas Becket, as Archbishop of Canterbury, but became exasperated when Thomas proved less malleable than he had expected.[9]

At a meeting with his knights in 1170 Henry rhetorically asked 'Who will rid me of this turbulent priest?' Four knights made haste for Canterbury and murdered Thomas at the steps leading from the crypt to the quire of his cathedral. Henry was penitent and Thomas was canonised in 1173, his tomb becoming a site of pilgrimage. Pilgrims who set out from London gathered on the south side of London Bridge at a hospice which became St. Thomas' Hospice for the infirm. There they would prepare themselves for the journey down to Canterbury. The shrine at Canterbury was destroyed on the orders of Henry VIII in 1538.

Although the street where the hospice stood remains St Thomas' Street, the advent of another hospital sponsored by the philanthropist Thomas Guy in 1721 eventually lead to St Thomas' Hospital moving to its present site opposite the Houses of Parliament. Today, Guy's and St Thomas' are both part of the same NHS Trust.

By the twelfth century, Islamic medical texts including those of Galen and ibn Sina had been translated into Latin and once more became available to European scholars. The study of anatomy advanced as dissection of the human body became permitted. Nevertheless, if contradictions to Galen's opinion were discovered, anatomists bent their own in order to fit. This confirmation bias towards the established opinions of an authority raises its head in research even today.

The Christian concept of salvation and life everlasting clearly had great appeal. Under the leadership of the Holy Fathers in Rome, the Church established a liturgy to facilitate man's relationship with God. The Office of the Dead comprised prayers and hymns for the souls of the departed and was conducted at funerals and at the beginning of November on All Souls' Day (All Hallows' Day, or Halloween), adjacent to All Saints' Day. Vulgate Psalm 114:9 exclaims: *'Placebo Domino in regione vivorum'* – I will please the Lord in the land of the living. The implication being that if the dear departed was of good report, they would rest in peace. The psalm was a means to that end and some families hired 'placebo singers' as an assurance. Problems arose when gatecrashers attended a funeral, ostensibly singing placebos but really in order to access the hospitality.

In France, largesse at funerals was particularly generous and it became obvious that much wailing and gnashing of teeth often did not represent grief at the departure of a loved one, so much as the anticipation of a feast. 'Placebo singers' became disparaged as being useless and deceitful. Geoffrey Chaucer wrote *Canterbury Tales* about the pilgrims travelling down to St Thomas' tomb at Canterbury in which the Parson referred to placebo singers as 'the Devil's Chaplains'. The Merchant told of an elderly knight, January, who was married to beautiful young May. His brother was a sycophant who never raised any concern at the union. Chaucer gave him the name *Placebo*.

Today the term 'placebo' still carries connotations of deception. That can be the case, but not necessarily, and is an issue considered further in later chapters.

The Renaissance: from the 15th to the 17th centuries

The Byzantine Empire fell in 1453 and Latin, Greek and Arabic medical texts could afterwards all be reconsidered and studied together. This renaissance of culture, arts and education was particularly expressed in Florence and Naples where the civic authorities formalised schemes to train doctors, lawyers, philosophers and theologians. The renaissance of new learning saw the development of the *studia humanitatis,* the humanities, including grammar, poetry and moral philosophy. [10]

Thomas Linacre (1460-1524)
On leaving school in Canterbury, Linacre studied medicine in Italy before bringing the 'New Learning' back to London where he founded the College of Physicians. By this means he sought to organise a system to licence physicians educated to degree standard, and to prohibit practice by non-licensed practitioners. Initially this scheme only covered a four mile radius of London and was under the jurisdiction of the Bishop. The radius was later extended to seven miles by Henry VIII who granted the College a Royal Charter in 1518. An Act of Parliament in 1523 extended the College's jurisdiction to the whole of England. Linacre also established readerships in medicine at Oxford and Cambridge.

Medicine in Europe began to exhibit two different aspects. The conservative, based on traditional authoritative Arabic medicine which was essentially Galenic, and a more liberal system encouraged by 'new learning' and the humanist approach of the Renaissance. By the 1530s the Belgian anatomist and physician Andreas Vesalius was able to carry out human dissection and show where Galen had been wrong. William Harvey was to have a similar impact on the understanding of physiology with his description of the circulation. Medicine slowly moved into the scientific era.

Paracelcus (1493-1541)
Born as Phillipus von Hohenheim in Switzerland, his adopted name 'Paracelcus' implied 'equal to Celsus'. Perhaps not unsurprisingly, colleagues regarded him as arrogant. He based his medicine on the traditional four Greek elements of earth, water, fire and air, and three spiritual substances – represented by mercury or quicksilver (the spirit and higher mental faculty), salt (the body) and sulphur (the soul). Together, these seven elements in various combinations gave matter its true form in harmony with the seven known planets and the seven major organs in man.

Seven has long been a 'magic' number – Ancient Egyptians regarded it as a 'god number'. There are seven days in a week; 4 x 7 gives the phases of the moon; there are seven classic crystal structures; seven liberal arts and sciences; seven wonders of the ancient world; seven tones in the natural musical scale; and seven discernible colours in the rainbow. Traditional Indian Medicine also described seven energy centres or 'chakras' in the body, with their associated 'meridians'. There are seven deadly sins, gamblers know the sums of numbers on opposite sides of a die equal seven, and that when rolling two dice, seven is the most probable total to be shown. And James Bond's number is …

Paracelsus made his medicines from plants and herbs using the techniques of alchemy which was widely practiced in the middle ages. The ancient Greeks' messenger of the gods, and god of illusion and deception was Hermes. During the Hellenistic period, philosophies based on Hermes combined with Thoth, the Egyptian god of magic and the result was Hermeticism. The combination of an esoteric and spiritual Hermetic philosophy with techniques of fermentation, distillation of 'essences' and refining which aimed to turn base metal into noble gold gave rise to alchemy (Arabic: *al-kimiya*, from *khemia*, hieroglyphic: *khmi*, black earth – that is, Egypt). We now know that such transmutation of metals is not possible by ordinary chemical means and alchemy has long had its day, but in the past many major figures studied alchemy, not least Isaac Newton. Paracelcus described how medicines should be made by fermentation and distillation using mercury (representing water – a plant's life essence); sulphur (fire – a plant's soul); and salt (earth – a plant's ashes). It would be a hundred years before chemistry was developed as a distinct discipline. Robert Boyle advanced his early alchemical research and introduced a more modern scientific approach in *The Sceptical Chymist*. Boyle (1627-1691), is now regarded as the first modern chemist. Chemistry as applied to the manufacture of medicines is 'pharmacy' (*pharmakon*, drug, medicine).

Paracelsus also commented on the qualifications of a good surgeon: He should have clear conscience, gentle heart and cheerful spirit; he should have greater regard for his honour than for money; he must not accept belief without understanding and must not scorn the workings of chance. He must not boast of knowing anything without experience and must never boast or praise himself. He should not practice self-abuse, or have a red beard. [11]

Paracelcelsians' claims to be able to access 'vital spirits' did not accord with developing rationalist medicine – their influence waned and they became referred to as quacks.

William Harvey (1578-1657)
Born in Folkestone, Kent, whilst Elizabeth I was still on the throne and Shakespeare was writing and acting, like Thomas Linacre, Harvey was educated at the King's School, Canterbury, then Cambridge University before qualifying in medicine in Padua in 1602. His works set in train a more questioning approach to medical science, and were a stimulus to Dr Richard Mead, who developed ideas which led to hypnotism. Harvey's description of the circulation of the blood in *De Motu Cordis* (1628) brought great fame and a position as physician to James I and Charles I. Initially many colleagues disagreed with his conclusions. Harvey himself was also concerned at the rumpus his views would cause – his manuscript started with a line from Virgil: 'All things are filled with Jove. But now the die is cast; my hope is in the love of truth and in the integrity of intelligence.'[12] His reticence was reflected two centuries later when Charles Darwin delayed publication of *On the Origin of Species*, fearing the opprobrium that might follow.

Harvey's book offered a mathematical analysis of the volume of blood in the body, challenging Galen's theory that blood was made in the liver and that there were two circulations. He carried out experiments on living dogs and reptiles, whose hearts beat slowly enough for more detailed study. His work was firmly based on experimentation and observation and it is not surprising that Francis Bacon, the populariser of empiricism, inductive philosophy and the scientific method became a patient. Harvey was the first to develop propositions about physiology on the basis of premises established by experimentation. Nevertheless, he continued to believe, as Galen, that mystical vital spirits had a role in life, even though they remained occult.[13]

Harvey's patient Charles I believed his own regal power was divinely ordained and that his authority was absolute. Parliament had a different opinion and Charles was executed in 1649. In 1653, Harvey left much of his fortune to the College of Physicians and established an Oration for the commemoration of benefactors of the College. This was accompanied by an exhortation 'to search out and study the secrets of nature by way of experiment, and also for the honour of the profession, to continue in mutual love and affection.'

Even so, the principles of medicine had been established by the works of Galen since the second century AD, and some doctors still declared they 'would rather err with Galen than proclaim the truth with Harvey.' Medical science slowly moved on, with a good shove from Francis Bacon and William Harvey.

The Enlightenment: From c.1650 through to c.1800

As the seventeenth century progressed, more philosophers and intellectuals began to use recognisably modern scientific methods to advance their knowledge. The writings of John Locke, Baruch Spinoza, Isaac Newton and François-Marie Arouet (*Voltaire*) were avidly studied. The invention of the printing press and developments in information technology during the sixteenth century enabled rapid dissemination of their new ideas. The political revolutions in America and Europe introduced the English Bill of Rights (1689), US Bill of Rights (1789) and the French Declaration of the Rights of Man and of the Citizen (1789). These rights arose from 'natural law' and not from superstition, religious doctrine, or the command of authorities and ruling princes. European princes, influenced by the principles of Age of Reason and Enlightenment, permitted religious toleration, freedom of speech and of the press. Although they supported developments in the arts and sciences, they usually retained ultimate authority – hence, *enlightened despotism*.

In the opinion of Immanuel Kant the Enlightenment was 'Mankind's final coming of age, the emancipation of the human consciousness from an immature state of ignorance and error. ...It always remains a scandal of philosophy and universal human reason that the existence of things outside us should have to be assumed merely on faith, and that if it occurs to anyone to doubt it, we should be unable to answer him with a satisfactory proof.' Kant wrote about scientific subjects throughout his life, raised the possibility that the influence of tides would cause the rotation of the earth to slow (which they do), and endorsed Emanuel Swedenborg's suggestion that the Milky Way was indeed a large disk of stars originating from a cloud of gas – a nebula.

Traditional Western Medicine, as espoused in various forms for over two thousand years, has given way to systems we find of value today as conventional orthodox mainstream medicine – now the norm in all cultures including those arising from ancient civilisations such as Indian, Chinese, Arabic, African and South American. The world of modern medicine is now of one culture – and that culture is based on the scientific method, irrespective of other more ancient traditional practices. There is no longer any distinct system of modern European or Western medicine, just scientific medicine.

Francis Bacon's great work *Novum Organon* emphasised the importance of scientific reasoning by an inductive process – from particular facts (based on evidence obtained from observation and confirmed by experimentation) to axiom to general law. Bacon emphasised that care had to be taken to avoid false ideas due to 'misuse of language; abuse of authority, peculiarity of the individual and traditions of the community.' Modern scientists, doctors and healthcare professionals continue to bear this in mind. Facts are established by observation and experimentation and no premise is accepted as true unless proven on that basis. Inductive reasoning will then lead to the discovery of physical facts as well as their causes.

In contrast, deductive reasoning, as used almost exclusively since the time of Aristotle, had accepted the generality of the situation as stated by an authority, magician, priest, guru, or wise teacher and then made conjectures as to the specifics. Critical assumptions were often based on nothing more than the imagination of their proponents. If the premises were true, and the argument was well made, the conclusion would be true – but many general assumptions were false and unsupported by evidence. The 'scientific method' continues to use deductive processes, but stimulated by Bacon, the inductive method has added probabilities to the mix.

The Lunaticks and the Industrial Revolution: 18th to 19th century

At the end of the eighteenth century, Britain's economy was still largely agricultural. Men with an intellectual bent met in coffee houses, societies and academic institutions for discourse, debate and dispute about science, ethics, the professions and politics. In 1660 an 'invisible society' was established in Oxford, then moved and was granted a charter as 'The Royal Society of London for Improving Natural Knowledge' under the patronage of Charles II in 1663.

In Birmingham, the Luna Society held monthly meetings for natural philosophers who had a particular interest in the application of science to medicine, transport, engineering and manufacturing. Meeting under a full moon to aid travel at night, it was active from 1765 until 1813. They were happy to be described as the 'Lunaticks' and became regarded as amongst the founders of the Midlands' Enlightenment and developing Industrial Revolution.

Amongst the Lunar Society's principal members, Erasmus Darwin was a family doctor who was also interested in botany and early theories of evolution. His grandson Charles became rather more famous fifty years later. The Rev. Joseph Priestley discovered oxygen and the Indian rubber eraser. Dr William Withering investigated the benefits of foxglove on the dropsy, analysed the active principle *digitalis*, and moved herbal medicine onto a more scientific plane.

These men all focused their minds on the applications of science. Practicalities required them to advance from ideas of superstition, rigid authority and deductive logic and embrace the modern scientific methods of experimentation, observation, analysis and induction.

The West Country had a problem with flooding in its tin mines, solved to a degree by Thomas Newcomen's invention of the first practical steam engine for pumping water in 1710. Newcomen is regarded as a forefather of the industrial revolution, certainly by the people of Dartmouth where he was born and worked, but it was Lunatick James Watt's invention of the condensing and rotary steam engine which got the revolution under way.[14] Benjamin Franklin was a corresponding member of the Society.

In the twentieth century, paradigms shifted a little more quickly: Wilbur and Orville Wright developed the first powered, controlled, heavier-than-air flying machine with the first twelve second powered flight on December 17th 1903. Only sixty six years later, on July 20th 1969, Neil Armstrong stepped onto the Moon.

In the field of health care, new practices, methods, equipment, operations and above all, new drugs, are constantly being introduced – and not always to good effect. There remains uncertainty about which treatments should become routine and which areas of research are important and most deserving of attention. The James Lind Alliance addresses these issues by establishing 'priority setting partnerships' with carers, clinicians and, most importantly, patients. The Alliance takes the name of ship's surgeon James Lind who pioneered clinical trials for research into the treatment of scurvy.[15,16]

The evolution of conventional orthodox medicine (COM)

Historically, most patients had care in the home, under the guidance of traditional 'wise women', 'cunning men', bonesetters and herbalists. In addition to their specific skills, magic and prayer were regularly invoked. Training as a physician was expensive and until the twentieth century, was largely based on apprenticeship. In the US, many who felt vocationally drawn to a career in medicine turned to cheaper 'irregular' schools where they, and their tuition fees, were welcome. Training was not always of an adequate standard. Only after Abraham Flexner published a damning report on the state of North American medicine in 1910 were there extensive reforms.[17]

During the nineteenth century, many criticisms of orthodox medicine were entirely justified. It was in that social climate that much medical care was offered by travelling 'medicine men' in circuses, fairs and medicine shows where the full panoply of misleading advertising and promotion was employed in order to gull the public.

Prior to the twentieth century, most orthodox doctors sought to suppress symptoms – often by 'heroic' bloodletting, purging and remedies containing heavy metals. This was the approach criticised by Samuel Hahnemann as being 'allopathic' (*allos*, other; *patheia*, suffering). The 'germ theory' of pathogenic medicine, caused by pathogens only gradually gained acceptance following its formalisation by Koch and the work of Pasteur and Lister in the nineteenth century (*pathos*, disease; *gen*, producing). It was hardly surprising that alternative systems of medicine developed in parallel.

Antoine van Leeuwenhoek (1632-1723)
A draper with a scientific bent, Leeuwenhoek improved the microscope. He made small powerful lenses enabling him to identify 'animacules', which today we call micro-organisms. He also identified red blood corpuscles and spermatozoa. His earliest correspondence with London's Royal Society appeared in its *Philosophical Transactions* in 1673. There was considerable scepticism about his suggestion of a single celled organism and the Society did not accept the findings until 1680 – whereupon they granted him its Fellowship.

Nicolas Andry (1658-1742)
The French physician Andry gave an account of the *Breeding of Worms in Human Bodies* in 1700. Andry referred to micro-organisms as 'worms' and suggested these were the cause of smallpox and other diseases.[18]

Ignaz Semmelweis (1818-1865)
In 1847, in the face of general scepticism about 'animacules' and whilst working as an obstetrician in Vienna, Hungarian Semmelweis put forward his theory that the cause of puerperal fever was contagion by micro-organisms, often brought in from other sick patients. He recommended careful hand washing with chlorinated lime – as did James Young Simpson in Britain and Oliver Wendell Holmes in the US. Semmelweis found no support amongst his continental colleagues, became depressed, was committed to an asylum and died after a beating. He has lent his name to the 'Semmelweis effect' – the tendency of doctors to reject new evidence because it contradicts their established beliefs.

John Snow (1813-1858)
When a severe cholera outbreak affected London's Soho in 1854, physician Snow examined not only individual patients who had the disease, but also the population as a whole. He concluded the outbreak was due to the water from a pump in Broad Street. At the time it was the widely held belief that such diseases were due to

miasmas (*miasma,* pollution by poisonous airs and vapours containing dangerous particles from decomposition). Initially, Snow struggled to have his ideas about the water supply accepted, though he brought the outbreak under control by removing the pump's handle. Subsequently Snow became regarded as being one of the founders of epidemiology – the branch of medicine which studies populations. The Royal Society for Public Health headquarters is at John Snow House and the *John Snow* is a public house in Broadwick Street, Soho.

Louis Pasteur (1822-1895)
Ten years after Snow, Pasteur proved that micro-organisms did not arise by 'spontaneous generation' but rather were carried on dust particles or in water. This led to Joseph Lister's (1827-1912) development of antiseptic surgery.

Robert Koch (1843-1910)
The anthrax bacillus was identified by Koch in 1877. Slowly the germ theory became accepted, coming to fruition with Koch's Postulates in 1890 – a series of tests to identify organisms causing diseases. Koch won the Nobel Prize for Medicine in 1905.

These eminent doctors applied the highest standards of scientific methodology available in their day, yet experienced much scepticism, cynicism and opposition to their theories. Change is never easy, and most physicians were content continue to practice as they had always done. Nevertheless, people did suffer from a wide variety of illnesses and injuries and did need attention. In the nineteenth century, lack of provision of care from regulated medical and other healthcare practitioners allowed unregulated practitioners to offer their services, opinions, advice, and products. Some knew perfectly well their remedies and treatments had no beneficial effect. They were clearly quacks and charlatans. Some honestly believed they were imbued with magical, spiritual, or even divine powers to heal. Some developed their own systems of 'medicine'. This enabled them to earn a living not only from treating patients but by selling courses for training others in their various proprietary techniques, by charging for registration of various 'qualifications', and by selling books, equipment and remedies.

This was not so very different from conventional orthodox medical systems, save that initially there was no higher authority to which these practitioners were accountable. Regular practitioners were accountable through the university and college system. Essentially, alternative systems of medicine were based on faith and not science. In the developing frontier states and territories of America, and in country areas of Europe, belief systems offered greater support and consolation for patients than the relatively ineffective remedies concocted by apothecaries at the behest of qualified physicians, let alone the extreme dangers of pre-twentieth century surgery.

The practice of medicine, whether conventional or alternative, involves techniques to deal both with the effects of pathological disease on the body and on emotions and the mind-spirit dimension of the patient. Hippocrates emphasised the importance of considering not only the disease the patient has, but also the patient that has the disease. The influence of spirits, energies and unexplained forces on animals, human health, emotional, and psychological well-being has always been recognised. Religions have paid particular attention to the spiritual dimension, but in early history there was often no clear distinction between priests who offered vicarious interventions with deities and magicians who conjured up spirits. The influence of magical approaches to health and wellbeing is still felt today.

Endnotes to Chapter 5

1. Barton J. Gershen, Word Rounds: *A History of words, both medical and non-medical.* Flower Valley Press, 2001.

2. Hermes, being also the god of deception and trickery, is also depicted with his caduceus in the logo of the International Brotherhood of Magicians.

3. Generally spelt 'sceptics' in the UK, 'skeptics' in the US.

4. Margaret Mead, *Abortion and the Hippocratic Oath.* www.Abort73.com 2010-09-03.

5. BMA News Review. July 2011.

6. www.PhilipCoppens.com/otator.

7. The term 'atom' was later to be used by John Dalton in his theories of chemistry, 1805.

8. Hence the symbol ℞ that doctors use to symbolise a prescription, which pharmacists use as a logo, and which I use to sign letters to my wife.

9. Becket was made Lord Chancellor in 1155, ordained as a priest on June 2nd 1162, and consecrated as archbishop the next day.

10. Raffaello Sanzio da Urbino's 1509 fresco of The School of Athens in the Stanza della Segnatura in the Apostolic Palace of the Vatican depicts Plato (said to resemble Leonardo da Vinci), hand pointing to the heavens and the world of ideas, and Aristotle, with outstretched palm between heaven and earth where his empiricist instincts lay. Renaissance humanists appreciated the room's overarching expression of the harmony between Christian teaching and Greek philosophy.

11. *Paracelcus – Selected Writings*, edited by Jolande Jacobi, Routledge & Kegan Paul, 1951, reported by William McKinlay, BMJ 2011;343;d8002.

12. M.E. Silverman, William Harvey and the discovery of the circulation of the blood. Clinical Cardiology 8, no.4, April 1985.

13. The poet John Donne considered the mysteries Harvey was revealing: 'Know'st thou how blood, which to the heart doth flow/ Doth from one ventricle to th' other goe?'

14. Eric Preston, Thomas Newcomen of Dartmouth. Dartmouth and Kingswear Society, Dartmouth. 2012.

15. Lind J. *A Treatise of the Scurvy.*1763. Edinburgh: printed by Sands, Murray, and Cochran for A. Kincaid and A. Donaldson.

16. www.lindalliance.org and www.jameslindlibrary.org.

17. Abraham Flexner. *Medical Education in the United States and Canada*, New York, Times/ Arno Press, 1910.

18. Andry also coined the term 'orthopaedic' from orthos, straight + paedion, child – describing how the bent limbs of rickety children might be treated. Hence the international symbol of orthopaedic surgery is a growing tree bound to a straight stake.

Chapter 6

Holism, Homeostasis and Harmony

The whole is more than the sum of its parts.
Aristotle

Out of clutter, find simplicity.
Albert Einstein

Always aim at complete harmony of thought and word and deed.
Always aim at purifying your thoughts and everything will be well.
Mahatma Gandhi

The universe is not required to be in perfect harmony with human ambition.
Carl Sagan

Proponents of complementary and alternative medicine regularly use terms such as 'holism', 'homeostasis', 'harmony' and 'balance' without always being clear exactly what they mean. There is a significant danger that patients and other individuals interested in camistry might be misled into making decisions about their care and wellbeing based on concepts which cannot be substantiated and are ephemeral at best. Camees have to consider just how these various terms arose, and what the implications of their use are.

In the fifth century BC, Leucippus and Democritus had considered that the universe consists of indestructible particles which could not be further cut. In his poem *On Nature*, Parmenides declared 'All is one, nor is it divisible.' In *Metaphysics,* Aristotle considered the concept that 'the whole is more than the sum of the parts' and warned of the fallacy of confusing the part with the purpose of the whole. Although the brain is where the thinking is done, brains do not think. People do the thinking.

In time, and as science developed, this approach gave way to Reductionism – 'The simple is the source of the complex.' A complex system can be explained by a reduction to its fundamental parts. Anthropology to biology to chemistry to physics to quantum mechanics.

Holism

The word 'holism' was coined in 1926 by South African soldier, statesman and scholar Jan Christiaan Smuts in *Holism and Evolution.*[2] He defined holism as 'the tendency in nature to form wholes that are greater than the sum of the parts through creative evolution.' His use of the term was modern, but the underlying principles were ancient. Albert Einstein opined that in the next millennium, two mind sets would direct human thinking: his own concept of Relativity, and Smuts' of Holism.[3]

During the First World War Smuts had formed the South African Defence Force. He became a Field Marshal in the British Army and helped create the Royal Air Force. This itself was a holistic creation – the Naval and Army Wings of the Royal Flying Corps becoming united as one. Nevertheless, he thought native Africans should not be given political power. In 1929 he advocated separate institutions for blacks and whites, and encouraged racial segregation in South Africa.

The term holism is now used in many branches of human endeavour including sociology, philosophy, economics, psychology, architecture, ecology and of course – complementary, condimentary and alternative medicine. Each uses the term with different emphasis and it is important to clarify the meaning of the term in the sense it is being used. Often it is used as a brand to market CAM practices, services and products with the implication that 'holistic healthcare' provides a benefit not available from orthodox practitioners or conventional medical practice. This is a useful marketing ploy but is false, and may mislead patients.

George Engle introduced the biopsychosocial (BPS) model of medicine to conceptualise psychosomatic phenomena and to reflect common experience that a disturbance on any one level – somatic, physical, psychic, or social – will affect all other levels.[4] This model suggests that thoughts, emotions and behaviours all have a significant role in disease and illness. The BPS model has been criticised as not fitting the definition of a scientific theory in that it cannot be tested but the BPS model forms the basis for many CAM practices and is being considered by more orthodox doctors who are now exploring the possibilities for a more humanistic person-centered medicine and healthcare.

The American Holistic Medical Association claims that disease is a result of physical, spiritual, social, and environmental imbalance. Few orthodox doctors would disagree, though the emphasis on each component may vary according to the fundamental principles behind the medical system used.

Camists use the term 'holism' to emphasise their particular approach and focus on the patient as a whole person – perhaps because the reductionist approach would invite comparison with the emperor with no clothes. Some imply that orthodox practitioners do not pay attention to the totality of patients' experience, and even that they do not care. But a holistic approach takes time, and quality time at that. Time to inquire into all aspects of physical, emotional, environmental, social, psychological and spiritual health. Time to listen attentively and conscientiously. Most conventional practitioners would be only too happy to be more holistic, if only they were granted the time.

Although 'the whole' may self evidently have qualities not possessed by its parts, that does not mean that its parts cannot be or should not be studied as such. If any sense is to be made of them, type I effects of treatments (due to the relationship with the practitioner) need to be distinguished from type II (due to the specific treatment).

Patients should not be misled into thinking camists have a monopoly of the holistic approach. Modern medicine is complex but modern doctors rarely work as individuals. We may specialise in one disease, in my case, of the musculo-skeletal system. And whereas I have replaced shoulders, hips, knees, ankles and big toe joints – specialism has led to younger colleagues now concentrating on only one joint. Nevertheless we are in a team working with other specialists, nurses, therapists, counsellors, and most importantly, family doctors. Our service is most certainly holistic. Given the propensity for terms such as 'holism' to confuse and mislead patients who do not appreciate its origin and meaning, orthodox healthcare practitioners need to be more open and robustly declare and affirm their own holistic approach. It is for this reason the work of the International Network for Person-Centered Medicine (INPCM) is becoming more recognised.

Homeostasis

Just as the concept of holism emphasises the harmonious relationship between body, mind, spirit and emotions, so at a molecular, cellular and system level, life forms achieve a balance between competing elements. Hippocrates (460 BC-370 BC) had formalised one of the earliest coherent systems of medicine and physiology, suggesting that four fluid 'humours', blood, phlegm, black bile and yellow bile, needed to be kept in harmony and balance for effective health and well-being. A balance which was influenced by external forces such as the seasons, environment and the cosmos, as well as internal influences such as ageing and emotions. Sir Clifford Allbutt, inventor of the clinical thermometer, traced humoral principles back to the ancient Egyptians. [5]

The French histologist Charles Robin (1821-1885) referred to the concept of harmony and balance occurring in the *milieu de l'interieur*.[6] Claude Bernard then regularly used this term in his own writing on the role of blood and other tissues. He described the 'perfection of the organism, such that the external variations are at each instant compensated for and equilibrated ... all the vital mechanisms have always one goal – to maintain the uniformity of the conditions of life in the internal environment.'[7]

Claude Bernard (1813-1878) is regarded as the founder of modern physiology and was the first French scientist to have a state funeral, but his ideas about the *milieu interieur* were not widely accepted until the twentieth century. He was also one of the first scientists to use *blind experiments* to reduce the chance of observer bias and the influence of placebo effects. In this context, 'blind' means that the researchers and subjects of the experiment are initially masked from information which might inadvertently influence them. This is now an important element of the scientific method in clinical trials.[8]

In a letter to his close friend Marie Raffalovich, Bernard discussed science, intuition and superstition and described what it meant to be a scientist:

> A scientist, if he is to have great ability, must have imagination but he must master the imagination and coldly probe the unknown. However, if he lets himself be carried away by his imagination, he will be overcome by vertigo and like Faust and others, fall into the chasm of magic and succumb to phantoms of the mind.[9]

The idea that the internal environment of a living organism is regulated to be stable and constant was termed 'homoeostasis' (*homoios*, similar; *stasis*, standing still). The concept was further developed by American doctor Walter Bradford Cannon and popularised in his book *The Wisdom of the Body* in 1932. [10]

Cannon described our bodies as being open systems which required specific mechanisms to maintain an internal steady state. For example: sugar concentration; temperature; acid-base balance (the concentration of hydrogen ions, pH); and all other vital physiological processes. Any variations leading to change are balanced through a feedback mechanism to restore the steady-state. Blood sugar is regulated by a number of chemicals including insulin, glucagons and other hormones, all with feedback mechanisms. Failure of any part of the homoeostatic mechanism can lead to dis-ease. Diabetes in the case of sugar.

Homoeostasis enables organisms to function within a broad range of external environmental conditions. The concentration of hydrogen atoms in normal body tissues is very tightly controlled to the range of pH 7.35 -7.45. Any variation from that is adjusted by a combination of kidney function, breathing and cellular respiration. It is virtually impossible to effect a change by any diet. pH itself is a measure of the concentration of hydrogen ions, and the scale ranges from 0 which is a high concentration of acid (e.g. gastric juices), to 14 which indicates a low concentration (e.g. bleach). Pure water is neutral with a pH of 7.0, and even that varies with temperature. Doctors regard pH 7.4 as being 'normal'.[11] pH is very important in maintaining an organism's function. Consideration is given here because many CAMs, diets and products sold to camees, are marketed with emphasis on pH. A small dose of understanding is necessary to avoid being quacked.

The fundamental principles of homoeostasis also apply in the wider environment. James Hutton, regarded as the father of geology, wrote in 1788 that he considered 'the Earth to be a super-organism, and that a proper study of it should be applied physiology.'[12] James Lovelock FRS has suggested the entire mass of living matter on any planet with life should be thought of as a 'homoeostatic super organism' – constantly changing via feedback mechanisms to achieve balance. Life is a necessary agent in its own survival. His seminal work *Gaia as seen through the Atmosphere* was published in 1972, and popularised in *Gaia: a new look at life on Earth* in 1979.[13] Lovelock noted the improbability that chemical soup could assemble life forms which would then evolve over billions of years into the systems we see today, but commented 'life on Earth was an almost utterly improbable event with almost infinite opportunities of happening. So it did.' In 2001 *Gaia* was re-published with the sub-text: *The Practical Science of Planetary Medicine.* Even book titles evolve!

Harmony

Originally the ancient Greek word *harmonia* referred to a 'concord or joining of sounds, usually agreeable and pleasant'. The word has etymological connections with *harmos*: a joint, and Latin *armus:* the upper arm or shoulder. The concept of joining different things together in balance and harmony developed in many traditional cultures. The Ancient Egyptians described the state of eternal harmony as *ma'at* – imperfections were due to human failings and could be restored though the intercession of the pharaoh. Ancient Chinese philosophers identified five elements or virtues to be found in nature: metal, wood, water, fire, and earth. All should be harmonized. The five elements corresponded with the five planets they had observed, five climates, five compass directions (including centre), five smells, spices, tastes, senses. Each of these elements was associated with the five principal viscera – heart, liver, spleen, lungs and kidneys. Five is an important number – Chinese prefer to avoid 'four'. In Cantonese the word *sei* means both 'four' and 'death'. Many Chinese buildings do not have a floor numbered four. Modern mentalists, who entertain by demonstrations of mind reading, openly declare we use our 'five senses to create the illusion of a sixth.'

The concept that nature harmonises and balances these various elements of an individual's make up has been applied in many different cultures down the ages. Disease was regarded as state of imbalance caused by disharmony both within the individual and between the individual and the environment, including the larger cosmos. Galen referred to *dyscrasia* (bad mixture and *eucrasia* (a synonym for harmony). To the North American Navajo, *hozhó* represents the importance of harmony between Mother Earth and Father Sky.

The aim of the traditional doctor was to restore a harmonious dynamic balance and equilibrium in terms of body and mind and spirit. After the Enlightenment, a more reductionist approach with emphasis on the pathological processes came to dominate regular orthodox medical thinking. There is currently a resurgence of focus on a person-centered medicine which recognises the importance of harmonising the main elements of body, mind and spirit. Juan Mezzich, President of the International Network for Person Centred Medicine, has described its work as seeking 'to articulate science and humanism in a balanced manner, engaging them at the service of the whole person.'[14]

Andrew Miles describes PCM as a system for the delivery of 'high-tech' scientific medicine within a humanistic framework and has written recently on its principal components.[15] The concept of PCM is noble, orthodox, holistic and harmonising – but formidable operational constraints within routine clinical practice may militate against its comprehensive introduction into health services. To date, the scientific method has not provided evidence such an approach actually has the benefits anticipated and here, it is time that will tell.

Endnotes to Chapter 6

1. This section first published in International Journal of Person Centred Medicine, Ed. Andrew Miles. Vol. 1, No. 3. September 2010.

2. Jan Smuts (1926). *Holism and Evolution.* New York. Macmillan.

3. In: *Jan Smuts-Memoirs of the Boer War* (1994). (eds. G. Nattnass & S.P. Spies. Introduction.

4. George Engel (1977). *The need for a Transitional Model.* Science. 196.

5. Albutt, Sir Clifford (1909). *The Fitzpatrick Lectures*, British Medical Journal 2 (2553).

6. Robin also discovered of the role of osteoclasts in bone formation.

7. Gross C.G. (1998). *Claude Bernard and the constancy of the Internal Environment.*

Neuroscientist. 4 (5).

8. The term 'blind test' was first used by William Stanley Jevons in *The Principles of Science* in 1874, but he was an economist and logician, and the term was not well recognised in medicine until the 1920s.

9. Ibid

10. Walter Cannon (1932). *The Wisdom of the Body.* New York. Norton. Mount Cannon in Glacier National Park is named after him.

11. For ease of explanation the technical details of hydroxonium ions (H_3O) and the fact that pH is not precisely the concentration or 'power' of H are set aside. pH is defined as the negative decimal logarithm of the hydrogen ion activity in a solution.

12. James Hutton (1788). *Theory of the Earth.* Transactions of the Royal Society of Edinburgh 1 (2).

13. James E. Lovelock (1972). *Gaia as seen through the Atmosphere.* Atmospheric Environment: 6 (8),

14. Mezzich, J.E. (2011). *The Geneva Conferences and emergence of the International Network for Person-Centred Medicine.* Journal of Evaluation in Clinical practice 17.

15. Prof. Andrew Miles (2009). *On medicine of the Whole Person: away from scientific reductionism and towards the embrace of the complex in clinical practice.* Journal of Evaluation in Clinical Practice 15 and personal communication.

Chapter 7

The evolution of scientific methods
and their application to medicine

If the enjoyment of happiness is a great good, the power of imparting it to others is greater.
Francis Bacon, Viscount St. Alban

Science is what we have learned about how to keep from fooling ourselves.
Richard Feynman

Science is not a body of facts. Science is a method for deciding whether what we choose to believe has a basis in the laws of nature or not.
Marcia McNutt
Editor, *Science*

Science has an annoying way of not finding what you were hoping for.
Fiona Godlee
Editor, *British Medical Journal*

For centuries, human understanding and knowledge was bound together as philosophy, myth, magic and medicine. Numerous techniques and methods were devised to enable the 'truth' to be studied with ever more accuracy and with ever greater probability of veracity – as agreed by all right thinking folks. Methods described as 'scientific' have long been used, but imperfectly. Gradually, methodology became formalised and consensus reached – mostly. At various times individual natural philosophers have been credited with advancing science by developing novel and practical methods for systematic inquiry.

An old proverb has it that 'It's hard finding a black cat in a coal-hole. Especially when there is no cat.' Sir Andrew Wiles, who proved Fermat's Last Theorem, has described science as 'Groping and probing and poking and some bumbling and bungling, and then a switch is discovered, the light is lit, and everyone says "Wow, so that's how it looks," and then it's off into the next dark room, looking for the next mysterious dark feline.'[1]

The reader should turn elsewhere for a thorough review of the history of science. Suffice it to say that knowledge derived from observation and study has always been considered a major component of the 'truth' – the verifiable reality of the world in which we live. The earliest sentient beings to evolve a consciousness relied on their imagination, emotion and intuition to give account of the world. Supernatural gods, spirits and vital forces were regularly invoked. Those who claimed abilities to intercede with supernatural and occult entities became respected as priests. Those who claimed abilities to conjure up spirits, demons and angels were magicians. Slowly, as more critical examination of the basis for their beliefs was undertaken and more comprehensive observations were made, methods were devised to move ever closer towards that elusive destination of 'truth'. There are different forms of truth, spiritual being one, but the key for healthcare is to establish *causal inferences*. That is, the extent to which one thing causes another – the extent to which the treatment has genuine therapeutic effect. This detail may not matter to a suffering individual but must be answered if other patients are to be advised and treated effectively and if group financial resources are to be committed. That is a task for all healthcare professionals and requires them to act with intellectual integrity and rigour.

One of the earliest medical textbooks, the Egyptian papyrus donated to the New York Academy of Medicine by Edwin Smith, dates from c. 1500 BC. Although it includes eight magic spells, the underlying principles of medical care are noticeably rational and scientific – based on systematic observation, analysis of evidence and testing of hypotheses.

Abu Ali al-Hasan ibn al-Haytham (Alhazen) (965-1039 AD)
Born in Basra, Alhazen commented: 'Truth is sought for its own sake. Finding the truth is difficult, and the road to it is rough.' He substantiated inductive conjectures with observation of experiments and rational mathematical analysis – an approach to gaining knowledge which became known as the 'scientific method'.[2]

Avicenna (c. 980-1037 AD)

Born in Uzbekistan, Avicenna's *Book of Optics* (1027) stated that premises should be established by raising questions and conducting experiments. Aristotle's deductive methods were often too dogmatic. In his famous *Canon of Medicine* Avicenna described principles of inductive logic and a scientific method which were later to be ascribed to John Stuart Mill who wrote *A System of Logic* in 1843.

Friar Roger Bacon (1214-1294)

Born in Somerset, some say Bacon was a student, then lecturer at Oxford. Bacon probably became a Franciscan friar. The Pope sought his views as to how Aristotle's science and philosophy could be incorporated into theology – Bacon suggested that conclusions derived from observation should be tested further by experiment. During the nineteenth century Bacon became regarded as having been the first modern experimental scientist. Contemporary interpretations of his work suggest that, although ahead of his time, the basis for much of his reasoning still relied on the philosophical and theological teaching of traditional authorities. Nevertheless Bacon used mathematics and was a champion of experimental study – suggesting 'thence cometh quiet to the mind'. Roger Bacon recognised the necessity for other independent workers to verify the results of any experiment and for the cycle of hypothesis, experimentation and observation to be repeated. His seven part work *Opus maius* led to him being called *Doctor Mirabilis* – Wonderful Teacher. The fifteenth century Digby Manuscript has Bacon tell us 'Without experiment nothing can be sufficiently known. There are two ways of acquiring knowledge, one through reason, the other by experiment...argument is not enough, but experience is.'

William of Ockham (various spellings including Occam. c.1288-c.1348)

Born in Surrey, William became a Franciscan monk and wrote extensively on logic, theology and physics and was called *Doctor Invincibilis* – Unbeatable Teacher. Theologically he argued that supra-individual universals, essences, or forms are the products of abstraction by the human mind and have no extra-mental existence. This led to his philosophical approach suggesting that 'Nothing ought to be posited without a reason given, unless it is self-evident, known by experience or proved by the authority of sacred scripture,' and 'What is done with fewer assumptions is done in vain with more.' This has been reworked by others as: 'Entities should not be multiplied beyond necessity.' This Principle of Parsimony suggests that when there are competing hypotheses, the one that makes fewest assumptions is most likely to get nearest to objective truth. So: given that many patients who are treated by camists report they feel better, consider whether this is most likely due to (a) activation of unidentified esoteric forces, innate intelligence, *yin*, *yang*, or spirits that are capable of affecting the flow of unidentified energies such as *qi* along imagined meridians and chakras; or (b) neuro-chemical activation by heightened response to expectation and suggestions that give rise to pleasurable feelings. You must be the judge.

The Parsimony Principle of reducing ideas to the core can be traced back to Aristotle and Maimonides before William – and has used by others since including Newton and Einstein. In 1852, Sir William Hamilton termed the principle as *Occam's Razor*. Modern doctors try to account for a patient's range of symptoms by identifying the fewest possible causes – diagnostic parsimony. Today's medical students are advised: 'when you hear hoof beats, think horses not zebras' – yet they have to beware not to miss the rare and unexpected. William Shakespeare had Hamlet tell us: 'There are more things in heaven and earth, Horatio, than are dreamt of in your philosophy.' Judgement and discretion is called for and that is why medical students are trained to be doctors and not computers.

Francis Bacon, later Viscount St. Alban (1561-1626) [3]

Francis (unrelated to Roger) developed 'a new and certain path for the mind to proceed in...which must be used for proving and discovering not first principles, but also the lesser axioms, and the middle, and indeed all. For the induction which proceeds by simple enumeration is childish.' In *Novum Organum Scientiarum* (1620) Bacon emphasised the importance of experimentation and the gathering of facts about a problem – the 'histories' as he called them, 'evidence' as we would say today:

> There are only two ways of searching into and discovering truth. The one flies from the senses and particulars of the most general axioms, and from these principles, the truth of which it takes as settled and immovable, proceeds to judgement and to the discovery of middle axioms. And this way is now in fashion. The other derives axioms from the senses and particulars, rising by a gradual and unbroken ascent, so that it arrives at the most general axioms last of all. This is the true way, but as yet untried.

Bacon took issue with the concept of Aristotelian deductive reasoning from axioms or unchallenged 'first principles'. That is, logical reasoning from the general to particular. This placed too much reliance on the validity of premises, which might themselves be false. If so, any conclusion would be false. For centuries, philosophers, priests and politicians conveniently overlooked this fact. In order to establish the initial premises more precisely, Bacon advanced an approach based on experiments and observations. Conclusions could then be inferred with a higher probability of being true. Bacon's emphasis on observation and inductive logic, building a case from the ground up, became further developed as the scientific method, and was put into practical effect by other philosophers of natural science such as his contemporary, Galileo Galilei (1564-1642).

Bacon's new system of inquiry led to a more reliable body of evidence. Bacon emphasised the importance of not leaping to conclusions and insisted on reporting negative instances, no matter how inconvenient. This calls for self-discipline, avoidance of dogmatic prejudice and intellectual integrity. Conclusions, formulated as a hypothesis, then have to be tested by further experiments. Only after applying an initial *inductive* process and moving from the particular to the general might the hypothesis be thought of as a general law of nature and capable of accurate prediction of particulars by the method of *deduction*.

In *Novum Organon,* Bacon set out an account of what today we would call 'research reporting bias' or 'publication bias' – the tendency for negative or inconvenient reports to be under-reported or even ignored altogether, whereas results supportive of the investigators' theories, prejudices or commercial ambitions tend to be over-reported and talked up. Kay Dickersin and Iain Chalmers have recently considered this significant problem which can dangerously lead to incorrect conclusions and false causal inferences.[4] They quote Albert Einstein: 'Academic freedom as I understand it means having the right to seek the truth and to publish and teach what is believed to be true. Naturally this right comes together with a duty not to withhold a part of what is believed to be true.' Austin Bradford Hill, the father of British medical statistics commented: 'A negative result may be dull, but often it is no less important than the positive; and in view of that importance it must, surely, be established by adequate publication of the evidence.'[5] Ben Goldacre's book on *Bad Pharma* sets out an account of the considerable reporting bias he found in analysing papers emanating from the pharmaceutical industry even today.[6] Bacon himself set out Aphorism XLVI of *Novum Organon:*

The human understanding draws everything else to be in harmony with, and to support, those things which at once please it. And, though it must be admitted that the force and the number of instances that occur to the contrary is greater, the understanding either does not heed to them or it disdains them – it distances itself from them and dismisses them – so that the authority of those previous beliefs remains inviolate. This is more or less of the reason for all superstitions such as belief in astrology, in dreams, in the fates and suchlike, in which men delight; they pay heed to those that come to pass but, on the contrary, when they are false – which happens much the more often – they neglect them and pass them over. And this evil creeps, persistently and most subtly, into the philosophies and the sciences, in which that opinion which is once accepted infects all the rest and reduces them to agree with it. Even in cases where delight and vanity were absent, an error ever present in, and peculiar to, human understanding is that it is more moved and excited by an affirmative than a negative; whereas, by all that is proper, each of these should have equal weight. But, on the contrary, in determining the truth of any axiom, the force of the negative has a greater influence.

That explanation of reporting bias which favours the positive has not been improved upon in four hundred years. Bacon is regarded as the father of modern empirical scientific methods which emphasise the importance of investigation, experimentation, observation – and honest reporting. Bacon served both Queen Elizabeth I, who knighted him, and James I who made him Viscount St. Alban. He was keen that natural philosophers studying science should meet together and co-operate in harmony. To that end, he recommended that King James should establish a institution or college for the study of experimental sciences. In the event it was left to James's grandson Charles II to patronise the Royal Society's foundation in 1660 – motto: *Nullus in Verba,* 'Take no-one's word for it.' Its founder members regarded Francis Bacon as their intellectual godfather:

Bacon is also said to have been the first to argue that one of the tasks of medicine was to prolong life. He divided medicine into three parts: preservation of health; cure of disease; and prolongation of life. The latter, Bacon wrote, 'is a new part and deficient, though the most noble of all.'[7]

Though he was Lord Chancellor, Bacon fell into debt and ended his career charged with corruption for accepting bribes. Such behaviour was not uncommon at that time but being caught led to public disgrace. Bacon's enthusiasm for experimentation may have led to his death from pneumonia, caught whilst he was out in winter studying the effects of cold and freezing on the preservation of meat. In *Brief Lives,* John Aubrey suggests he had been stuffing a chicken with snow.

René Descartes (1596-1650)

In *Rules for the Direction of the Mind* (1619), Descartes sought to set aside the traditional Aristotelian system and suggested that 'perfect knowledge must necessarily be deduced from first causes.' Descartes thought he could establish those first causes simply by his own reasoning from first principles.

He established scientific thinking as the basis of rational thought and insisted on precise definition of *quantities*. All nature could be explained in terms of reduction to elementary particles. However, he proposed reality existed in two categories: *res extensa* of the physical universe and *res cogitans* of the mind. This was a more metaphysical approach than that of Francis Bacon and although Descartes was a renowned philosopher and made significant contributions to mathematics and its application to science, it has been Bacon's experimental approach which has became established as fundamental to the modern scientific method.[8]

Descartes pondered what it is to 'know' anything and how he himself could be certain of anything. Mathematics seemed to provide the greatest certainties, and he developed methods of applying algebra to geometry. Analytic geometry still uses x-y co-ordinates named Cartesian after him. He sought to establish incontrovertible true simple mathematical statements, such as a straight line being the shortest distance between two points, and then built on this by logical steps and using deduction to construct 'the world' he was studying. Because the basic premises were true, so were the conclusions. Descartes established the basic facts by reason, and in philosophy his approach developed as Rationalism – *Cogito ergo sum*.[9]

Descartes' division of reality into two independent realms – mind and matter, subject and object, observer and observed – is an idea known to us now as Cartesian Dualism. Albeit the two realms are interdependent in a 'real substantial union.'[10] Nowadays most philosophers place emphasis on basic evidence being established by experimentation, observation and empirical experience. Most scientists now regard the mind as the outcome of the physicochemical activity of the brain, not as a discrete entity.[11] In *The Concept of the Mind* (1949) Philosopher Gilbert Ryle regarded Descartes as having made a 'big categorical mistake' in speaking of mind as a substance – 'the dogma of a ghost in the machine'.

Intensive work continues to unravel the mystery of the mind, and its close cousin, the human spirit. A novel contribution to the mind-body-spirit debate which still engages enthusiasts for camistry was made by Clarence Lewis in *Mind and the World Order.* Lewis used the term *qualia* (singular *quale*) to describe what it is like to have the character of a particular mental state. Experiencing pain, smelling grass, seeing a colour – subjective, qualitative impressions. 'There are recognizable qualitative characters of the given, which may be repeated in different experiences, and are thus a sort of universals; I call these "qualia." The quale is directly intuited, given, and is not the subject of any possible error because it is purely subjective.'[12]

Qualia describe the character or experience of 'what it is like.' American philosopher and cognitive scientist Daniel Dennett advises 'Qualia is an unfamiliar term for something that could not be more familiar to each of us: the way things seem to us.'[13] Many people find the world seems to them to have an immanent transcendent quality which leads them to add 'spirit' to the mind-body construct.

Sir Isaac Newton (1642-1727)
Like Bacon and Descartes, Newton established his knowledge by avoiding bias, prejudice and delusion but unlike Descartes, his method was more inductive. Newton was determined to seek out the true causes of observed effects. *Principia Mathematica* (1687) set out his *Four Rules of Reasoning* including cause and effect analysis and a version of Occam's Razor. 'In experimental philosophy we are to look upon the propositions collected by general induction from phenomena as accurately or very nearly true, notwithstanding any contrary hypotheses that may be imagined, till such time as other phenomena occur, by which they may either be made more accurate, or liable to exceptions.'[14]

Newton's rules emphasise that a true scientist should not be dogmatic but change opinion in the light of experience.[15] In *Opticks* Newton wrote: 'Hypotheses have no place in experimental science.'[16]

William Cullen MD FRS (1710-1790)
Cullen studied in Glasgow, served as a ship's surgeon, then became Professor of Medicine in Glasgow and Edinburgh. He taught in English rather than in the customary Latin and was famed for his *Lectures on the Materia Medica* (1761). Amongst his students, William Withering discovered the use of digitalis, extracted from the foxglove; John Brown developed his own, rival, Brunonian medical system; and Benjamin Rush returned to America where he did much to ensure humane treatment for the insane, as well as contributing to the colony's independence as a member of the Continental Congress.

Cullen emphasised the importance of 'the nervous power' on health, recognising that electric or ethereal power was transmitted down nerves and affected every organ. He advised that 'operation of medicines depends somewhat on their own nature, but as much on that particular modification of the system to which they are applied. Temperament is the general state of the system, the variety of temperaments is prodigious. The ancients had confined them to four.'

He wrote of *impressions* of different strengths and that 'pleasant sensations are generally of a middle force of impression. The reflex sensations of pleasure and pain are mutually exchangeable by repetition. Thus tobacco, certainly at first very unpleasant, by custom is rendered very soon agreeable. According to the state of the body, the same thing feels cold at one time, and warm at another. Pleasing objects also vary in the same manner.' Cullen described how he gave some patients placebos in order to placate them, knowing full well their condition itself would not be affected.[17]

Cullen also lectured on diet and nutrition, recommending 'we use no acrid substances in our food; or if we do, they are only employed as *condimenta*.' He distinguished between agreeable plants used for food and acrid plants used for medicine. He wrote about virtually every order of Linnaeus' plant taxonomy – on *Hypericum perforatum*, St John's Wort: 'there are many well vouched testimonies of its virtues, particularly of its diuretic powers. This oil is much recommended in epileptic and maniac cases though, I confess, I do not understand how it can act.'

Cullen's lectures on the use of *cinchona* bark to treat malaria and agues were translated into German by Dr Samuel Hahnemann. Hahnemann carried out further experiments and testing (German, *pruefung*), though the standard of science was poor with no controls and with results no one else could repeat. Hahnemann then went on to devise his own alternative system of medicine as *Homeopathy*. Neither Cullen nor Hahnemann actually carried out properly observed controlled experiments to establish the evidence on which a firm scientific opinion could be established. They both simply reported the opinions of ancient sages and added their own – substantiated by philosophy, not physiology. Whether Hahnemann was aware of Cullen's use of placebos is not recorded.

William Hunter FRS (1718-1783)

Hunter studied medicine in Edinburgh under William Cullen and developed a prestigious practice as an obstetrician in London. His paper, *On the Structure and Diseases of Articulating Cartilages* noted that 'If we consult the standard chirurgical writers from Hippocrates down to the present age, we shall find that an ulcerated cartilage is universally allowed to be a very troublesome disease; that it admits of a cure with more difficulty than to carious bone; and that, when destroyed, it is not recovered.' An observation no less correct today.

Hunter's Anatomy School in Windmill Street in London's Soho was adjacent to the Middlesex Infirmary which developed as The Middlesex Hospital before being incorporated into University College Hospital in 1987. In the middle of the twentieth century, the medical school's students of human surface anatomy again appreciated presentations in Windmill Street – the famous burlesque theatre only closing in 1964.

John Hunter FRCS FRS (1728-1793)

John assisted his elder brother William in the Anatomy School and then spent three years as an army surgeon on the Continent. On return to London in 1763 he set up a private practice but also became renowned for his teaching. Much of this was based on his remarkable museum. He emphasised the value of understanding structure and function, not only of humans, but of all animals. His observations were meticulously recorded and he stressed the importance of experimentation. When Edward Jenner wrote to him saying he was thinking of experimenting on a hedgehog, Hunter replied 'But why think about it – why not try the experiment?' And later: 'Dear Jenner, I am puffing of your tartar as the tartar of all tartars, and have given it to several physicians to make trial, but have had no account yet of the success.' The Royal College of Surgeons of England has placed a tablet over his grave recording their 'admiration of his genius…and their grateful veneration for his services to mankind as the Founder of Scientific Surgery.' The Hunterian Museum at the Royal College of Surgeons in Lincoln's Inn Fields is highly regarded and all are welcome to visit. Entry is free.

John Haygarth FRS (1740-1827)

Haygarth carefully applied the scientific method to all aspects of his medical practice. Born in Yorkshire he studied medicine in Edinburgh, London and Paris and spent thirty years as a physician in Chester, being particularly concerned with reducing the mortality rate of smallpox. This he did by promoting the new methods of inoculation, often in the face of intense opposition. His *Inquiry How to Prevent the Small Pox* was published in 1784, brought international fame and Fellowship of the Royal Society.

Throughout his career Haygarth carried out research firmly based on experimentation and observation. On retiring to Bath in 1798 he found many patients in that fashionable resort were spending considerable sums purchasing Perkins' Metallic Tractors. These patented six centimetre long metal wands were said to be made of esoteric and secret alloys. Placing them on the afflicted part, they would then be drawn away, thus removing malign forces. Haygarth made painted wooden copies of the tractors and compared the effects of the wooden tractors with the metal variety on a series of patients with rheumatism. To ensure their opinions about any benefit from the treatment were unbiased, patients were not told whether or not they had received the 'genuine' or 'sham' treatment. Naval surgeon James Lind had carried out clinical trials to find a cure for scurvy fifty years before, but Haygarth can be credited with conducting the first *placebo-controlled clinical trials*.

The word placebo was first used in its modern medical sense in 1772, to describe pills made of sugar or flour – known by the physician to be worthless. Haygarth's book *On the Imagination as a Cause and as a Cure of Disorders of the Body* (1800) was the first to set out a placebo effect in scientific analysis – a *single-blind clinical trial* meaning that the patient had no knowledge as to whether the treatment was genuine or sham.[18] Developments along these lines led to *placebo-controlled double-blind trials*, first reported in Russia in 1832 to test the effectiveness of homeopathy. To avoid bias affecting results, not only was the patient denied knowledge of whether or not they had received a placebo or remedy, but so too the experiment's observer until the conclusion of the experiment. These trials demonstrated homeopathy was no more effective than placebos.

Haygarth's experiments, showing the metallic tractors were no better than sham 'fictitious' wooden ones, nevertheless demonstrated 'to a degree which has never been suspected, what powerful influence upon diseases is produced by mere imagination. Medical practitioners of good understanding, but of various dispositions of mind, feel different degrees of scepticism in the remedies they employ. One who possesses the largest portion of medical faith will be of greatest benefit to his patients.'[19]

Sir William Herschel KH FRS (1738-1822)[20]
Herschel was not a doctor, but trained as a musician, found fame as an astronomer, and lived in Bath at the same time as Haygarth. He serves as a paradigm of dedication, attention to detail and perspicacity which are the hallmarks of a good scientist and he was an inspiration to Darwin. Herschel developed reflector telescopes with concave metal mirrors to improve the standards of observations. Clouds of gas known as nebulae had been identified in the mid eighteenth century but were assumed to be part of the Milky Way. It was Herschel who placed them at vast deep space distances from our own galaxy. A number of astronomers had previously observed Uranus, but it was Herschel who first identified it as a planet in 1781. As it was twice as far from the sun as Saturn, the known solar system immediately doubled in size. Its orbit did not comply perfectly with predictions based on Newtonian mechanics, and it was proposed there must be another planet even farther out. Neptune was discovered in 1846. That is how science works.

Herschel gave serious consideration to *The Construction of the Heavens* (1785) and told the Bath Philosophical Society that science required a delicate balance of observation and speculation: 'If we indulge of fanciful imagination and build worlds of our own, these will vanish like Cartesian vortices. Adding observation to observation, without attempting to draw conclusions and explore conjectural use would be equally self-defeating.'

William Falconer FRS (1744-1824)
Falconer was appointed physician at Chester Infirmary in 1767. He then moved to the Bath General Hospital in 1770 and is buried in Weston. He wrote extensively on Bath Waters, gout, hip disease, diet, climate, the pulse, poisons, and passions. His paper to the Bath Society in 1786 described experiments on constipation and showed that ordinary Somerset rhubarb was clinically as effective as the expensive Turkish variety which was generally preferred by wealthy patrons. Following the scientific manner introduced by his colleague Haygarth, Falconer based his opinion on observation of two groups of patients, one acting as control.

Bath was fashionable and its waters and remedies sought by the great and good. To relieve bowel complaints, Prime Minister William Pitt (the Younger) took the waters at Bath in 1806, but gout made matters worse. John Haygarth prescribed drops of Paregoric Elixir, then cascarilla, and finally, after consulting Falconer, rhubarb.[21] The news of Napoleon's success at Austerlitz did not help Pitt's spirits, and he died within the month.

William Whewell FRS (1794-1866)

Whewell (pronounced 'Hyule') is best known for his *History of the Inductive Sciences* (1837) and *Philosophy of the Inductive Sciences* (1840). He was a poet, Professor of Mineralogy, of Moral Theology and of Casuistical Divinity. From the earliest times the study of science was very much a part of philosophy and carried out by 'natural philosophers'. The poet Samuel Coleridge was a good friend of Sir Humphrey Davy and enthusiastically attended his lectures at the Royal Society, encouraging his friend Whewell to come up with a new term to describe these 'men of science'.

To replace 'natural philosophers' or 'men of science' Whewell coined the neologism 'scientist'. Initially he introduced the term anonymously at a meeting of the British Association for the Advancement of Science. At first he used it satirically: 'Some ingenious gentleman proposed that, by analogy with *artist* they might form a word *scientist*... there could be no scruples since we already have such words as *economist* and *atheist.*' Other colleagues used it as a term of abuse.

By 1840 in *The Philosophy of the Inductive Sciences,* Whewell was prepared to admit creating 'a name to describe a cultivator of science in general. I should be inclined to call him a *scientist* – he is a mathematician and physicist or naturalist.' Whewell also coined 'ion', 'anode' and 'cathode' for Michael Faraday; 'consilience' (to mean the unification of knowledge and branches of learning); and 'physicist', as a man of physics as distinct from 'physician'.

Whewell sought a balance between establishing scientific truth through pure empirical observations and the subjective contrary 'which we may call ideas and perceptions'. 'Fundamental Ideas' arose from the mind itself, not simply from observations. He regarded the mind as an active participant in the progress towards truth. This balance between the extremes of pure empiricism and ideal realism was not too dissimilar to the approach of Francis Bacon – although Bacon had laid emphasis on the importance of empiricism and the inductive approach, whereas previously, rationalism based on dogmatic ideas had held sway.

A scientific hypothesis is a proposition, an assertion, a starting point for reasoning. Hypotheses can originate from experience, analogy or intuition, but should not be regarded as 'truth' until proven by experiment. Even then, only true to a degree of probability. Whewell opined a hypothesis should predict consequences which can tested, and he introduced criteria for testing scientific hypotheses.

John Stuart Mill (1806-1873)

The philosopher, economist, administrator and Member of Parliament, took forward ideas on empiricism which had been developed by John Locke and David Hume.

Mill's ideas captured the imagination of the public. Apart from influential works on liberty, utilitarianism and principles of government, he set out proposals for scientific methods and a *System of Logic* (1843) which were at some variance with those of Whewell. Mill and Whewell had a robust debate about these matters which much enlivened contemporary philosophy as they argued whether science would be better served by inductive methods of reasoning or hypothetical deductive methods. Whewell asserted that 'heuristic devices' of hypothetical assumptions could account for observed data and allow a scientific law to be deduced. Mill did not agree and demanded experimental proof. This presaged Karl Popper's concept of *falsifiability* as a test of good science.

Mill's philosophy encompassed social, political, ethical and religious dimensions. He felt there was a tendency in 'supernatural religion' to hinder the development not only of intellectual but also moral nature. Religion's appeal is to self-interest rather than to disinterested and ideal motives, and can stand in the way of the critical evaluation of social norms.[22] For 'religion' we could today substitute 'alternative medicine.'

Mill's Methods of induction continue to provide stimulus to the development of scientific routines for establishing causes and effects. This is important when trying to get to grips with CAM, as many patients declare that because they have experienced benefit after a treatment, the benefit was caused by the treatment. Not necessarily so. Correlation does not imply Causation. To believe that 'after this, therefore because of this' (*post hoc, propter hoc*), is a logical fallacy.

Sir Karl Popper CH FRS (1902-1994)
Born in Vienna with Jewish grandparents, Popper was brought up as a Lutheran, became a Marxist, and then a social liberal, emigrated to New Zealand in 1937, then England in 1946, where he became Professor of Logic and Scientific method at London University. He was knighted in 1965, elected Fellow of the Royal Society in 1976, and made Companion of Honour in 1982.

Popper moved on from observation, experimentation and induction. In *The Logic of Scientific Discovery* of 1934 Popper emphasised that to establish knowledge and truth, the scientific method required *empirical falsifiability*. Stimulated by Einstein's theories of space-time and suggestions that events might appear simultaneous in one frame of reference, but not another, Popper proposed the principle of *falsification* was more relevant than induction. Observations and experiments were all very well, but are themselves 'theory laden'. Better not to go from observation via induction to generalisation. No matter how many positives might be found, there may still be some unobserved negatives. As when a black swan was unexpectedly found by Captain Cook, and as suggested at the sub-atomic scale by Heisenberg's Uncertainty Principle. Popper suggested that a better way for science to proceed was to look for exceptions, single instances, which might falsify a given hypothesis. This approach is unlike non-scientific or pseudo-scientific methods which remain adherent to authoritative but untested and non-falsifiable opinions.

Popper emphasised the importance of demarcation—sorting the scientific from the unscientific. The unfalsifiable are unscientific – any claim that an unfalsifiable theory can be proved true by scientific method is pseudo-science.

Popper was particularly keen to expose the pseudo-scientific nature of Karl Marx's *Theory of History* and Sigmund Freud's *Theory of the Psyche*. Popper's critical rationalism led to the *peer review procedures* which are an essential part of the modern method. Any hypothesis that is put forward is tested to destruction. That is, peers are expected to be critical about each other and do all they can to demonstrate the falsity of any proposed hypothesis. If critical trial and review does not identify a false premise, there can be greater confidence in the proposition being true. But only probably.[23]

Thomas Kuhn (1922-1996)
Kuhn's *The Structure of Scientific Revolutions* (1962) suggested that science, and the methods used to arrive at rational scientific truths, moves forward not incrementally but rather in fits and starts which he described as 'paradigms' (pattern, example). 'New scientific truth does not triumph by making opponents see the light, but rather because its opponents eventually die, and a new generation is familiar with it.'

Clearly there is no one 'scientific method' but rather a group of ideas, practices, and principles which assist in reducing the probability of falsehood to a level where results are regarded as 'true'. The methods (plural), try to make sense of the messy place in which we live – and the messy lives we lead.

Albert Michelson (1853-1931) and Edward Morley (1838-1923)
Along with most physicists of the late nineteenth century, Michelson and Morley assumed the obvious – light waves travel across the vacuum of space in a medium termed the 'luminiferous ether'. Experiments carried out by Michelson in 1881 produced negative results, and no support for this theory. The results were not filed away, as has been the case with negative CAM and drug trial results, but rather Michelson continued work on the problem with Morley. The result was 'the most famous failed experiment in history.' It had to be accepted that there was no evidence for the existence of the ether. In years to come there were calls for 'more research', but it plainly has to be acknowledged that the ether does not exist. This outcome was a major stimulus to Albert Einstein who published his theory of Special Relativity in 1905 – with no ether required.

Albert Einstein (1879-1955)
Einstein is the most easily recognisable scientist of the twentieth century, yet even he was not right every time. When he developed his field equations for general relativity which includes gravity, he could not get the two sides to balance out unless he incorporated a 'cosmological constant'. Not long after publication in 1916, Edwin Hubble showed the universe is expanding and there is no need for such a constant after all. Einstein was mortified. Feeling he had made 'the greatest mistake of my

life', he removed the constant. Later study has suggested a small positive constant is in fact needed in the necessary mathematics which describe an expanding universe, but the point for us is that Einstein was prepared to admit he had been wrong at the time, and move on. Not all camists show similar integrity in relation to research on their favourite CAM.

Michelson, Morley and Einstein present paradigms of professional practice expected of serious scientists. Their approach to discovering truth should be compared to those of practitioners of pseudo-science, camists, and *wudoka* who follow the path of *wu*.

'The Scientific Method™' does not exist, but methods used by scientists are the best we have for getting to the 'truth'. Harriet Hall, former USAF jet pilot and surgeon, and now the *SkepDoc* points out: 'True believers will never give up their favourite treatment because of negative evidence; they will always want to try one more study in the hope that it will vindicate their belief. They see science as a method they can take advantage of to convince others that their treatment works. They don't see it as a method of finding out whether their treatment works.'[24]

For all science's acknowledged imperfections, wrong turnings and even falsehoods, it is a major logical fallacy to suggest that just because science is not perfect, non-scientific methods provide a better path to rational truth and understanding.[25] Saying 'You also, you are no better' is the *tu quoque* fallacy. A pointing finger is pointless.

Those *wudoka* who prefer the paths of nothingness, have to reach an accommodation with modern scientists. There is no 'war' – no 'attacks' are called for, and we all have to respect each other's position, but there can be no expectation that a compromise can be reached. There is a Million Dollar Prize for the camist who can offer plausible proof of their system's clinical efficacy.[26]

Science tries to explain how it is. Camistry explains how some people would like it to be.

Endnotes to Chapter 7

1. Stuart Firestein: *Ignorance. How it drives Science*. Oxford University Press. Oxford. 2012.

2. Alhazen. *Critique of Ptolemy,* translated by S. Pines, *Actes X Congrès chinaceanal d'histoire des sciences,* Vol 1, Ithica 1962.

3. Related to neither Friar Roger Bacon, nor to Francis Bacon OM, the twentieth century painter – though the latter's approach to the 'truth' is a considerable stimulus to those of artistic temperament.

4. Kay Dickersin, Iain Chalmers. *Recognising, investigating and dealing with incomplete and biased reporting of clinical research.* J. R. Soc. Med. 2011: 104.

5. Austin Bradford Hill. Discussion of a paper by DJ Finney. *J. Roy. Stat. Soc.* 1959;119.

6. Ben Goldacre. *Bad Pharma.*. Fourth Estate. London 2012.

7. Ellis R.L., Heath D.D., Spedding J. *The Collected Works of Francis Bacon,* Routledge 1996. As noted by Murray Enkin et al in *BMJ* 2011;343:d8008.

8. Aristotle held that to ask whether the *psuchē* (soul, spirit, essence) and the body are one thing or two is an incoherent question. *De Anima* II.i.

9. '*Je pense donc je suis.*' Better known in its Latin translation: *Cogito ergo sum.* 'I think, therefore I am.' René Descartes (philosophically). Also: 'I am, I said', Neil Diamond (lyrically).

10. René Descartes. *Sixth Meditation.* AT VII 80.1: CSM II 56.

11. Or do they? See Maxwell Bennett, Daniel Dennett, Peter Hacker, John Searle. *Neuroscience and Philosophy.* Columbia University Press. New York. 2007.

12. Clarence Irving Lewis 1929. *Mind and the World Order: Outline of a Theory of Knowledge.* Dover reprint, 1956.

13. Daniel Dennett. *Quining Qualia* in A. Marcel and E. Bisiach, eds, *Consciousness in Modern Science*, Oxford University Press 1988. Ase.tufts.edu. 1985-11-21. Retrieved 2010-12-03. Dennett defines 'To quine' as a term for denying the existence of something real. A satirical definition, taking the name of analytical philosopher Willard Van Orman Quine in vain. Enjoy.

14. The original text had nine rules.

15. Newton's own theory of gravity remained paramount until Einstein theorised, and Eddington proved, that light itself can be bent by large masses. Space-time warps. Newton is still good enough if you wish to travel anywhere in the universe, except at close to the speed of light – at which point your mass will become infinite and your length in the direction of travel, zero. Tricky.

16. Paul Daniels' real name is Newton Edward Daniels. That's magic!

17. The term 'placebo effect' was not used regularly until the twentieth century.

18. John Haygarth. *On the Imagination as a Cause and as a Cure of Disorders of the Body.* R. Crutwell, Bath, 1800

19. Ibid.

20. KH: Knight of the Hanoverian Guelphic Order, bestowed on Herschel by the Prince Regent – like Herschel, a Hanoverian.

21. Cascarilla: a bitter tonic from the bark of *Croton eleuteria,* an aromatic West Indian shrub. Paregoric Elixir: a tincture of camphor with opium. 'Paregoric' from a Greek form of oratory in which distraction of attention featured – a not uncommon technique of medical practitioners. More recently, the term implies 'anodyne'.

22. Fred Wilson. *John Stuart Mill*. Stanford Encyclopaedia of Philosophy.

23. 'I am, therefore I do.' Karl Popper; 'I do, therefore I am.' René Descartes; 'Do be do be do.' Frank Sinatra.

24. Harriet Hall: http://www.skepdoc.info/

25. The *tu quoque* fallacy (Latin: you too, or you also): An appeal to hypocrisy is heard all too often as an attempt to discredit science. Science's faults and inconsistence do not discredit the general method, nor criticism of pseudo-science. *Tu quoque* responses suggest conclusions are not supported by the premises of the principle argument. That may be logically fallacious. This is a form of the *ad hominem* argument – the person or idea might be inconsistent, but that does not invalidate the argument. Associating a person's faults or ideas with the validity of their argument is logically fallacious.

26. James Randi Educational Foundation. www.randi.org. The offer is for a demonstration of any psychic, supernatural, or paranormal ability under satisfactory observation. This includes water with memory, release or balancing of supernatural energies, engagement of vital forces and similar. Camists should apply, magicians should not – the illusions are too easy to reproduce.

Chapter 8

Quality in healthcare

It is a capital mistake to theorise before one has data. Insensibly one begins to twist facts to suit theories, instead of theories to suit facts. **Sherlock Holmes**[1]

The term 'Quality in Health Care' is a term regularly invoked but used variously and vaguely. Usually there is no definition of what is meant or how the term is being applied.

The definition of quality by Chambers Dictionary is: 'the degree or extent of excellence of something'. 'Excellence' is described as being of 'exceptional quality'. Tautology in action. The Oxford English Dictionary has: 'an attribute, property, special feature; the nature, kind, or character of something; the degree or grade of excellence possessed by a thing.'

Measuring the Quality of Healthcare

Without measurement, management is meaningless. Experiments cannot be planned, there can be no meaningful outcome assessments, false causal inferences will be made and resources wasted. The reluctance of practitioners to identify and admit when they are wrong may lead to patients making bad healthcare choices. Healthcare measurement and analysis is critical for the advance of good science and wellbeing. We need metrics not myths.

John Graunt

Market research for his haberdashery business led to publication of *Natural and Political Observations upon the Bills of Mortality* in 1663. Thomas Cromwell, Master of the Rolls, had established national records of deaths in the 1540s, but because each parish priest had his own method of recording, comparison was impossible. Graunt's work came to the attention of The Royal Society but as he was a mere tradesman he was not initially welcomed as a member. The support of King Charles resolved that difficulty and Graunt became a charter member of the Society, though it preferred to give credit for the development of statistics to Graunt's friend, the more aristocratic Sir William Petty. Impressed by Francis Bacon's rational and mathematical approach to philosophy, Petty joined the Invisible College which met to consider experimental investigations. Regarded as an intellectual, he was knighted in 1661 and was a founder member of the Royal Society. Samuel Pepys recorded these goings-on contemporaneously and modern historians now regard Graunt's *Political Observations* as the origin of quantitative and probabilistic data analysis. Petty used Graunt's life tables and death rates to explain financial losses and established statistics as an important tool for economics and politics. Petty's *Political Arithmetic* (1687) recommended that governments should not interfere overmuch in the economy, any more than a physician should meddle with a patient. Karl Marx makes references to Petty's work in *Das Kapital,* expressing concern that workers could become alienated from society.

In 1749 the Swedish National Register of Births, Deaths and Marriages was established, and was a major stimulus for the subsequent collection of population data throughout Europe. At that time the Swedish government thought their population was twenty million. It turned out it was only two million – which somewhat alarmed social and military planners.

Sir John Sinclair

Sinclair was the first to use the word 'statistics' in English. In *A Statistical Account of Scotland* (1791) he advised: 'By "statistical" is meant in Germany an inquiry for the purposes of ascertaining the political strength of a country or questions respecting matters of state – whereas the idea I annex to the term is an inquiry into the state of the country for the purpose of ascertaining the quantum of happiness enjoyed by its inhabitants, and the means of its future improvement; but as I thought that a new word might attract more public attention, I resolved on adopting it ...'
[2] The term 'political arithmetic' fell into disuse. Even now, what we need is more correct political arithmetic and less arithmetic political correctness.

Outcomes research has to be based on adequate statistical power. Bias and chance all too easily intrude into comparisons of healthcare treatments. Anecdotes of 'personal experience' may well not apply to anyone else, or at any other time. The pleural of anecdote is not data.[3] Because any result might be due to chance, at least one hundred patients need to be studied to test the significance of even a medium difference between two treatments. If any fewer patients have been studied, remain sceptical about the value of the research.

Sir Ronald Fisher

The eminent statistician recommended that if the probability of a given result being due to chance is 5% or less, that should be regarded as being worthwhile and 'statistically significant'. Each researcher can choose their own level of significance but should justify their choice – Fisher's suggestion has become the norm. In statistics, 'significance' does not mean important, but rather indicates the likelihood that any given result occurred by chance. Results are described as being 'statistically significant', or not, and expressed in percentages or 'probabilities'. For example, 5% is a probability of 0.05.

For the purposes of this book we need go no further, save to warn the reader against being taken in by glib 'statistics' and false information. Scepticism and statistics have to go hand in hand. Robert Matthews warns: 'Ronald Fisher gave scientists a mathematical machine for turning baloney into breakthroughs, and flukes into funding.'[4] Sleight of tongue and semantics can reverse any meaning and totally mislead the unwary, particularly if commercial instincts impinge and a charlatan wants to take advantage of the gullible. Darrell Huff's classic *How to Lie with Statistics* is essential reading for those who are going to use statistical methods. And statistics apply to populations, not individuals.

Camees should always consider the probability that their chosen CAM will satisfy them no more than a placebo would. If a medically qualified doctor endorses a CAM, they are required to be honest, truthful and comply with General Medical Council guidelines to ensure patients are fully informed about all aspects of the intended treatment. If a practitioner does not properly inform the patient about the improbability of the intended treatment having an effect beyond the placebo, the patient cannot give informed consent to having treatment.

Graunt's life tables, Petty's *Political Arithmetic* and Sinclair's statistics were a stimulus to more critical analysis of healthcare quality. In the latter half of the eighteenth century Edinburgh Infirmary started publically reporting whether patients left hospital 'cured, relieved, incurable, died, or dismissed by desire or for irregularities.' Statistics became used more effectively in other branches of medicine and science.[5]

Reverend Thomas Bayse FRS

A Presbyterian minister who also studied mathematics, Bayse's *Introduction to the Doctrine of Fluxions* asked how certain can we be about uncertainty, explored the mathematical association between cause and effect and considered 'prior probability' – Bayse's Theorem.[6,7] Alan Turing used the theorem when devising a computer to decode Enigma and so do spam filters on computers. Fortunately, and bearing in mind the 'average' never characterises complex phenomena, for regular practical healthcare purposes, simple non-Baysean statistics suffice – probably.[8,9]

James Lind

Appointed ship's surgeon in 1740 when Britain was at war with Spain, Lind went with Commodore George Anson's squadron into the Pacific via Cape Horn. The expedition was a disaster. Of the nearly two thousand marines and sailors who had originally set out, less than two hundred survived. Typhus, cholera and scurvy were a major causes of death but the Admiralty had no idea what to do about it. Lind carried out research on scurvy, using twelve patients, two in each of six groups given different treatments: cider; elixir of vitriol (alcohol, ginger and sulphuric acid); vinegar; sea water; oranges and lemons and a purgative. Working directly with patients, and trying the effects of these different remedies, Lind established the first well recorded *clinical trials* in 1747.

A year later Lind left the Navy and started a practice in Edinburgh where he took the next step in what we now refer to as evidence-based medicine. The results of his own clinical trials were reviewed with the few other available studies and in 1753 Lind published *A Treatice of the scurvy in three parts, together with a critical and chronological view of what has been published on the subject.* This approach is now termed a *systematic review.* Lind concluded oranges and lemons were best, but being hard to obtain in the West Indies, the Royal Navy used limes. Hence the American term for the British as 'Limeys'. Lind emphasised:

> My opinions are not founded on private observations, or on any one particular case, which might prove an exception to a general established principle in practice. They are the result of some thousand patients, whose cases are still preserved in the hospital. Remedies more absolutely certain might perhaps have been expected from an inspection of several thousand patients. Partial facts may, for a little, flatter with hopes of greater success; yet more enlarged experience must evince the fallacy of all positive assertions in the healing art.[10]

Lind supported Sydenham's recommendation that malarial agues should be treated with cinchona bark. Samuel Hahnemann also experimented on this bark, though ended up diluting the therapeutic molecules out of active existence.

Reverend John Wesley

The Anglican priest also published *Primitive Physic: or an easy and natural method of curing most diseases* in 1747. Care from a physician was unaffordable for most and his congregation needed help. Like Lind, Wesley recommended oranges for treating scurvy, but they were expensive. For those who could not afford them Wesley suggested the patient should 'live on turnips for a month.' For consumption he recommended: 'In the last stage, fuck a healthy woman daily. This cured my father.'[11] No wonder Wesley's *Primitive Physic* has outsold all his others.

Miss Florence Nightingale OM RRC FRSS

Born in the Italian city from which she took her Christian name, at home in England Florence insisted on being taught mathematics. In 1837 she experienced a strong sense of vocation which she recorded in a letter to her sister: 'God called me in the morning and asked me if I would do good for him.' She decided to become a nurse. At that time, such tasks were deemed too menial for a woman of her background, but she was determined and travelled widely in Egypt, Greece and Germany whilst establishing useful relationships with influential politicians. She had no formal training in nursing, for there was none. Her father came to terms with her ambitions and was able to provide her with an allowance whilst she worked as Superintendent at London's Institute for the Care of Sick Gentlewomen (dismissing most of the staff), before moving to the Middlesex Hospital.

In 1854 Nightingale led a small nursing team to the Scutari Barracks in the Crimea, where the British Army was fighting the Russians. At that time, ten times more soldiers died from illnesses and infections than from war wounds. By the simple expedient of improved sanitation and hygiene, death rates fell. Nightingale began collecting statistics, setting down whether patients left the hospital 'recovered, disabled or dead'.

Nightingale was the first woman to be made a Fellow of the Royal Statistical Society (1858), of the American Statistical Association (1874) and became the first female member of the Order of Merit. In 1908 she became only the second woman to be honoured as a Freeman by The City of London. [12] Her own fifty year invalidity is regarded by some as evidence of her manipulative personality.[13]

Nightingale enthusiastically took up the 'pie chart', which had been developed by political economist William Playfair and used this to present her statistical analyses of death and disease rates.[14] In particular Nightingale developed the polar area diagram, a circular histogram. Her statistics went a stage further than simple tables of mortality that Graunt had devised – she considered soldiers who survived and returned home, but also noted if they were disabled. This is of contemporary concern, as evidenced by charities such as the *British Legion*, *Help for Heroes* and *Combat Stress*.

Evidence-based medicine (1997) has been defined by Sackett and colleagues as: 'The conscientious, explicit and judicious use of the current best evidence in making decisions.'[15] This requires statistical analysis – Florence would be pleased. The Nightingale Collaboration was founded in 2011 to 'challenge questionable claims made by healthcare practitioners on their websites, in adverts and in their promotional and sales materials by bringing these to the attention of the appropriate regulatory bodies.'[16]

Trends in the management of quality in healthcare

Medicine continually evolves. Systems based on superstition and metaphysics have been superseded, but problems remain. Some of those who have made particular contributions to improvement in healthcare quality include:

Samuel Christian Hahnemann (1755-1843)
Hahnemann recognised the poor quality of treatment and the harm being done by the physicians and remedies of his day. He abandoned conventional bleeding, polypharmacy, purging and emesis with toxic heavy metals. The quality time and trouble he took to discuss patients' concerns became a major challenge to the prevailing orthodoxy. Although his system of *Homeopathy* was widely derided and not accepted by the mainstream, consciences were pricked and change was encouraged. Had Hahnemann incorporated a more scientific approach to his own researches and avoided metaphysics, he might have had greater influence.

Abraham Flexner (1866-1959)
Flexner was not a medical doctor but had a great impact on American medical education in the twentieth century. He is probably Louisville's most famous son after Muhammad Ali. In 1905 Flexner went to study the German university system and wrote a critical book about American higher education. Although not generally well received, its insights were recognised by the American Medical Association and in 1908 the AMA asked the Carnegie Foundation for the Advancement of Teaching to fund a review by Flexner into education in North American medical schools.

Medical Education in the United States and Canada (1910), the Flexner Report, castigated most schools. As a result, nearly half the orthodox medical schools had to shut or merge, with pressure on the schools for eclectic, osteopathic, chiropractic, homeopathic, Thomsonian, naturopathic and other non-orthodox medical systems. Flexner regarded the non-orthodox as schools of quackery and charlatanism. One disgruntled osteopathic school sued Flexner and the Carnegie for libel but had to withdraw. American medicine was obliged to reform.[17]

In 1912, the Congress of Surgeons of North America declared 'Some system of standardisation of hospital work must be developed to the end that those institutions having the highest ideals may have proper recognition and others be stimulated to raise the quality of their work. In this way patients will have some means of recognising those institutions devoted to the highest ideals of medicine.' In 1918 the American College of Surgeons pointed out: 'All hospitals are accountable to the public for their degree of success, and if this initiative is not taken by the medical profession, it will be taken by the lay public.'

In 1959 his obituary in the New York Times suggested 'no other American of his time has contributed more to the welfare of his country and of humanity in general.' The Flexner Report continues to be cited as the catalyst for the rapid improvement in medical education seen in North America during the twentieth century.

Ernest Amory Codman (1869-1940)
Codman qualified in medicine from Harvard and became a surgeon, but he was not a happy bunny. He realised that for all the acclaim accorded to eminent colleagues, nobody actually knew what the outcomes of their ministrations were. In 1803 Sir Thomas Percival had suggested that there should be a register of surgeons' outcomes but little had been done. Codman was determined to do something about 'outcomes research' and he developed a system of charting and collecting data on every patient treated, with at least one year follow up. All complications were recorded and published. Many physicians decided Codman's system of recording 'end results' was not helpful – to their own reputations. Codman suggested: 'Every hospital should follow every patient it treats long enough to determine whether the treatment has been successful, and then to enquire "if not, why not" – with a view to preventing similar failures in the future.' [18]

Codman was also a founder of the American College of Surgeons and its Hospital Standardization Program. In its first review, 692 hospitals in the New York area were inspected. Only 89 passed muster and the results were burned in a fireplace of the Waldorf Astoria where the review meeting was held. The original standardization programme has evolved and become the Joint Commission on Accreditation of Healthcare Organisations (JCHAO). At its annual conference in 1997, Dr Avedis Donabedian was awarded the first individual Ernest A. Codman Award for exemplary contributions to quality improvement and patient safety.

Walter Shewhart PhD (1891-1967)
Physicist, engineer and statistician, Shewhart developed 'statistical control charts' to analyse variations in industrial output and non-compliance with set standards. He devised a simple four step method to reduce variation in a manufacturing process and improve quality. The steps of this process have become known as the Shewhart, Audit or PDCA (plan-do-check-act) cycle. Shewhart is regarded as the 'father of statistical process control':

The 'Audit Cycle' is in fact an upward spiral which has gradually become a *sine qua non* in conventional healthcare – much as Francis Bacon had set down in his *Novum Organum* of 1620: hypothesis, experiment, evaluate, repeat. Efforts to improve quality implicate the whole healthcare institution and system, including government, and so in the early 1990s the term Total Quality Management (TQM) was lifted from commercial and business practice. This was too 'managerial' for many in healthcare, and the term Continuous Quality Improvement (CQI) became more fashionable. 'Politicians must encourage the highest standards of health service by their refusal to give credence to unscientific data and invalid quality management methods.'[19]

W. Edwards Deming PhD (1900-1993)

Like Shewhart, Deming was a physicist and statistician. He recognised the problems caused by error in scientific measurement in industry and developed Shewhart's ideas further. At the end of the Second World War Deming helped the US Department of the Army carry out a census in Japan. By training engineers and managers in statistical techniques he made a major contribution to Japan's industrial recovery and subsequent reputation for high quality products. These systems have encouraged more integrative approaches towards cooperative involvement of clinicians, patients and managers in reducing variations and complications and improving quality.

Professor Sir Austin Bradford Hill FRS (1897-1991)

After spending four years dealing with his own tuberculosis, Bradford Hill's work with the Medical Research Council in the 1940s established the use of streptomycin for the treatment of TB and is regarded as being the first 'Randomised Controlled Trial' (RCT).

Nobel Prize winner Sir Peter Medawar emphasised: 'Exaggerated claims for the efficacy of a medicament are very seldom the consequence of any intention to deceive; they are usually the outcome of a kindly conspiracy in which everybody has the very best intentions...The controlled clinical trial is an attempt to avoid being taken in by this conspiracy of good will.' [20,21]

Evidence produced by RCTs is more credible with larger patient groups, and better still if trials use placebo control groups. If other investigators can produce comparable results, the credibility of the evidence will be accepted. These are high standards, but not essential. Sometimes investigators simply have to do the best they can. It is very hard to have effective placebo control groups for CAMs, though without them judgement of any evidence for CAM effectiveness requires a large bucket of salt and active scepticaemia. And we all know salt is not good for you.

Randomised controlled trials are not essential in assessing CAMs, but some sort equivalent clinical evaluation is. Without them, how is anyone, including camists, to know what works? Simply obtaining anecdotes from acolytes will not do. 'It seems to me...' simply does not meet the standard of evidence required to develop public policy.[22]

Professor Archie Cochrane CBE (1909-1988)

'Archie's experience as a medical officer to prisoners of war made clear to him the importance of care when there is no hope of cure, and reinforced his interest in testing unsubstantiated claims about the effects of medical treatment.'[23]

As Cochrane himself said about his instructions as a medical officer:

> I had considerable freedom of choice of therapy: my trouble was that I did not know which to use and when. I would gladly have sacrificed my freedom for a little knowledge. I had never heard of 'randomised controlled trials', but I knew that there was no real evidence that anything we had to offer had any effect on tuberculosis, and I was afraid that I shortened the lives of some of my friends by unnecessary intervention.

Cochrane trained in Public Health and became an epidemiologist and Director of the Medical Research Council's Epidemiology Research Unit. Influenced by Bradford Hill's Randomised Controlled Trials, Cochrane tried to identify which treatments did more harm than good and how to care if cure was impossible. His book, *Effectiveness and Efficiency* (1972) became seminal and Cochrane was lauded internationally.[24] He commented 'It is surely a great criticism of our profession that we have not organised a critical summary, by speciality or sub-speciality, adapted periodically, of all relevant randomised clinical trials.'[25] After his death an international alliance was created to remedy this omission – The Cochrane Collaboration. Camistry has yet to adopt a similar critical approach.

Avedis Donabedian (1919-2000)
Donabedian identified 'Seven Pillars of Quality' in 1990, and went on to describe how quality could be assessed in respect of three principal dimensions: *Structure* – not only physical facilities, equipment and staffing numbers, but also staff qualifications and ability; *Process* -what actually goes on; *Outcome* – as determined by clinical indicators, outcomes review and audit. In each of these dimensions, a multitude of standards can be used. The balancing effects of benefit, risk and cost should also be incorporated. In 1984 Professor Robert J. Maxwell, then Director of London's King's Fund College, set down a basic set of criteria for quality assessment, based on Donabedian's work.[26]

Professor Paul Meier (1924-2011)
Born in New Jersey, Meier wrote a paper describing a method of accounting for missing data in statistical analysis. He submitted this to the American Statistical Association, only to find that Edward L. Kaplan had a similar paper but with different wrinkles. Kaplan and Meier were told to work together, thrash out their differences and produce a single account. Four years later the Kaplan-Meier curve of mortality and survival was introduced in the *Journal of the American Statistical Association.*[27]

Meier's obituary in the British Medical Journal held that this article is the fifth most cited of any academic paper.[28] Meier was particularly interested in randomisation, noting 'for a fairly long time randomisation was not thought of highly. I defended randomisation every chance I got ... if you use randomisation you could find out stuff you really need know.'[29]

Codman, Cochrane and Meier were concerned that when it came to assessing the value of their treatments, health professionals often did not have a clue what they were talking about. The scientific method was being more regularly applied, but systematic data collection, analysis and reporting was poor for most of the twentieth century. The principles of statistical control and analysis, which developed in US industry and then jump started the recovery of the Japanese economy after the Second World War, steadily began to have an impact.

Donald Berwick KBE MD FRCP (b.1946)

A Harvard trained paediatrician, Berwick proposed that continuous improvement methods used in industry could be applied in healthcare. His article is another on the list of 'seminal', and stimulated wider interest in these methods.[30]

As President Emeritus of the Institute for Healthcare Improvement, Berwick has been a major stimulus to quality improvement in the NHS, and has been appointed an honorary Knight Commander of the Most Excellent Order of the British Empire. Which would entitle him to be styled as 'Sir' were it not for George Washington.

Towards a partnership approach to quality in healthcare

The concept of 'continuous improvement' became established in Japan during the 1950s as *kaizen* – a way of thinking and working which evolves within an organisation, involves every employee, and with a facilitative and non-authoritarian management. *Kaizen* should not be confused with the style of management encountered all too often in the NHS – that of *tanaka*.[31]

The BMA Clinical Audit Committee's *A Partnership Approach to Quality* (1994) considered a number of definitions of 'quality'. Whilst patients were the most important determinant, there were other groups who used different definitions and standards at different times. These included other healthcare professionals, the purchasers of services, the providers, the public at large, and politicians. The BMA consensus definition of 'Quality in Health Care' was coherent with that of the US National Institute of Health and captured features of particular importance to clinicians: 'Quality in health care is the extent to which desired outcomes are achieved and undesirable outcomes are avoided.' 'Quality' can then be determined by the degree of conformance with stated standards.

All definitions of 'quality' have validity but require clarification of the meaning intended. Politicians are frequently vague in order to avoid being wrong footed, and often decline to give a definition. In which case, how can anyone know what they are talking about? They are very reluctant to face up to the reality that scarce healthcare resources need allocating rationally – that is, rationing. Politicians do not like statistics because they are difficult to explain to their customers – the voters. Different statistical methods are needed in different circumstances. Tough. Quality in healthcare is fundamental to modern living and the opinion of Professor Robert Maxwell should be heeded: 'Once any physician settles for something less than the best he or she can do, the fundamental professional ethic is in danger. If doctors ever cease to aspire to the best they know, they become hacks not serious physicians, surgeons or whomsoever. An NHS composed of hacks or frustrated and disillusioned professionals is on a slippery downward slope.'[32]

1995 saw the National Centre for Clinical Audit (NCCA) set up under a contract between the Department of Health and a consortium of organizations with an interest in health care led by the BMA and Royal College of Nursing.[33] NCCA's contract concluded in 1998, and its work was superseded by the National Institute for Health and Care Excellence: 'NICE guidance supports healthcare professionals and others to make sure that the care they provide is of the best possible quality and offers the best value for money. We provide independent, authoritative and evidence-based guidance on the most effective ways to prevent, diagnose and treat disease and ill health, reducing inequalities and variation.'

The management of health systems requires attention to the detail of quality – but that can only be based on the firm science behind treatments and remedies offered. These are high demands, but if patients are to receive the best possible care, that is the alternative to health and wellbeing systems based on superstition and pseudo-scientific opinion.

The Cochrane Collaboration

The first 'systematic review' carried out by independent researchers is credited to Duke University psychologists J. B. Rhine and J. G. Pratt who published *Extra-Sensory Perception after Sixty Years* in 1940. 145 ESP experiments from 1882 to their own were collated and analysed.[34] In 1976 Gene Glass introduced the term 'meta-analysis' to describe this approach.[35] In 1992 the Cochrane Collaboration was established in London to take forward Cochrane's principles: in order to provide meaningful analysis and information for healthcare decisions, the results of all available studies and randomised controlled trials should be pooled and systematically reviewed. [36]

Sir Iain Chalmers, the Collaboration's first director, had been deeply affected by his experience working in Palestinian refugee camps as a newly qualified doctor, where he came to recognise the futility, ineffectiveness and harm caused by some established treatments: 'That shattering experience induced in me a chronic *scepticaemia* and insistence that therapeutic claims should be informed by reliable research evidence.' The Collaboration is now a network of 28,000 people in 100 countries. Its website declares: 'We work together to help health care providers, policy makers, patients, their advocates and carers, make well informed decisions about healthcare, based on the best available research evidence, by preparing, updating and promoting the accessibility of *Cochrane Reviews* – over 5,000 so far, published on line in the *Cochrane Library*. Our work is internationally recognised as the benchmark for high quality information about the effectiveness of healthcare.' [37]

Evidence-based medicine. E.B.M.

'Evidence-based' means just that – based on evidence. Even stories, myths, anecdotes and opinions that 'It seems to me...' , 'I just know...', or 'It worked for me...' constitute 'evidence', albeit weak. (Latin: *evidens,* perceptible, clear, obvious, apparent, ground for belief). To be helpful to patients and the conventional professions, 'evidence' should be well grounded. Recommendations based solely on tradition, anecdote or authority should be set in context. 'Evidence' in healthcare implies that it has been acquired using scientific methods of experimentation and observation which is plausible, reproducible and which has a high level of agreement amongst educated, trained and knowledgeable medical scientists and health care professionals acting ethically. 'Evidence' can never be perfect and there will be doubts, controversies and disagreements amongst the orthodox professions – but scientists and practitioners will at least do the best they can to make accurate observations, conduct detailed analyses, draw rational conclusions and expose themselves to critical peer review.

There is a hierarchy of evidence – from that regarded as most valuable down to least: Systematic expert reviews; Meta-analysis; Randomised Double Blind Placebo-controlled Clinical Trials; Randomised Controlled trials; Cohort Studies; Case Controlled Studies; Physiological Studies; Faith – intuition and opinion that 'it seems to me...'

That is not to say the 'least' studies have no value, but before a patient is subjected to any intervention, it is essential to have a good reason for believing it might be of benefit – and randomised trials provide the greatest probability of meaningful and rational knowledge. As Sir Michael Rawlins emphasised when Chairman of NICE: 'Decision makers need to assess and appraise all the available evidence irrespective as to whether it has been derived from RCTs or observational studies, and the strengths and weaknesses of each need to be understood if reasonable and reliable conclusions are to be drawn.' He drew attention to the advice of Bradford Hill who developed RCTs, namely: 'Any belief that the controlled trial is the only way would mean not that the pendulum had swung too far but that it had come right off the hook.'[38]

In 1980 the BMJ expressed concern that medicine was experiencing a 'flight from science'.[39] Increasingly patients were being treated by alternative medicine - meditation, acupuncture, and a galaxy of special diets. Much of the appeal of alternative medicine lay in the setting in which it was given. Practitioners gave their patients time, courtesy, individual attention, and they listened. Healing was not necessarily the same as curing, and a compassionate healer who did nothing to arrest the disease process could nevertheless relieve symptoms.[40] Whatever the merits of alternative medicine, the majority of camees were people seeking a solution to an unresolved long-term problem, had become disillusioned and had lost confidence in conventional medicine.[41] The BMA felt that while alternative medicine may comfort, the responsibility of the medical profession was to types of care that can be assessed scientifically.[42] The alternative is, well – alternative.

In the late 1980s, papers from David Sackett, Gordon Guyatt and others at McMaster

University formalised the whole process of obtaining, analysing, and acting on best available evidence. The term 'Evidence Based Medicine' was introduced in 1991, and Sackett's *Evidence Based Medicine* (1992) has become a standard textbook.[43] Sackett, who was bedridden with polio as a child, went on to become Director of Oxford's Centre for Evidence-Based Medicine and first chairman of the Cochrane Collaboration. He was made an Officer of the Order of Canada and died aged eighty in 2015.

Extraordinary claims require extraordinary good plausible evidence if they are to be accepted. Following extensive preliminary research on toxicity and effectiveness in the real world of patient care, RCTs are a final step in analysis.[44] They provide the best method of discrimination between treatments, though less powerful methods may have to suffice. RCTs do not provide 'the answer', 'the proof' or 'the truth' but do inform rational understanding.

The practice of 'EBM' is not homologous. There are many methods and principles sheltering under that broad umbrella. Studies of individual patients' experience can certainly be included. Sackett emphasised: 'The practice of evidence based medicine means integrating individual clinical expertise with the best available external clinical evidence from systematic research.' EBM is not the final answer for giving patients an honest appreciation of the treatments they are considering. It is the best we can do at present. With apologies to Winston Churchill's insights, BMJ Editor Fiona Godlee acknowledges EBM may be the worst system for clinical decision making, except for all the other systems that have been tried.

Some doctors are suspicious that 'EBM' can be hijacked by health economists, managers and politicians in order to ration healthcare – resulting in a return to the days of 'empiricist quackery'. Others are concerned the personal touch may be lost in the science. Sackett called them 'old farts'.[45, 46, 47]

Patient-centred medicine
The term 'Patient-Centred Medicine' was introduced by psychiatrist Dr Edith Balint in 1969 to describe how GPs could move from their more traditional approach concentrating on illness and pathology and, by understanding the patient as a 'unique human being', could support patients with emotional, psychological and spiritual problems.[48] Some authors and practitioners find the concept of *centeredness* helps promote good quality practice. 'The unifying themes of "centeredness" favours the social, psychological, cultural and ethical sensitivity of the practitioner-patient relationship.'[49]

Good patient-centred practice respects patients' autonomy and that requires patients are given enough information to ensure properly informed consent and evidence-based patient choice – anything else is unethical, paternalistic and a throwback to the old days when health practitioners simply told patients what to do. The question arises as to whether all proponents of 'integrative medicine' and 'patient centred care' have actually explained to their patients what is involved, and that alternatives to scientific-based medicine may be used. Quality may be compromised and substituted, not only by pseudo-science but by pseudo-care. Patients need to check and read behind the promotional and marketing material of any courses, conferences or care programmes in which they may be interested. No quack will raise their wings and admit they are intending to mislead or deceive their potential audiences, clients or patients, but they will protest vehemently at close examination of their real aims and will avoid answering searching questions. No one ducks like a quack.

Endnotes to Chapter 8

1. The fictional detective who used factual induction. As recorded by Dr James Watson and reported by GP Dr Arthur Conan Doyle.

2. John Sinclair. *Statistical Account of Scotland.* Vol XX.

3. Ray Wolfinger claims he originally said the inverse: 'The pleural of anecdote is data' – but had said it as a rejoinder to put in place a student who had referred to 'mere anecdote'. Wolfinger acknowledges that the phrase has morphed since 1969, but now makes more general sense. http://askville.amazon.com/original-source-quote-plural-anecdote data/ AnswerViewer.do?requestId=1415780.

4. Robert Matthews. Sunday Telegraph, 13 September 1998.

5. G.B. Risse. *Hospital Life in Enlightenment Scotland.* Cambridge University Press, 1986.

6. Bayse's Theorem: $P(A \mid B) = P(B \mid A). P(A). P(B)^{-1}$

7. When I lecture on the principles of quality improvement in healthcare, I demonstrate using a bag containing ten black and ten white balls. After nine black balls in a row have been drawn, and shown, I point out that I am a magician. With that information the probability that the next is also black changes, as I can obviously determine the colour drawn at will. Prior knowledge on this point would have helped estimates. Guesses have a place, and may be inevitable, but the better the information about prior premises, the better the calculation and answer.

8. Doctors have long recognised the value of statistics. In 1828 Charles Hastings established a quarterly journal, *The Midland Medical and Surgical Reporter and Topographical and Statistical Journal.* In 1832 he founded the forerunner to the British Medical Association, entreating colleagues to practice *'With head and heart and hand'.* That remains the Association's motto today.

9. West B. *Homeostasis and Gauss statistics; barriers to understanding natural variability.* Journal of Evaluation in Clinical Practice. 16 (2010).

10. James Lind: *'A Treatice of the scurvy in three parts, together with a critical and chronological view of what has been published on the subject'* 1772 edition; U. Tröhler. *James Lind and the evaluation of clinical practice.* 2003 and JLL Bulletin: *Commentaries*

on the history of treatment evaluation: www.jameslindlibrary.org. In the 19th century, another British trained naval surgeon, Takaki Kanehiro, conducted controlled trials on Japanese sailors suffering from beri-beri, proving diet was the problem – now known to be thiamine deficiency.

11. John Wesley. *Primitive Physic.* Facsimile of 14th edition. The New Room, Bristol. 2003. Page 45, para.191. www.newroombristol.org.uk. Also note John Wesley's *The Desideratum, or Electricity made plain and useful,* 1759.

12. Like 'chairman', 'ombudsman' and 'fellow' – 'freeman' is non-gender specific.

13. In BMJ 2012; 344:e2317, Theodore Dalrymple recommends that F.B. Smith's *Florence Nightingale: Reputation and Power* (London, Croom Helm,1982) is worth studying. Also see: Rosemary Leadbetter, Oxford Brookes University; *Florence Nightingale,* www.medicinae.org/e01.

14. William Playfair (1759-1823), developed the bar chart and line graph used today in economic analyses. He was also regarded as a scoundrel.

15. David Sackett (1934-2015). *Evidence-Based Medicine* New York: Churchill Livingstone 1997.

16. www.nightingale-collaboration.org.

17. Abraham Flexner 1915. National Conference on Charities and Correction, 1915, 584-588.

18. Ernest Codman 1914, quoted by Flook E.E.; Sanazaro PJ. *Health Services Research, and R & D in perspective.* Ann Arbor, MI: Health Administration Press, 1973.

19. Richard Rawlins, *Paradigm Regained: Toward a partnership model for quality.* Journal of the Association for Quality in Health Care, Spring 1994. As a regional co-ordinator for the National Joint Register, I pressed for greater commitment from government to support good quality data collection. In 2013 after reviewing newly available outcome data, NICE demanded that many varieties of metal-on-metal hip prostheses no longer be used.

20. Peter Medawar. *Advice to a Young Scientist.* Harper & Row. New York 1979.

21. Doll R; Hill AB (1954) *Smoking and Carcinoma of the Lung.* British Medical Journal 2 (4682).

22. *Test, Learn, Adapt.* Cabinet Office, London.14/6/12. www.cabinetoffice.gov.uk/sites/default/files/resources/TLA-1906126.pdf.

23. Sir Iain Chalmers. www.jameslindlibrary.org/illustrating/articles/archie-cochrane.

24. Archie Cochrane. *Effectiveness and Efficiency.* Nuffield Provincial Hospitals Trust London, 1972.

25. Archie Cochrane. *Medicines for the Year 2000.* Office of Health Economics. London.

1979.

26. Robert J. Maxwell. *Quality Assessment in Health.* BMJ 1984.288.

27. Kaplan EL, Meier P. *Nonparametric estimation from incomplete observations.* Journal of the American Statistical Association.1958; 53.

28. Paul Meier. *Obituary.* BMJ, 3 September 2011 volume 343.

29. Sir Richard Peto. New York Times. August 11th 2011, www.nytimes.com.

30. Donald Berwick. *Continuous Improvement as an Ideal in Healthcare.* N. Eng J. Med. 1989 Jan 5;320(1).

31. *Tanaka:* Take All Names And Kick Ass. Which is why I became chairman of the Advisory Council of the King's Fund Organisational Audit which sought to establish high standards of 'structure' and management in the NHS. KFOA transformed and became the Health Quality Service.

32. Robert J. Maxwell. Director, King's Fund College. The Lancet, 26 October 1985.

33. Declaration of interest: I was Chairman of the BMA's Clinical Audit Committee and BMA representative to the Management Board of NCCA.

34. I wrote on their work for my entry examination to medical school – in which I revealed how the same results for ESP could be demonstrated by magicians. Now, including myself.

35. Glass GV 1976. *Primary, secondary, and meta-analysis of research.* Educational Researcher, 5.

36. www.cochrane.org.

37. Dr Prathap Tharyan, Director of South African Cochrane Centre and Network.

38. Sir Michael Rawlins (no relation). *On the evidence for decisions about the use of therapeutic interventions.* The Harveian Oration ; The Royal College of Physicians of London, 16 October 2008.

39. Leading article. *The Flight from Science.* BMJ 1980; Jan 5th p.1. 280:12.

40. Smith T. *Alternative Medicine.* BMJ 1983;286.

41. www.nhshistory.net/chapter_4.htm.

42. Report of the Board of Science. BMA, London: 1986.

43. Guyatt G, Cairns J, Churchill D et al. *Evidence Based Medicine. A new approach to teaching the practice of medicine.* JAMA 1992; 268.

44. Sackett DL, Strauss SE, Richardson WS, Rosenberg W, Haynes RB. *Evidence-based medicine: how to practice and teach EBM,* 2nd ed. Edinburgh and New York: Churchill

Livingstone, 2000.

45. Fitzpatrick M. *The Tyranny of Health: Doctors and the Regulation of Lifestyle*. Routledge. 2000.

46. Simon Singh and Edzard Ernst. *Trick or Treatment?* Bantam Press. London. 2008.

47. Bruce Charlton, Andrew Miles. *The rise and fall of EBM*. Q. J. Med. 1998; 91.

48. Julian Hughes, Claire Bamford, Carl May. *Types of centeredness in health care*. Medicine, Health Care and Philosophy (2008) Vol 11, 4.

49. Andrew Miles, Juan Mezzich. *The care of the patient and the soul of the clinic: Person-centred medicine as an emergent model of modern clinical practice*. International Journal of Person Centred Medicine, Vol. 1, No. 2. (2011).

Part Two:
Principles and Practice of Camistry

Chapter 9

Tripe, Piffle, Poppycock and Balderdash - Codswallop, Twaddle and Tosh.
Alternatives to modern evidence-based scientific medicine: Supplements, Complementary, Alternative and Integrated Medicine.

There is nothing, no matter where you read it or who says it, unless it agrees with your own reason and common sense.
Gautama Budda, 5th century BC

Of late years a class of practitioners has arisen, which, in so far as it is constituted of persons 'duly qualified' may be designated sectarian; nevertheless, it is made up for the most part of charlatans. It comprises those who, whether duly qualified or not, practise medicine upon the basis of some exclusive dogma or principle, or with reference to some exclusive remedial agent. Legitimate medicine is catholic and eclectic; it has neither exclusive dogmas nor creeds; it requires its members to seek knowledge from every available source, and apply it in every available mode as may be demanded by the circumstances of the practitioner or the patient; the object of the exercise of the art being the relief or cure of the patient as promptly, safely, and pleasantly as possible, without any formal restriction as to the means or mode.
Dan King, 1858[1]

CAM is a political/ideological entity, not a scientific one. It is an artificial category created for the purpose of promoting a diverse set of dubious, untested or fraudulent health practices.
Steve Novella[2]

Reasoning will never make a Man correct an ill Opinion, which by Reasoning he never acquired.
Jonathan Swift[3]

No rational argument will have a rational effect on a man who does not want to adopt a rational attitude.
Sir Karl Popper

Still a man hears what he wants to hear
And disregards the rest.
Paul Simon, *The Boxer*

Science: 'The intellectual and practical activity encompassing the systematic study of the structure and behaviour of the physical and natural world through observation and experiment.' (Oxford English Dictionary. Latin: *scientia*, knowledge; from proto-Indo European, *skei*, 'to cut up'). That is, 'science' is what we know by distinguishing one thing from another – one of the earliest tasks of a human baby.

The earliest physicians, magicians, priests and philosophers did their best to care for their patients – with limited knowledge, intuition and powerful imaginations. The ancient Greeks slowly introduced more rational approaches, questioning authority and encouraging closer attention to experimentation and observation.

In his seminal work *The Structure of Scientific Revolutions* (1962), Thomas Kuhn suggested that scientific advances are not gradual and incremental but rather that the established order continues until a revolution in thought occurs. Kuhn describes how he was confronted with 'unanticipated problems about the differences between natural scientists and social scientists. Attempting to discover the source of that difference led me to recognise the role in scientific research of what I have since called "paradigms". These I take to be universally recognised scientific achievements that for a time provide model problems and solutions to a community of practitioners.' (*paradiegma*, pattern, example).

Scientists may initially show disdain about a new theory and regard any new findings as mere anomalies, but if they can be shown to be plausible and the results are reproducible by other scientists, doubts will be set aside and the new theory accepted. Nowadays paradigms are being shifted all over the place, as new insights are shared amongst a culture, society, or group of scientists and knowledge moves to a new and different level. Kuhn again: 'Scientific development is a succession of tradition-bound periods punctuated by non-cumulative breaks.' [4]

During the nineteenth century healthcare became better organised, established scientific authority and instituted regulations for practice. Nevertheless, most patients still had to rely on home remedies and patent remedies comprising unknown ingredients, often toxic – all heavily promoted by exaggerated advertisements. Qualified doctors were an expensive luxury. Their education was poor and the 'heroic' traditions of purging, bloodletting and polypharmacy were often worse than treatments offered by itinerant quacks. Most 'medicine' was designed to suppress symptoms – cures had to be left to nature.

Today all countries of the world have medical and healthcare systems with doctors regulated by one authority or another. Medicine practised by such practitioners is now regarded as conventional, orthodox and mainstream – other systems have to be regarded as unorthodox and as alternatives to evidence-based scientific medicine. All modern medicine is evidence based. Who would wish otherwise? Some people prefer the alternatives as being more aligned with their own values, beliefs and philosophical inclinations. That is, their faith.

Camistry, the practice of healthcare interventions for which there is no plausible evidence of effect beyond the placebo, is seen in a multitude of guises, some of which are considered in this section on *Principles and Practice of Camistry. Placedo* is coined in order to reflect interests in the esoteric. Derived from *placere* – the Latin for 'to please' and *dō*, Japanese: 'the way'. *Placedo,* practised by *placebists,* considers the 'way' or path to better understanding of placebo effects. This approach may be appealing to many sensitivities.

Supplements

'Supplements' are widespread in the fields of CAM practices and commercial interests are expanding rapidly with significant profits to be made. (Latin: *supplere,* supply; *supplementum,* something added to supply a deficiency). In 2012 the UK supplement industry was valued at £385M. For that reason any reporter or commentator hinting that a 'supplement' may have little or no value runs the serious risk of a legal challenge. Placebists who wish to avoid litigation have to be very circumspect in how they comment on the issue of dietary supplements.

Dietary supplements are described by their promoters as providing nutrients, vitamins, minerals and other chemicals which may be missing from the patient's regular diet, or not be absorbed properly. If so, we would be dealing with a disease and an orthodox practitioner's assistance should be sought. Conventional practitioners certainly prescribe supplements when it is clear patients are deficient of vital chemicals. Decisions are rarely a matter of black and white – grey shading allows manufacturers to produce a wide variety of 'supplements', not all of which would be prescribed by orthodox practitioners. The terms 'food supplement' or 'nutritional supplement' are synonyms. *Nutraceutical* is a term more recently introduced to promote marketing and sales of unregulated drugs and supplements by hinting they are pharmaceuticals. The term has no legal meaning in the US or UK.

In spite of there being international regulations covering codes of practice, healthcare is a market all too easy for quacks and charlatans to enter. In the United States, the Dietary Supplement Health and Education Act 1994 stated that 'dietary supplements' may contain vitamins, minerals, herbs, and amino acids, and preparations of these chemicals. The US Food and Drug Administration categorises dietary supplements as foods, not as drugs. If a manufacturer wishes to sell a product as a pharmaceutical they have to achieve the high standard of FDA approval. Unlike dietary supplements, pharmaceuticals have to demonstrate their efficacy as well as safety. It is unlawful to market a supplement as a treatment to cure a specific disease or condition and packaging must identify the contents as being a dietary supplement.

Scientific evidence to demonstrate effectiveness is sparse. Marketing abounds with contingent phrases such as '…may be of benefit …' and '…can be used …' Of course they may be, of course they can be. But the evidence of actual effect on illness is substantially lacking. Marketing of supplements is nothing if not imaginative and borders on the realms of science fiction. At times authorities have to consider mis-selling and fraud.

The world of science fiction has long overlapped with quackery and orthodox medicine. As a distinct genre of literature, science fiction is of relative recent origin. In 1871 Edward Bulwer-Lytton, an enthusiast for homeopathy and water cures, wrote *Vril, The Power of The Coming Race* with the now classic opening sentence: 'It was a dark and stormy night ...' He described how a powerful all-permeating energy fluid, 'Vril' conferred the powers of healing and of telekinesis by the Vril-ya people, who lived in subterranean passages.

The story was all fiction but included much apparently genuine science, and some people came to believe that Vril probably was a real magical force but that a conspiracy of *Illuminati* kept this knowledge hidden and occult. This seems to have been the view of Madam Helena Blavatsky, who developed a career as an occultist and spiritualist medium. In 1875 she founded the Theosophical Society in order to integrate spiritualism and science.

Theosophy influenced the Vril Society, also known as the Luminous Lodge, which some claim was founded to study Rosicrucianism, the Illuminati and elements of Hindu mysticism. These occult orders taught psychological techniques to enable a race to be developed superior to any other on earth. The Vril Society seems to have had members in common with the Thule Society, which was a study group for inquiries into Germanic antiquity – Thule being lands of the farthest north. In the 1920s these Societies were the first European groups to use the swastika as a symbol linking Western with Eastern occult practices. The swastika had originated as sacred symbol in the early religions of the civilisation in the Indus Valley and the design has appeared in many civilisations down the centuries. It was claimed some members of the Nazi party joined the Vril and Thule Societies.

Edward Bulwer-Lytton himself was content to have his work regarded as fiction. But imagine how things might have been if he had claimed his work was the result of 'divine revelation' – if he had created a commercial healthcare business or College of Vrilism. If such an initiative ran into problems with government authorities, the Church of Vrilism could be founded, with practitioners acting pastorally and tending to their flock. Quite how its practitioners could be distinguished from quacks seeking to defraud patients is hard to imagine.

The European Union's Food Supplements Directive 2002 set standards of safety and purity. The products can be labelled with health and nutrition claims, but not as cures for specific diseases. The European Court says its standards are necessary and appropriate to protect the public interest. Since 2008 all manufacturers of products making health claims have had to submit evidence to the European Food Safety Authority (EFSA). Of more than 44,000 claims submitted, only 248 have been authorised. For example, EFSA has rejected claims that glucosamine and chondroitin 'help support healthy joints', a position endorsed by the US National Institutes of Health in 2014.[5]

In 2012 the *Chicago Tribune* reported: 'Federal inspections of companies that make dietary supplements – from multivitamins and calcium chews to capsules of Echinacea and bodybuilding powders – reveal serious and widespread manufacturing problems in a $28 billion industry that sells products consumed by half of all Americans. In the last four years, the US Food and Drug Administration has found violations of manufacturing rules in half of the nearly 450 dietary supplement firms it has inspected, according to agency officials. "It's downright scary" said Daniel Fabricant, head of the FDA's Division of Dietary Supplement Programs. "At least half of the industry is falling on its face".' [6]

A significant business sector has grown up to provide 'supplements' and sell a wide variety of remedies and chemicals. These do not meet the necessarily high standards for regulation as medicines and cannot legally be sold as such, but imaginative marketing men and women have come up with a wide variety of descriptors to get around this inconvenient obstruction to the commercial success of 'Big Charma' (Complementary Health and Remedy Manufacturers). Supplements are real chemicals, and they have real type II physiological effects. They are not simply placebos, though if sold or prescribed as part of a constructive therapeutic regime, type I placebo effects are also seen.

For treating influenza, Cochrane Collaboration reviews have concluded that Echinacea, zinc, steam inhalation, vitamin C, garlic, antihistamines, Chinese medicinal herbs, intranasal corticosteroids, intranasal ipratroprium, Pelargonium herbal extract, saline nasal irrigation, increasing fluid intake, and anti-virals are all ineffective, have questionable benefit, or are associated with significant adverse effects.' [7, 8]

The Consumer Association's wants to see 'All supplement manufacturers comply with the EU Register of Health and Nutrition Claims…and all confusing and exaggerated claims removed from packaging.' Although this chapter has considered Big Charma, the conventional pharmaceutical industry is not without its critics – read Dr Ben Goldacre's *Bad Pharma* and be prepared to be amazed.

Organic

Real Secrets of Alternative Medicine principally considers issues of health and well being but an associated matter is our food and sustenance. Here we have to consider the evidence for 'organic' products in much the same way as those for 'health and wellbeing' and 'supplements'. There is the same potential for us to be fooled and misled by marketing.

A Stanford University study of four decades of research has found no evidence that meat, fruits and vegetables labelled as organic contain more nutrients and have a lower risk of contamination with *E. coli* or other harmful bacteria than regular food. [9]

Critics have been concerned that the term 'organic' is a marketing ploy, designed to gull people into paying more for food and sustenance than necessary. It is ironic that more time and effort has been devoted to defining just what constitutes 'organic' than to demonstrate that there are advantages to consuming the products of this chimera. As always, *caveat emptor.*

Condimentary, Complementary, Integrated and Syncretic Medicine

The placebist wishing to assist camees make wise healthcare choices can but encourage a conscientious and comprehensive review via the Internet before any purchase. Bear in mind that as conventional, orthodox and mainstream medicine continued to develop on the basis of scientific evidence-based precepts, so systems of medicine which did not subscribe to scientific principles became described as 'alternative'. Most have developed as autonomous healthcare systems with idiosyncratic methods of diagnosis and treatment.[10]

Not unsurprisingly, non-medical practitioners of camistry wish to have the professional status of conventional orthodox healthcare practitioners. Those who do not believe in CAMs, but practice them nonetheless, are of course quacks and charlatans. Rather than set out their stall transparently as 'alternative', many camists prefer to describe themselves and their practices as 'complementary'. Use of this term is intended to imply the systems can be used alongside, in conjunction with and offer 'completion' to regular orthodox medicine. That is what 'complementary' means. Such distinction is spurious and misleading. If a particular practice works, orthodox health care practitioners will use it. It will be subject to scientific critique and will change as indicated. It is arrogant to suggest modern medicine needs the addition of 'complements' to its therapeutic regimes. If there is no plausible evidence of effect on a pathological disease or physiological system, a therapy should be regarded as being either worthless, or as an 'alternative' system based on faith.

Complements have to work and have clearly demonstrated effects beyond placebo effects, or the term is meaningless. It is best to regard these alternative systems of medicine as *condimentary*. A condiment imparts flavour, adds to the pleasure of food, is nice to have, will be appreciated and patients report 'benefit' (Latin: *condimentum,* spice, seasoning, sauce). Condimentary medicine and therapies may get the philosophical, metaphysical, emotional and spiritual juices flowing but have no significant effects on the underlying pathological processes.

Condimentary medicine captures the principles of balance and harmony in all things. Galen's medical system of the four humours provided a basis for personalities. Avicenna referred to this balancing of humours as *Quwwat-e-Mudabbira* – the 'healing power of nature' or 'vital force'. He taught that the 'humours' were derived from the diet and that they could be brought into balance by adding a dash of an appropriate condiment to food – mustard, peppers, salt, sugar etc. Tom Nealon has suggested that a sanguine person wishing to be more phlegmatic might like to try hot pequin chilli sauce. He suggests the naga jolokia pepper is dangerous because it acts on opposite humours simultaneously. At four hundred times hotter than Tabasco, Nealon claims Robert Oppenheimer described it as 'a destroyer of worlds' when 'he put too much on his *huevos rancheros* one quiet morning in Los Alamos'. [11]

Following trends in America, many camists are now referring to CAM systems as 'functional', perhaps to disguise the lack of science behind such practices. Another term which has come to particular prominence is 'integrated medicine' ('integrative' in the US). The US Institute of Medicine uses the term to indicate 'integration of physical, psychological, social, and preventive factors which are known to be effective for the achievement of optimal health'. Note the phrase 'known to be effective'. CAM proponents, including those associated with the UK's new 'College of Medicine' use the term, confusingly, to suggest that alternative medical systems (which have no known plausible effects on specific diseases) should be more closely integrated with conventional orthodox medicine and health care systems. This newcomer to the field of alternative medicine should not to be confused with the four hundred year old UK Colleges of Physicians. The motives of its enthusiasts may be altruistic and they may have a genuine belief that modern scientific medicine should be conducted in close association with pseudo-scientific systems. Perhaps they simply enjoy the company of 'like-minded souls'. Possibly their motives are more prosaic and commercial, naming their college to enhance marketing and mislead patients by presenting an acceptable face of the otherwise unacceptable. Many conventional medical and healthcare students want courses on CAM, perhaps hoping to enlarge their subsequent practice by diversification. Many medical schools are happy to provide such courses – for a fee.

'Twas ever thus. Traditional Western Medicine itself arose out of commercial schools which provided their proprietors and staff with a living. But at issue here is the basis on which modern medicine and healthcare is taught and practiced – intellectual honesty and probity. CAMs are not rational evidence-based systems and suggestions for 'integrated' medicine are nothing more than a marketing ploy – a 'bait and switch' operation in which a customer is lured into a purchase on the basis of a promise of one thing, only to find another is delivered – a standard operating procedure amongst confidence tricksters. [12]

It is essential that the terms 'integrated' or 'integrative' are clearly defined. Their use when referring to integration of CAM with COM must be distinguished from the term when used to describe the integration of conventional practices – and of health care with social care. There is a real difference, but unless the usage is made clear, those promoting the integration of CAM with COM may mislead patients as to their exact intentions. In the sixteenth century, Francis Bacon warned that using the same word in different ways led to deception by 'false idols'.

The US National Center for Complementary and Alternative Medicine (NCCAM) started as the Office of Unconventional Medicine in 1991 with $2M of discretionary US Government funding. Its current budget is about $125M a year with about thirty per cent of the total research budget focussed on pain management.[13] Its Director,

Dr Josephine Briggs, started a blog in 2012 and in the first she set out the Center's objectives: 'to bring rigorous science to the broad array of health practices that have arisen from outside of mainstream medicine'. A hard task, as most of the modalities studied are highly implausible and would break well established laws of physics if proven to be effective. Dr Briggs' second post considered: *'Integrative – What is in a Word?'* She suggests that 'from one end, "integrative medicine" offers a holistic, gentle, patient-centered approach that will solve many of our Nation's most pressing health care problems. At the other end, "integrated care" represents an invasive rebranding of modern equivalents of "snake oil" by practitioners who raise unrealistic hopes and promote approaches that are not sensible, supported by evidence, or proven safe'. Nevertheless, in 2015 the Center changed its name to National Center for Complementary and Integrative Health, moving further down the path of denial and obscuring its real objectives – which now seem to be the encouragement of the insurgency of irrational ideas into conventional medicine. Does this represent a failure to face reality? Denial? An attempt to deceive and mislead the public? You must be the judge.

It is worth heeding infectious disease specialist Mark Crislip's insight: 'If you integrate fantasy with reality, you do not instantiate reality. If you mix cow pie with apple pie, it does not make the cow pie taste better; it makes the apple pie worse.'[14] In other words – if you integrate pseudo-science with science it does not make science more rigorous and does not make sense of non-sense.

CAMs cannot be 'integrated' without undermining and adulterating the basic tenets of conventional practice. Patients want more personal attention and practitioners who want to oblige may find the concept of *wudo* engages their sensibilities and provides opportunities for promoting the 'way of *wu*' as being 'integrative' (Chinese: *wú*, nothing, nothingness and also 'spirit medium; shaman; magician; witch doctor'; Japanese: *dō*, way or path). Aristotle is cited as one of the first 'holistic' physicians who believed in the oneness of mind, spirit and body. Irrespective of philosophical perspectives, much is made of camistry being 'cost effective' though that depends on a CAM having a demonstrable effect on disease processes, not just on patients' emotional and psychological responses to disease.

Enthusiasts for 'Integrative Medicine' present a false dichotomy claiming that 'health and healing involves more than pills and surgery' and that conventional medicine cannot adequately heal many chronic conditions. Quite so, but that is no reason to use implausible non-evidenced based faiths. Rather, modern medicine must improve, and that does not mean by incorporating 'traditional' or outmoded treatments such as 'energy medicine'. The popularity of public faith in a treatment is no indicator of its scientific value – *argumentum ad populum* (appeal to the people) is a fallacious argument. Camistry is an expensive way of assuaging anxieties. There will be a crisis in medicine if CAM is confused with COM medicine. The failure of some enthusiasts to distinguish between style and substance, practice and practitioner, therapy and therapist, weakens the valuable effects their efforts might otherwise promote.

Meanwhile the health think tanks, the King's Fund and the Nuffield Trust, reported to the Department of Health and the NHS Future Forum on *Integrated care for patients and populations: Improving outcomes by working together*.[15] As the authors point out: 'The ageing population and increased prevalence of chronic diseases require a strong re-orientation away from the current emphasis on acute care towards prevention, self-care and care that is well coordinated and integrated.... Integrated care means different things to different people... To understand whether integrated care has been successful, it is first necessary to define the goals of integrated care and to ensure that these are what patients, service users and their carers actually want'. Nigel Hawkes writing in the BMJ commented: 'while the report says that measuring the experiences of patients should be given 'urgent priority', it has few suggestions about how to do this'.[16] Nowhere in the twenty page report is there any suggestion of integrating CAM with COM. The terms 'complementary and alternative' do not appear.

Some otherwise orthodox doctors claim there is benefit to be had in 'the science of integrative oncology'. By which they mean camist practices such as homeopathy, acupuncture, herbalism, chiropractic, reiki and other energy systems are integrated with orthodox treatments for cancer. The attention of an empathic practitioner, compassion, dietary and lifestyle advice undoubtedly has benefit on the 'body, mind and spirit' and should be provided by orthodox practitioners, but the issue as to whether the camist practices themselves have any effect on pathology is often conveniently overlooked. Conflation of good comprehensive orthodox care with camist techniques packaged as 'integrative oncology' is unnecessary. Camistry cannot be integrated with orthodox systems any more than one religion can be integrated with another. Orthodox medicine and camistry can work together in a general sense – and should do so if it can be shown that patients benefit. That is collaboration and cooperation, not integration. It may be that the attempts of camists to 'integrate' – without going to the trouble of meeting the standards of orthodox professional training, qualification and practice prevents a more honest, open and constructive atmosphere of cooperation. The reader must be the judge.

Conventionally qualified camists must look to their own consciences and explain how they may be distinguished from quacks who seek to defraud. Anyone with the responsibility for, or who wishes to influence the use of the public's health care resources, has to make serious decisions as to whether any care offered on the basis of belief, and with little or no evidence of efficacy, should be funded from the public purse or not.

Health insurers will have to consider whether they should use their clients' premium contributions to fund therapies that have no plausible evidence of efficacy. Clients could then have a choice of policies with or without access to camistry, and with different premiums. A number of companies are now more closely defining the care for which they will or will not reimburse their clients – BUPA has recently said it will no longer reimburse for homeopathy. The fact that policies are available to cover CAM should not be seen as endorsement of camistry or as evidence that CAMs are efficacious. Patient choice is paramount, and must be fully informed. A critical issue is the failure of companies to adequately explain their policies and criteria to their clients. As ever, patients must be the judge. Retreats and spas where a calm, attentive and empathic ambience prevails can relieve stress and increase feelings of wellbeing. Such resorts and facilities, providing a variety of 'holistic therapies' based on 'traditional medicine', manipulation, homeopathy and herbs, do result in patient benefit from type I placebo effects, but we come back to the central issue – type II effects on specific disease processes are not affected, effectively.[17] Claims to harmonise *yin* and *yang*, enhance *aura*, realign *chakras* and rebalance *doshas* cannot be substantiated. Insurance premiums should reflect this.

Inevitably, camists and those who support CAM seek greater approbation, validation and wider acceptance – hence attempts to 'integrate' CAM with COM medicine. The Prince of Wales created his Foundation for Integrated Health in 1993, secured £900,000 funding from the Department of Health in 2005 but saw it enter administration in 2011. Its key directors and supporters then founded the 'College of Medicine' – which has been described a College of Quackery because so many of its initial Council were associated with pseudo-scientific CAMs.[18] Prince Charles has long had faith in unconventional therapies, telling the BMA in 1982:

> Perhaps we just have to accept it is God's will that the unorthodox individual is doomed to years of frustration, ridicule and failure in order to act out his role in the scheme of things, until his day arrives and mankind is ready to receive his message; a message which he probably finds hard to explain himself, but which he knows comes from a far deeper source than conscious thought.

HRH continues to endorse 'integrated medicine' as explained on his web site: 'The Prince is a keen advocate of integrated healthcare. This means taking a wider, preventative approach to healthcare by addressing the underlying social, lifestyle and environmental causes of disease.' Good – we would all support that. That is how the government, NHS and medical organisations use the term 'integrated', but he goes on: 'In this system of integrated medicine patients, protected by a sound regulatory environment and the support of the National Health Service, have access not just to conventional medical treatment but to proven complementary care and therapy.'[19] The Prince has repeated his call for camistry in the Journal of the Royal Society of Medicine.

The Prince is using the term 'integrated' to imply that un-scientific 'complementary' care should be integrated and syncretised with modern medical and NHS healthcare practice. This creates a problem – heading back to the days of superstition. At least he appears only to support 'proven complementary care' and by definition 'complementary medicine' is not proven. If it was it would be 'conventional medicine'. The Prince is not prepared to share any evidence he has that homeopathic remedies have any effect at all and that consultations with a homeopath provide anything other than type I placebo effects on feelings and emotions.[20]

CAMs are not simply expressions of care, compassion and a holistic approach to healing. They express different beliefs about disease, health and wellbeing and are faith based belief systems. CAMs may be mutually contradictory, yet a number of camists will claim they are trained, qualified, and practice a variety of techniques based on these varied beliefs. Being 'trained, qualified and regulated' is meaningless if there is no substance to the practice. Indeed, patients and the public may be misled as to the value of the practice if they ape the orthodox. Is this the intention? You must be the judge.

Syncretism (syn; together with) derives from first century Cretans who, when facing a mutual enemy, set aside the antipathy between their different federations and integrated their forces. The term can be applied to the combination of any different beliefs or schools of thought, even if contradictory. Mostly used in relation to religions, syncretism has also been used in politics, psychology, mathematics and the arts (where the term 'eclecticism' is usually applied).

Syncretism may be a constructive concept for philosophies and religions, but in the realm of science, seeking to infiltrate non- or pseudo- scientific precepts with those established by the scientific method is clearly harmful to both. The non-scientific may become impotent and whither. The scientific may be adulterated and diluted. Syncretism is doomed to fail, as it cannot deliver what the majority of patients want – to get as close to their idea of truth as possible. Honesty should prevail. Anyone who wants alternatives to conventional medicine should be able to have them, but in an open and transparent therapeutic *milieu* and with a good understanding of their non-scientific alternative nature. They may of course also choose conventional medicine. Their choice.

In 2010 Professor of Education John C. McLaughlin claimed to have discovered 'a new version of reflexology, which identifies a homunculus represented in the human body, over the area of the buttocks…as with reflexology the map responds to needling as in acupuncture and gentle suction such as cupping…' McLaughlin was invited to present his findings at an international conference. He then admitted his paper had been a hoax and expressed concern that the term 'integrated medicine' is being used to smuggle alternative practices into rational medicine by way of lowered standards of critical thinking. [21]

The principal challenge for those who wish to integrate or syncretise their alternative systems with orthodox systems is to answer – just how do they ensure proponents are not hoaxers, quacks or fraudsters?

Contemporary CAM in context

In 2000, the House of Lords Select Committee on Science and Technology identified three main systems of complementary and alternative medicine.[22] Guides provided by the Prince's Foundation for Integrated Health and the British Complementary Medicine Association, identify many more. All provide the patient with alternative systems of medicine to that established as conventional, orthodox, mainstream medicine by credible, plausible, reproducible and evolving scientific principles. The websites of these various alternatives are worthy of review and further study, and the next chapter sets out brief accounts of some of the better known.

A review of homeopathy serves as a good paradigm of how alternative systems of medicine have moved away from convention and orthodoxy, and developed as distinct and alternative systems. Bear in mind that conventional medicine itself has always changed in the light of further and better information – eventually.

All policies in respect of homeopathy, whether established by medical authorities such as the BMA or Government itself, need to take account not only of current practice but also of the context from which the system of 'homoeopathic medicine' emerged. Homeopathy is a distinct philosophy – placing faith in the system of medicine founded on the work and principles established in Germany by Samuel Hahnemann (1755-1843). Trained in the conventions of his time, for good reasons Hahnemann took issue with much of the orthodox medicine of his day and abandoned conventional medicine. Currently, the fundamental belief of homeopaths is in a different, antithetical system of science and results in homeopathy remaining a practice that cannot be integrated with conventional systems. It is an alternative system and, by its own definition, a faith.

Some patients want the choice of an alternative system. Taxpayers may also wish to exercise their choice – and may choose not to fund time spent with practitioners of alternative medicine, condimentary medicine or pseudo-scientific medicine. They may choose not to fund expenditure on unproven remedies. Patients should not be denied their choice of an alternative health system by attempts to integrate the alternative with the orthodox. Hahnemann's work to improve the lot of his patients and avoid the side effects of the conventional remedies of his time should be applauded.

Driven by the application of the scientific method with regular critique, the application of statistics and other methods for evidence based health care which openly acknowledges when treatments or medicines have been found wanting – conventional orthodox mainstream medicine is constantly changing and developing. The General Medical Council expects today's registered doctors to act with integrity and 'provide effective treatments based on the best available evidence.' CAM has not made comparable progress with their own ethics and practice.

To place homeopathy and other CAM in context, the European conventional, orthodox, mainstream medical profession of the mid eighteenth century needs consideration. Doctors did not then appreciate that illnesses were caused by specific diseases, which in turn might be due to microorganisms, by cancers or by deterioration of individual tissues and organs. Most of the signs and symptoms which are now grouped together and called a syndrome or specific disorder, had not then been identified. In the eighteenth century there was no universal consensus as to how care might be accomplished and many systems were proposed. Today there remains controversy about details, but the fundamental approach of a scientific, rational, evidence based underpinning of conventional orthodox medical practice is internationally accepted as providing the greatest probability of achieving desired outcomes. Conventional medicine is also required to be holistic and take into account environmental, emotional and spiritual aspects of health. Some enthusiasts for camistry imply that 'holism' is ignored by conventional medicine. That is a false dichotomy, and those who promote such an idea are ignorant or mischievous.

From time immemorial, different countries, cultures and communities have developed different traditional medical systems. These were intimately bound with the philosophy, theology, cosmology, astrology, alchemy, thaumaturgy, metaphysics, ethics, psychology and politics of the time and culture. Some took a deep hold and have lasted millennia. Others faded after a brief enthusiasm. The principle on which Hahnemann founded his particular system – *similia similibus curentur,* 'let likes be cured by likes', appeared in ancient Chinese and Indian medical writings of four thousand years ago. Further development followed with Hippocrates (460-377 BC) who held there were two ways of curing – by the 'similars' and by the 'contraries'. Aulus Celsus (1st century AD) and Galen of Pergamum (129-199 AD) recommended use of 'contraries'.

In the Middle Ages the second Hippocratic principle, that 'opposites cure opposites' by achieving balance and harmony, was known as 'The Law of Hippocrates'. Systems using 'similars' were developed further by those attracted to vitalism, including the philosopher St Thomas Aquinas and the alchemist, astrologer and physician Phillipus von Hohenheim who styled himself 'Paracelcus'.

Vitalism holds that the functions of a living organism are due to a vital spirit, spark or energy, equated by some as the 'soul' – as distinct from mere physicochemical reactions. Paracelsus also opined that 'resolute imagination is the beginning of all magical operations.' In Scotland, Dr John Brown (1735-1788) based his medical systems on the idea. As a student in Edinburgh, Brown had studied under the eminent Dr William Cullen whose teaching was still largely based on the Hippocratic 'four humours'. Brown was tutor to Cullen's children, but after being stricken with gout, began doubting Cullen's medical system. Brown's degree was initially refused. He continued attacking Cullen's theories and in 1786 moved to develop a practice in London, dying penniless two years later. Nevertheless, the Brownian medical system became particularly popular in German speaking Europe. In 1802 cavalry were needed to stop a riot between Brownian and non-Brownian medical students at the University of Göttingen.

John Brown, Dr Erasmus Darwin (Charles' grandfather) and other contemporary men of science were attempting to unify grand scale concepts within a specific 'medical system'. Brown's fundamental principle was that of 'excitability' – a basic quality in living matter – a capacity to perceive and be able to respond to outside events. Brown's system enabled a doctor to restore imbalances and maintain balance between outside stimulation and inherent excitability. These ancient ideas are seen even today in 'energy medicine' systems.

German philosopher Immanuel Kant argued In *The Critique of Pure Reason* (1781) that using reason without experience of observation and experimentation leads to illusions. This philosophy came to be known as Transcendental Idealism and was developed by Fichte, Schelling, Hegel and others. At that time orthodox medicine lacked the systematic structure set out by other sciences and a number of different and competing 'medical systems' developed. Philosopher F.W.J. Schelling studied Brown and described 'nature' as being an organic whole. Some physicians found this approach appealing as they felt healing was impossible without the body, mind and soul being in harmony. Schelling's works set out how matter is infinitely divisible and all nature's forces are interrelated, 'The whole is larger than the sum of its parts.' Not so far from today's Gaia hypothesis.

Schelling sought to establish a new intimate, mystical relationship between man and nature. His approach became part of the development of the philosophical tradition of German Idealism. Schelling encouraged natural philosophers to move from their empirical results and to consider the larger meaning of natural science. He expanded his ideas in lectures on *Naturphilosophie* in 1804. This was a semi–mystical view of science and the world – the nature of truth is to be discovered by thought and intuition. Such considerations underlie much of Goethe's philosophy. In time, many found these ideas too speculative and as modern scientific methods developed, so interest in Schelling's writings waned.

Slowly, stimulated by the scientific principles introduced by the Enlightenment, orthodox medicine developed, statistical analysis exposed fault lines, and personalities and politics came to play a part in more scientific, rational and ultimately generally acceptable and improved medical and healthcare practices. A brief review of yellow fever serves as an example:

Yellow fever is caused by a small strand of RNA virus which only lives in primates (including humans) and mosquitoes which carry it from animal to animal. It seems to have spread from Africa during the sixteenth century, and by the 19th was regarded as one of the most dangerous of the infectious diseases. Most people recover but 15% go on to suffer from recurring fever with liver damage causing jaundice and gastrointestinal tract damage causing 'black vomit'. One in five of this group die. Those who survive have lifelong immunity – which is achieved nowadays by vaccination.

A yellow fever epidemic affected Philadelphia in 1793. Doctors could do little. Not even Dr Benjamin Rush who, with the support of Benjamin Franklin, trained in medicine in Edinburgh before returning to Philadelphia and developing a reputation as an eminent physician. In Edinburgh he had studied the work of John Brown and took forward the idea of 'excitability' to his own later contributions in psychiatry.

During the yellow fever epidemic Rush saw more than a hundred patients every day and based much of his treatment on significant bloodletting coupled with purgatives of mercury – a practice styled as 'depletion theory'. Bloodletting and purging with mercury had been recognised as basis of much medical practice from antiquity.

Rush had a very dominant personality and may have been a manic-depressive. Henry Knox, Secretary of War, noted 'Rush bears down all before him.' Rush is credited as being the founder of American psychiatry. Political activist Alexander Hamilton studied the death rates and found that patients treated by Rush with his depletion methods did worse than those cared for more modestly. Hamilton, born British in the Caribbean, was the first United States Secretary of the Treasury, and was aide-de-camp to George Washington during the Revolutionary War. Hamilton's criticism was shared by others. Rush seems to have overestimated the amount of blood in the circulation by 100% which may account for his belief in 'heroic therapeutics' and that the removal of 300mls of blood four times in a day would be beneficial. As this represents a quarter of an adult's circulating blood volume, death through loss of blood would not have been far off.

William Cobbett, as a conscientious journalist, considered it his duty to advise the public. Having settled in Philadelphia after the Revolution, his *Porcupine's Gazette* was widely read, although Washington expressed concern at the coarseness of language and 'want of official information on many factors'. Cobbett fiercely attacked Rush's use of bloodletting, describing him as 'The Bleeding Physician of Philadelphia'. He wrote that 'Times are ominous indeed, when quack to quack cries purge and bleed.' Today, Cobbett would have his own blog.

Rush suffered a sense of humour failure, and feeling his reputation had been sullied, sued for libel – the first medical libel lawsuit in the United States. In 1797 Rush was awarded $5000, an extraordinarily high sum for those days, now worth $3M. Cobbett's use of municipal records of death rates and mortalities suggested that during the 1797 epidemic Rush had a 60% mortality rate, whereas he was claiming only 10%. Proper statistics were not more usually applied to the assessment of medical treatments until later in the nineteenth century and Rush offered no proof of his outcomes beyond saying his treatment seemed to him to 'work'. President George Washington probably died because of epiglottitis, but letting of about a third of his blood volume during his terminal illness would not have helped. On the grounds that such treatment had previously 'worked' for him, Washington himself initially demanded that his estate overseer, George Rawlins, commence the bleeding before the doctors arrived.

Much of Cobbett's attack on Rush was driven by political considerations, Rush being a Republican whilst Cobbett, Hamilton and Washington were Federalists. Rush was confident his style of practice was perfect for a new democratic form of government. Medicine should be freed from the tyranny of the over-learned and simplified so that the principles and treatments could be taught to almost everyone. He felt a healthy public would be politically and socially healthy and that 'the point of medicine, like Christianity itself, was to overcome nature by means of Christ's redemptive gift and restoration of man to his original, perfect state.'

Training in alternative medical systems

One of the most attractive features of CAM is the very fact that it is 'alternative' and satisfies alternative ways of thinking. Most practitioners have received some form of training in their chosen CAM modality and to that extent are 'qualified'. Those qualifications will of course not meet the standards required for registration with the orthodox healthcare professions. As time passes, camists have sought to gain greater credibility and to validate their chosen profession by improving the education of its members. But rather than require members to train and qualify as an orthodox professionals and then to develop a special interest in camistry, a number of camists have sought to develop their own degree courses *ab initio*, and to have these validated at regular universities. Inevitably there have been expressions of concern by scientists, doctors and organisations such as *Sense about Science,* that such qualifications are spurious and that to award an academic degree as a Bachelor of Science for pseudo-scientific studies is not appropriate and may be intended to be deliberately misleading. Initially, by misleading the students who undertake the courses – subsequently, misleading their patients. Integrity has left many campuses.

Dr David Colquhoun, Professor of Pharmacology at University College London, has expressed concern at the number of state-funded British universities which still have 'science' courses in complementary and alternative medicine in spite of not being evidence-based. 'It may seem harmless and even a welcome alternative to traditional perspectives. But teaching people that homeopathy is evidence-based when it is not, and encouraging students to distrust the scientific method, not only runs counter to reason, but can be dangerous. In extreme cases – such as the prescription of herbal remedies for potentially fatal diseases such as AIDS – it can kill. Steve Jobs for example might still be alive if he had not initially decided to treat his cancer by diet, rather than radiotherapy.' [23] Currently, some homeopaths claim they can cure Ebola and even AIDS.

One thing is certain – these subjects are not science. Quite why these universities offer courses in these subjects granting the degree of Bachelor of Science, unless the intention is to deliberately mislead students, is unclear. Vice-Chancellors have been asked – they have not replied.[24] Nor has there been any explanation for the present government's disinclination to refer the issue of homeopathy for assessment by the National Institute for Clinical Excellence. It is the responsibility of NICE to assess cost effectiveness of treatments offered by the NHS in England and Wales. Commissioners of healthcare need to know whether they should fund homeopathy.

In the absence of a NICE assessment, the default conclusion must be that homeopathy should not be funded by the public purse in England and Wales. In the absence of evidence to the contrary, registered medical practitioners who endorse funding for homeopathy may be considered fraudulent. They are using public funds for remedies with no evidence of effectiveness. Their consciences must be the judge.

Real Secrets offers a stimulus to more extensive study and understanding of issues surrounding camistry. Placebists do not seek to persuade camees to set aside their interest in *wudo* or any particular CAM, nor to avoid use of any remedy, treatment or procedure they wish. A conscientious placebist simply encourages study of the origins, context and developments of CAM and leaves it to the camee to ensure they understand the issues, to draw their own conclusions, make their own choices and give fully informed consent to treatment. Certain CAMs have attracted more attention than others and are used more extensively – they are considered next.

Endnotes to Chapter 9

1. Neurologist Dr Steven Novella. www.sciencebasedmedicine.org/index.php/National-health-interview-survey-2007-cam-use-by-adults.

2. Dan King. *Quackery Unmasked,* 1858. https://en.wikisource.org/wiki/Quackery_Unmasked/Chapter_XIV.

3. Swift's quote (1721) has variants such as: *'You cannot reason a man out of what he never reasoned himself into'.*

4.. Thomas Kuhn, *The Structure of Scientific Revolutions.* University of Chicago 1962, and Postscript, Second edition 1970, paragraph 7 page 208.

5. C. Kent Kwoh et al. *Effect of Oral Glucosamine on Joint Structure in Individuals With Chronic Knee Pain: A Randomized, Placebo-Controlled Clinical Trial.* Arthritis & Rheumatology. Volume 66, Issue 4, pages 930–939, April 2014. http://onlinelibrary.wiley.com/doi/10.1002/art.38314/abstract4 and *Don't believe the Hype,* Which? Consumers Association. London September 2013.

6. www.chicagotribune.com/health/ct-met-supplement-inspections-2012063.

7. Murdoch D.R. *et al. Effect of vitamin D3 supplementation on upper respiratory tract infections in healthy adults: the VIDARIS randomized controlled trial.* JAMA. 308:1333-1339, 2012. http://jama.jamanetwork.com/data/Journals/JAMA/24997/joc120088_1333_1339.pdf.

8. Linder J. *Vitamin D and the cure for the common cold.* JAMA 308:1375-1376, 2012.

9. http://www.nytimes.com/2012/09/04/science/earth/study-questions-advantages-of-organic-meat-and-produce.html?_r=1.

10. HL paper, Session 1999-2000. 12, (2000) The Stationery Office, London.

11. Tom Nealon. www.hilobrow.com/2010/10/09/de-condimentis-4.

12. David Colquhoun *BMJ* 2011;343:d4368.

13. www.NCCAMresearchblog.nih.gov.US.

14. 'Orac': www.scienceblogs.com/insolence/2012/06/20 & Mark Crislip: *Perpetual Motion* www.sciencebasedmedicine.org/index.php/perpetual-motion-more-on-the-bravewell-report. February 24th 2012.

15. The King's Fund/Nuffield Trust, London, January 2012.

16. Nigel Hawkes. BMJ 2011;343:d8344.

17. The Duchess of Cornwall is reported to have spent weeks in 2010 and 2012 at the Soukya Centre, India where Royal suites cost $1000 a night (*Daily Telegraph* 29th October 2012, p. 2). This 'Holistic Healing Centre' is owned by Dr Isaac Mathai – 'MD Homeopathy from the Hahnemann Post-graduate Institute of Homeopathy, London'. This is actually at 42-44 High Street, Slough, Berkshire, not in London. No entrance examination is required for students. Mathai now runs a chain of homeopathic clinics in Bangalore. Therapeutic programmes include those for Stress Management, Rejuvenation, Detoxification, Smoking Cessation and Anti-ageing. Conditions treated include acne, alcoholism, arthritis, anxiety, cancer, chronic fatigue syndrome, cirrhosis of the liver, osteoporosis, and sexual diseases. 'The fundamental principle underlying Holistic Treatment is that the natural defence and immune system of an individual when strengthened, has the potential to heal and prevent diseases.' At present there is no plausible evidence of the effectiveness of any of the medical systems offered in achieving those laudable objectives. Rest and relaxation is likely to be of benefit.

18. *British Medical Journal*, 16th July 2011, vol. 343 p. 110.

19. www.theprinceofwales.gov.uk. FAQs.

20. Given the Prince purports to support evidence-based medicine, I have written and asked him. His secretary advises he does not enter into debate on the subject. The BMA Representative Meeting of 2015 had a request for this information on its agenda. How can progress be made if the evidence the Prince has remains covert?

21. John C. McLaughlin, *Integrative Medicine and the point of credulity*. BMJ 341, December 2010.

22. House of Lords paper, Session 1999-2000 12,(2000). The Stationery Office, London.

23. David Colquhoun. www.telegraph.co.uk/science/science-news/9051103. Jobs had a pancreatic neuroendocrine tumour. With conventional treatment, the median survival over the past ten years for patients who develop carcinoid syndrome has improved from two years to more than eight years.

24. Nick Ross, President of HealthWatch-UK. Personal communication.

Chapter 10

Homeopathy

The one who heals is right.
Samuel Hahnemann, 1796.

Homoeopathy has proved lucrative, and so long as it continues to be so will surely exist – as surely as astrology, palmistry and other methods of getting a living out of the weakness and credulity of mankind and womankind. It always does very great harm to the community to encourage ignorance, error, or deception in a profession which deals with the life and health of our fellow creatures.
Oliver Wendell Holmes Snr, 1842[1]

Like all quackeries, homeopathy has been supported by the shallow, weak and credulous, on one side, and the charlatan and the rogue on the other. Such alliances are invariably broken when either the eyes of the one are opened, or the rapacity of the other is not gratified.
The Lancet, 1857

If it is still insisted that the number and respectability of the supporters of Homœopathy are proofs in its favor, we might urge, with much more propriety, the truth of Divination, Sorcery and Witchcraft. The believers in these delusions have been far more numerous, and their attestations far more imposing. Hahnemann and his disciples toiled and labored for twelve long years to find the common source of all the numerous streams and rivulets of human ills, and when they had arrived at the supposed goal, and gazed in delirious exultation upon the mystic fountain, the chimera vanished and left them in total darkness. All the thinking, reasoning, strong-minded, common-sense men of Great Britain, reject Homœopathy – and besides the paupers, it has little or no support except from a few of the higher classes who think it beneath them to think at all about medical systems, and who consequently know little of the merits of any, and are likely to adopt that course which promises most with the least means. Men of indifferent attainments, itching for notoriety, often became homeopathy's advocates. It makes little or no progress among men of learning and

talents – where reason and not fashion is the guiding star; but is often seen in all its mushroom glory where the vain and fickle-minded give direction to public opinion.
Dan King, 1858[2]

Dr Samuel Christian Hahnemann (1755-1843)

Hahnemann was a caring doctor who devised his own idiosyncratic system of medicine as an alternative to the poor quality of orthodox medicine of his time. Biographers suggest he was a pedantic, rude and exacting young upstart, and very unpopular with patients and colleagues alike: 'Hardly a day passed without some complaint against him. As a doctor he was intolerant in his attitude to both colleagues and patients.'

Born in Meissen, Germany, he was brought up in a lurid atmosphere filled with superstition of spirits, witches, ghosts, hobgoblins, devils and the wildest delusions. Afra Dickh had been convicted of witchcraft and hanged in Fürsteneck only fifty years earlier. Hahnemann was a serious student, becoming fluent in five languages by the age of twenty. He initially studied in Leipzig but had no funds and did what he could to make a living as a translator. For two years he worked as a librarian to the Governor of Transylvania and became a member of a Masonic lodge in Hermannstadt. At that time, much of Freemasonry was involved in studying the occult, alchemy, the medical sciences and spiritism. One of Hahnemann's biographers has commented: 'from his schooldays onwards he had followed Descartes, Spinoza and Leibnitz – and then proceeded to vitalism and to the naturalism of Schelling and Hegel. He advanced beyond this to spiritism and for a while lost his way in occultism.'[3]

Hahnemann returned to the fold and was awarded his doctorate in medicine by the University of Erlangen in 1779 but became disillusioned with the harmful effects of treatments then being used by orthodox practitioners. Hahnemann wrote: 'Precious and fragile human life, so easily destroyed, was frequently placed in jeopardy at the hands of these perverted people, especially since bleedings, emetics, purges, blistering plaster, fontanels, setons, caustics and cauterisations were also used.'[4] He was critical of polypharmacy which involved forty or more ingredients in a single prescription and was outraged when Leopold II of Austria died after four bleedings in 1792.

One of the first books Hahnemann wrote was on secrets which would prevent and cure an epidemic of scarlet fever which was killing hundreds of children in Germany. With the purchase of his book and its secret, came 'a little powder free of charge which contains enough to render several thousand people immune from scarlet fever.' It did no such thing, but as it contained minute amounts of belladonna, Hahnemann had a run in with the medical authorities.

Hahnemann next claimed to have discovered a 'new salt' which he sold at £7 per kilogram. Chemists then identified this was in fact salt of boric acid worth forty pence a kilo (today's prices). They were not amused, but Hahnemann proclaimed 'I am incapable of wilfully deceiving. I may however, like other men, be unintentionally mistaken.' Over the next fifty years Hahnemann intentionally developed his own alternative system of medicine which he called *Homœopathy*. Patients undoubtedly benefitted as Hahnemann's system avoided the heroic bloodletting, poisoning and purging of other physicians.[5]

Hahnemann's writings were influenced by German Idealism and Freiedrich Schelling's *Naturphilosophie*, reflecting Hahnemann's belief that he was 'God's chosen instrument for the healing of mankind.' Schelling had suggested 'the more unsubstantial matter becomes by dilution, the purer and more effective could be its spirit-like and dynamic functions.' The subsequent development of experimental natural science had a destructive impact on the credibility of these theories; nevertheless, when Hahnemann translated Cullen's *Materia Medica* he learned that the bark of Peruvian cinchona trees could be used to treat malaria. Samples had been brought to Europe from Peru, named after Countess Anna Chincon, and by 1656 cinchona's use in curing fever was noted in the records of a doctor in Northampton. Linnaeus named the genus *Chincona officinalis* and nearly thirty species have since been described. The active alkaloids of quinine and cinchonidine were isolated in 1818 and it is now known these kill the plasmodium parasite which causes malaria. Hahnemann experimented by taking progressively larger doses of cinchona. He found the symptoms of malaria were reproduced – cardiac irregularity, headache, red cheeks, limb weakness, with cold fingers and feet. He became ill – yet when he then diluted the doses he felt better. Hardly surprising. Further experiments followed and his definitive theoretical work *The Organon of Rational Healing,* later re-titled *The Organon of the Healing Art,* was published in 1810. The title *Organon* reflected the name given to the standard collection of Aristotle's six works on logic, and Francis Bacon's *Novum Organon* (new tool).

The principles advanced by Hahnemann were: (i) That a spiritual, non-material, vital life force imbues us all. He claimed diseases were 'solely spirit-like (dynamic) derangements of the spirit-like power (the vital principle) that animates the human body.' (ii) That most diseases are caused by morbid derangements of the vital force. 'It is only the pathologically untuned vital force (miasm) that causes diseases'. The principal miasm which caused critical infections was due to an itch which he called *psora*. In the Organon, Hahnemann advised 'This Psora is the true and fundamental cause that produces all the other countless forms of disease ...' (iii) That the choice of medicines and remedies should be chosen for the similarity of their effects on healthy subjects rather than on the symptoms of the disease. This is the *similia principle* that 'Like cures like' with the effects of medicines established by experiments or 'proving' on healthy people. Small doses of medicines should be given in single doses and not in complex mixtures which might cause 'aggravations'.

The similia principle is often referred to by homeopaths as *The Law of Similars* but is not a law in any sense known to a scientist. A scientific law is defined as an analytic statement of universal and invariable facts of the physical world and is subject to change in the light of further evidence. Down the centuries, other writers have referred to the 'similia principle' as being nothing more than superstitious 'sympathetic magic' – suggesting living things have an essence that can be transferred. There is no scientifically plausible mechanism to support the suggestion that a small dose of a substance will treat symptoms it might cause at higher doses. Vaccines are not in this category because they do contain measurable doses of dead organisms or their proteins and their mechanism of action is well-established and part of the immune response. Hahnemann's fallacy of believing that because one thing (feeling better) follows another (taking a remedy) they are causally related has dogged studies of homeopathy ever since. The logical fallacy of believing that 'after this, therefore because of this' is considered elsewhere.

Hahnemann tested potential remedies on himself and other healthy (male) associates. This method continues today, but the German word *pruefung* used by Hahnemann (meaning 'testing' or 'examination') has been translated into English as 'proving'. Both languages derive their words from the Latin *probare*, to test, but whilst in modern English usage 'probability' means 'likelihood' – 'proving' today caries a connotation of certainty which Hahnemann did not intend. The British Homeopathic Association states: 'Hahnemann deduced that an illness could be treated with a very small amount of a substance that, in larger quantities, could cause that illness. These experiments were called proving and led him to observe and describe the basic principles of homeopathic medicine.' Some may be misled into thinking there is an element of scientific truth in the procedure of 'proving' that is not merited (OED: to prove – to demonstrate the truth or existence of something by evidence). Any claims that Hahnemann 'proved' anything are deliberately misleading. The German for 'to prove' is *beweisen* and that is not the word Hahnemann used. There is no reason why homeopathic writings in English should not refer to the investigations as 'testing', 'experiments' or even 'research', as the German *pruefung* translates but invariably homeopaths use the terms 'proof', 'proving' and 'provers' with the misleading certainty that implies. Moreover, as Anthony Campbell has pointed out: 'Hahnemann's method of conducting his proving, though extremely meticulous and painstaking, did nothing to eliminate the effects of suggestion. The subjects knew what medicines they were taking and what effects they might experience.'[6]

Hahnemann fourthly asserted that the more remedies are diluted, the more effective they become – *The Law of Infinitesimals*. This was not an original conceit. Hippocrates had advised: 'A physician must use as little intervention as possible in restoring health.' In the sixteenth century an Irish alchemist Butler had ministered to James I and obtained wonderful cures of headache by a single drop of olive oil into which he had dipped a magic pebble said to have been obtained from the Philosopher's Stone. Butler's hermetic magic and 'infinite' medicine were endorsed by John Babtista van Helmont, an alchemist, physician and disciple of Paracelcus. As van Helmont's treatises were held in considerable esteem, Butler's technique of using infinitesimal doses became more widely investigated in Europe.

Following the indisputable logic that small doses of 'medicine' were more beneficial than large, Hahnemann went on to use progressively smaller doses, prepared with violent shaking by rapid strikes of the container on a leather bound Bible between each dilution. He deemed this 'succusion' was essential to his method and resulted in 'potentization' or 'dynamization'. (Latin: *succutere*, to shake). He called the ensuing remedies 'potencies'. Hahnemann claimed the more dilute the remedy, the higher the potency and the greater its effectiveness. He accepted that diluting medicines normally weakened them but held that dynamization released astonishing powers – the 'energy' which he regarded as essentially spiritual. Eventually he claimed there was no need for patients to take the medicine; it was enough if they merely smelt them. Potentized medicines were the 'vital force' in a bottle. At this time natural scientists were studying magnetism and Hahnemann hoped the vitalistic healing force he had identified would be confirmed in like manner. That has not come to pass.

Hahnemann's *Organon* contains three hundred pages but infinitesimal doses are not mentioned until page 204, and then only in notes. Nevertheless Hahnemann's followers regarded his 'discovery' as being one of the greatest in medicine. Hahnemann describes his method of preparing vegetable remedies:

> To obtain the hundredth degree of potency, mix two drops of alcohol with equal parts of the juice of the plant, and then mix this with one hundred drops of alcohol, by means of two strokes with the arm from above *downwards;* by mixing in the same way one drop of this dilution with one hundred drops of alcohol, you obtain the ten thousandth degree of potency, and by mixing a drop of this last dilution with another one hundred drops of alcohol you obtain the millionth degree. This process of spiritualisation or dynamization is continued through a series of thirty phials up to the thirtieth solution. This thirtieth degree should always be used in Homeopathic purposes. [7]

Hahnemann initially advised succusion by ten downwards strokes, but later only two 'least the remedy be made too potent'! (Organon page 316). But why thirtieth degree? Bear in mind that Hahnemann was developing his system at a time of much interest in occult practices, mystical revelations, and hermetic philosophy throughout Europe. These themes were also of interest to the Freemasons as they developed their systems for personal growth. When Hahnemann was initiated into Lodge St. Andreas, Hermannstadt in 1777 he would have noticed the motto of Freemasonry – *Aude Sapere*, taken from Horace: 'Dare to be Wise.' Hahnemann used this motto on the title page of *The Organon.* The thirtieth was the key degree to which a Freemason could be exalted; the age at which Jesus is said to have commenced his public ministry (Luke 3:23). Hmm…

The potency scales are usually presented as centesimal, with a base of 100, not as decimal, base 10 as in normal arithmetic (Latin: *centum; C,* a hundred). Hahnemann ruled the standard potency of homoeopathic medicines should be the 30th centesimal (30C), a dilution of 1 in 10^{60} – one divided by one, followed by sixty zeros: 1/1000, 000,000,000,000,000,000,000,000,000,000,000,000,000,000,000,000,000,000,000. Today, homoeopathic remedies are prepared by taking an original substance, grinding them to powder and mixing with an equal amount of distilled water or alcohol for up to six months in a process of 'trituration' (Latin: *trituare,* to grind). The result is the 'mother tincture'. One drop of this is then added to 99 drops of water or alcohol and violently shaken for a minute before being succussed by rapping against a hard surface. It is held that this succusion 'spreads the remedy's energy and vibrations throughout the preparation.'[8] This procedure is then repeated, nowadays by machinery – one unit of solution plus ninety nine of solvent – 'potentizing' the solution. As Hahnemann put it: 'potentization unlocks the natural substances. It uncovers and reveals the specific medicinal powers lying hidden in their soul.'[9]

Thirty such procedures (1 unit of 'mother tincture' of the substance plus 99 of solvent: dilution of 1 in a 100), repeated 30 times gives a 30C preparation. Cinchona, aconite, mercury, bryonia, belladonna, sulphur, Hypericum are amongst hundreds of such 'remedies'. Some homeopaths use other scales of dilution such as 1 in 50,000 (termed LM). Why they cannot simply use regular mathematical notation has not been explained and has lead to allegations they intend to mislead patients.

As for such extreme dilutions – Ben Goldacre invites us to imagine a sphere of water with a diameter of 150 million kilometres – the average distance from Earth to the Sun. An eight minute journey at the speed of light. A sphere of water of that size, with one molecule of the substance in it, would represent a 30C dilution.[10] Homeopaths not infrequently use dilutions of 200C. Wikipedia advises: 'the dilution advocated by Hahnemann for most purposes, on average, would require giving two billion doses per second to six billion people for 4 billion years to deliver a single molecule of the original material to any patient.'

A letter from one consultant physician employed by a NHS Trust who was asked to see a lady suffering from facial neuralgia states: 'I am going to start her on some homoeopathic medication, initially giving her Magnesia phosphorica 30C.' Then, two months later: 'She's had a good response and says her pain has improved by 50%. I have increased the potency *(dilution)* of her medication to Magnesia phosphorica 200C...' Six weeks after that: 'she has not made any further progress with the facial neuralgia, I think she is a little more symptomatic than she was last time. I have changed her medication today giving her Sanguinaria 30C...' Note that he says 'medication' – that is, 'medicine'.

200C is ten followed by four hundred zeros – 10^{400}. There are only about 10^{80} atoms in the observable universe, at most, 100^{100} (one googol). This consultant, employed by the NHS, was fraudulent. He claimed that he gave this patient, funded by the NHS, a preparation so dilute it could not have contained a single magnesium phosphorus molecule, even if the universe is five times the size of that we can observe.

This physician no doubt claims that the original molecule left some vague and indeterminate 'spiritual energy' behind. Even so, what he most certainly did not do is provide the patient with any medication of magnesia phosphorica as he claimed.

That is fraud – of the patient and of the NHS who paid for his ministrations. Why the government allows the NHS to conspire in such deceit is unclear. Why the GMC does not consider such doctors as being unfit to practice is likewise to be explained. In 2010 the official journal of the British Society for Rheumatology published a paper from Dr George Lewith's department at Southampton University: *'Homeopathy has clinical benefits in rheumatoid arthritis patients that are attributable to the consultation process, but not the homeopathic remedy.'* The remedies they used were made to the LM potency.[11] In a subsequent letter to the same journal of June 20, 2011, the authors commented 'the use of LM potencies is standard practice in patients with inflammatory pain conditions to ensure symptoms are not unduly aggravated (by standard homeopathic remedies); the facility to use this potency was therefore both ethically and clinically appropriate.' For traditional homeopaths, 1 LM potency, is 1 in 50,000.[12] LM is actually the Roman numeral for only 950, so more perspicacious and numerate homeopaths refer to the 'LM' potencies as 'Q' (for quinquagintamillesimal). Others stick to the quite inaccurate designation. There is no evidence this makes the slightest difference.

Hahnemann himself suggested 'In earlier instructions, I specified that a whole drop of liquid in a given potency be added to 100 drops of wine spirit for higher potentisation. But meticulous experiments have convinced me that the dilutions of 100:1 are much too narrowly limited to develop the powers of the medicinal substance properly and to a high degree, by means of a large number of succussions, unless one uses great force.'[13] Hahnemann did not publish the results of his 'meticulous experiments' and they have not been confirmed by anyone since. Moreover, one drop added to a hundred gives a dilution of 1 in 101, not 1:100, and is not a 'centum'. Hahnemann's mathematics was awry – by a factor of 0.99% for the first dilution, and 29.7% for 30C. Oh dear. Fortunately this makes not the slightest difference.

In 1811 Amedeo Avogadro published his theory that the volume of a gas is proportional to the number of atoms or molecules in it, regardless of the nature of the gas. This was during Hahnemann's lifetime, but it may not have come to his attention. It is now accepted that at a dilution greater than $1:10^{23}$ a solution probably no longer contains a single molecule of the original substance. This is at about the 12th centesimal homeopathic dilution or 12C.

Hahnemann explained dynamization along the lines of the 'force' and 'energy field' as had been demonstrated by Anton Mesmer in his theories on 'animal magnetism' in 1779. Mesmer formalised an occult magic art that had been used for centuries by shamans to bring people under their spell and used the induced trance like state to heal patients. Hahnemann compared the similarities between the practice of homeopathy and mesmerism in the 6th edition of *The Organon:*

> I find it yet necessary to allude here to animal magnetism, as it is defined, or rather Mesmerism. It is a marvellous, priceless gift of God ... by means of which the strong will of a well-intentioned person upon a sick one, by contact and even

without this and even at some distance, can bring the vital energy of the healthy mesmeriser endowed with this power into another person dynamically. The above mentioned methods of practicing mesmerism depend upon an influx of more or less vital force into the patient. [14]

Hahnemann's own explanations for the results he achieved were metaphysical, taking a cue from the esoteric and Kabbalistic teachings of Paracelsus. The Principle of Contagion has long been relied upon by practitioners of sympathetic magic – contact between two objects will result in continued effects even after they have been separated. Dilution gradually separates the active principle from a homeopathic solution until there is nothing active left, yet the effects remain, so it is said by modern homeopaths, due to water having a 'memory'. Hahnemann felt that the diseased parts of the ill patient were particularly susceptible to his remedies, and patients had increased sensitivity to mystical energies. Currently, homeopaths invoke quantum mechanics, 'vibrations', and 'resonance'. This is why there is an account of the origin of the Universe, and us, in this book. Some homeopaths claim that water can 'remember' substances that have been potentised. Many homeopaths are in denial, others accept that the remedies represent a metaphysical quality which is beyond rational explanation. But if homeopathy is metaphysical, it is a philosophy and belief system – a faith and not a natural science which can be incorporated into modern medicine. In 1834 Dr Armand Trousseau admitted giving his patients bread pills, telling them they were homeopathic remedies and achieving comparable results.[15] Fabrizio Benedetti suggests this was the first use of inert placebos to assess effectiveness of a medical treatment. Would that Hahnemann had been so conscientious and used controls in his own tests.

French immunologist Jacques Benveniste published a paper in *Nature* (1988) in which he suggested high dilutions of substances in water could leave a 'memory'.[16] Most scientists did not find these results plausible. James Randi, the magician who is concerned about honesty and integrity in science, suggested the research had not been carried out properly. It emerged that Benveniste had not carried out the crucial original tests himself, but had left that step to assistant Elizabeth Davenas, and she had known which test tubes contained homeopathic preparations and which were genuine controls. No other scientist has been able to reproduce Benveniste's results. Nor was Benveniste himself able to, in spite of a million dollars being offered by the James Randi Educational Foundation for anyone who can convincingly demonstrate an effect, including homeopathy, which is not scientifically explicable. Moreover, it had not be made clear that the work had been partially funded by a large homeopathic remedy manufacturer. In 1998 Benveniste wrote a paper for the *Anomalist:* 'On the role of stage magicians in biological research.' The magician he had in mind was The Amazing Randi.

In 2009 Dr Luc Montagnier who shared the Nobel Prize in physiology or medicine in 2008 for the discovery of HIV, claimed that DNA emits weak electromagnetic waves that cause structural changes in water that persist even in extremely high dilutions. Contrary to claims of camists, Montagnier says his work offers no support for homeopathy. In any event the scientific community currently regards these claims as implausible and is highly critical.

Two important principles have to be considered when reviewing research of this type: extraordinary claims demand extraordinary evidence; and research must be done in such a manner that fraud is not possible. The philosopher Thomas Paine, born in England, an immigrant to America and Founding Father of the United States advised:

> If we are to suppose a miracle to be something so entirely out of the course of what is called nature, that she must go out of that course to accomplish it, and we see an account given of such miracle by the person who said he saw it, it raises a question in the mind very easily decided, which is – is it more probable that nature should go out of her course, or that a man should tell a lie? We have never seen, in our time, nature go out of her course; but we have good reason to believe that millions of lies have been told in the same time; it is therefore, at least millions to one, that the reporter of a miracle tells a lie.[17]

A particularly influential critique of homeopathy came from Dr Oliver Wendell Holmes Sr. (1809-1894), whose son became the Acting Chief Justice of the Supreme Court of the United States. Dr Holmes trained in Boston and Paris, and qualified from Harvard Medical School in 1836, where he later became a professor and Dean. As a student, Holmes had been a member of the 'Puffmaniacs' who met to socialise, talk – and smoke. Holmes also achieved significant fame as a poet and writer.

Holmes had earlier studied with the pathologist Pierre Louis who had demonstrated the futility of bloodletting. Louis emphasised how important it was that a physician allows nature to take its course, as diseases 'regressed to the mean'. That is, tended to recover in any event, unless the physician interfered too much – the *méthode expectante.* Holmes suggested 'that if all the *materia medica,* as now used, was tossed into the sea – it would be all the better for mankind – and all the worse for the fishes.'[18] William Crosswell Doane's poem *Lines on Homeopathy* had it: 'Stir the mixture well lest it prove inferior/ Then put half a drop into Lake Superior/ Every other day take a drop in water/ You'll be better soon/ Or at least you oughter!'[19]

In 1842 Holmes lectured the Boston Society for the Diffusion of Useful Knowledge and published *Homœopathy and Its Kindred Delusions*. This should be required reading for all interested in homeopathy. The paper is certainly critical, but the issues that Holmes raises do have to be seriously considered by anyone considering use, support for or practice of this alternative system of medicine.[20] Holmes advised:

> When a physician attempts to convince the person, who has fallen into the Homœopathic delusion, of the emptiness of its pretensions, he is often answered by a statement of cases in which its practitioners are thought to have effected wonderful cures... Such statements made by persons unacquainted with the fluctuations of disease and the fallacies of observation, are to be considered in general as of little or no value in establishing the truth of a medical doctor and all the utility or method

of practice.

Those kind friends who suggest a person suffering from a tedious complaint, that he 'had better try Homœopathy,' are apt to enforce their suggestion by adding, that 'at any rate it can do no harm.' This may or may not be true as regards the individual. But it always does very great harm to the community to encourage ignorance, error, or deception in a profession which deals with the life and health of our fellow creatures. Whether or not those who countenance Homœopathy are guilty of this injustice towards others has to be considered.

To deny that some patients may have been actually benefited through the influence exerted upon their imaginations, would be to refuse to Homœopathy what all are willing to concede to everyone of those numerous modes of practice known to all intelligent persons by an opprobrious title. So long as the body is affected through the mind, no audacious device, even of the most manifestly dishonest character, can fail of producing occasional good to those who yield it an implicit or even a partial faith. The argument founded on this occasional good would be as applicable in justifying the counterfeiter and giving circulation to his base coin, on the ground that a spurious dollar had often relieved a poor man's necessities.

Hahnemann regarded Olfaction as the culmination of his life's work – 'even the smelling of remedies may produce immediately direct and decided therapeutic effects.' Holmes noted Hahnemann's opinion that 'the smell of the rose will cause certain persons to faint' and claim that therefore homeopathic doses could hasten recovery. Hahnemann had cited Byzantine historians who recorded 'that the Princess Eudosia with rose-water restored a person who had fainted.' [21] Even today rose-water is passed round the table at dinners of the Worshipful Society of Apothecaries, on the grounds that a dab behind the ear will be refreshing. It works.
Dr Worthington Hooker reviewed Homœopathy for the Rhode Island Medical Society prize in 1851 and commented:

Believe nothing which is incredible except on evidence which is overwhelming... homœopathy's mode of observation is capable of establishing no facts, and is therefore of no practical use; and the treatment of disease, based upon this mode of observation, must therefore be utterly absurd.

Hahnemann's ideas did actually provide a safer system to the quite awful state of orthodox medicine in the eighteenth and nineteenth centuries. Orthodox doctors of Hahnemann's time had little more to offer than the purging, bloodletting, and use of toxic heavy metals which had been the staple of conventional medical practice for centuries. Physicians still sought to balance the four Hippocratic humours with the four elements of earth, air, fire and water. Some incorporated the 'fifth essence' of Aristotle and Paracelsus, the quintessence of a 'vital force'. Toxic lead, phosphorus, arsenic, antimony and mercury were all regularly used. Because conventional physicians prescribed medicines to counteract symptoms, Hahnemann referred to the orthodox medicine of his day as 'allopathy' (*alloin,* different; *pathos,* disease). He termed his own system 'Homœopathy' because he used ultra dilute doses of medicines, which in greater strengths would actually cause comparable symptoms (*homoios,* similar, like). Today, homeopaths still refer to orthodox doctors as being 'allopaths', though the days of prescribing medicines purely on the basis that they produce symptoms opposite to that produced by the disease itself are long past. That term is now anachronistic, unhelpful, pejorative and indicative of lack of understanding.

Homeopathy beyond Hahnemann

Homeopathy is not homogenous. There are different forms, different expressions. Some ideas have taken hold, others discarded. 'Homeopathy is not a seamless unity but consists of a rather loose amalgam of ideas that can only be understood if they are viewed historically.'[22]

Medical science has moved on, homeopathy has not done so and has become a cult and belief system. The early disciples of Hahnemann were men of slender attainments, whose standing and qualifications did not entitle them to much eminence in the medical profession, but whose vanity and ambition found full scope in Homœopathy. Hahnemann declared his favourite student was Clemens von Boenninghausen who took up homeopathy in the belief that pulsatilla remedies (windflower) had cured his tuberculosis. Boenninghausen made the classic mistake of failing to disassociate correlation from causation. He graded remedies on the strength of their relationship with symptoms, publishing a 'repertory' of helpful remedies in his *Therapeutic Pocketbook* (1846). He 'trialled' high potencies of 200C in animals (though with no controls), and promoted the idea of 'contraindications' which has been developed further as 'polarity analysis'. This reflects other ideas in alternative medicine such as that of *yin* and *yang*. It is claimed 'the polar modalities are a direct reaction of the vital force to any pathological disturbance.' Boenninghausen was not medically qualified, but the King of Prussia granted him a licence to practice as a physician.

In the United States of America, doctors began using homeopathy in the early nineteenth century. Constantine Hering (1800-1880) qualified as a doctor from Leipzig in 1826 and established his practice in Philadelphia where he founded the Homoeopathic Medical College of Philadelphia. As a promotion, two hundred and fifty students marched through Philadelphia in 1893 with banners aloft accompanied by a brass band. Regular students taunted them: 'Sugar pill, sugar pill/ Never cured and never will.' With the advent of millions of immigrants there was a crying need for medical care, but the 'regulars' made it very difficult for all but the wealthy and connected to enter the medical profession. Homeopathic schools were less demanding, and open to women. By 1900 there were twenty-two purely homeopathic general hospitals, and by 1914, fifty-six together with thirteen mental asylums with two thousand beds each.

Hering had been brought up as a Swedenborgian and enthused about Hahnemann's homeopathy which complemented that sect's religious beliefs. Emanuel Swedenborg (1688-1772) was a distinguished Swedish scientist, mining engineer, statesman and philosopher who in his fifties came to believe he had contacts with the spirit world in dreams and in person. He believed he had experienced new religious revelations and claimed that Jesus had opened his spirit so that he could freely visit heaven and hell and enter into conversations with angels and demons. His ideas seem to have had an influence on William Blake and Samuel Coleridge. Like Hahnemann, Swedenborgians emphasised the importance of vitalism and spiritual impulses.

In 1908 all the homoeopathic colleges in Chicago were merged as the Hering Homoeopathic Medical College, with Eclectic physician Dr James Tyler Kent (1849-1916) as Dean. In his *Lectures on Homœopathic Philosophy,* Kent claimed the teachings of Swedenborg and Hahnemann corresponded perfectly. He held that homeopathy was founded on divine authority and that disease resulted from transgression of this order. 'It is law that governs the world and not matters of opinion or hypothesis...Let us acknowledge the authority.' Kent used no potency (dilution) less than 30C and commonly used 2000C. Kent's approach was regarded as 'high potency' and his recommendations were set out in his *Repertory to the Homœopathic Materia Medica.* His approach was anti-scientific and his version of homeopathy was authoritarian, metaphysical, and based on divine order. He continued to hold that illness was due to *psora* – an internal state which predisposed patients to disease. Other Homeopaths were more content with 'low potency' – up to 6C, and they became the significant majority in America. So much so that during the 1940s many became ever closer to orthodox doctors, set aside their colleges of homoeopathic medicine, and became integrated with regular orthodox medical training and practice. In 1911 the government closed Hering College, and many other homeopathic colleges throughout the USA, as they were not up to conventional medical standards which by now were becoming definitively scientific.

Margaret Tyler (1857-1943), born and raised in a family of homeopaths, qualified as a doctor from Edinburgh in 1903 and studied the Kentian homeopathic system in America. On her return to England in 1907 she and her mother founded a scholarship for other doctors to train in America under Kent. The inheritance from her father Sir Henry funded the Tyler Wing at the London Homeopathic Hospital.[23] Sir Henry's title (and wealth) was inherited from his father – he was a baronet, not a peer as some American accounts would have it.

Kentianism became the homoeopathic orthodoxy in Britain, with James Kent's *Repertory* as the authority. An early Tyler scholar was John Weir (1879-1971) who qualified as a doctor at Glasgow in 1907 and became consultant physician at the London Homoeopathic Hospital in 1910. Weir was physician to George V, Edward VII (who knighted him in 1932), Edward VIII, George VI, and Elizabeth II. George VI was such an enthusiast for homeopathy he named his racing horse *Hypericum.* Also known as St John's Wort, homeopaths use 30C preparations of Hypericum as a treatment for depression. It is not possible to say whether the King's referral to orthodox physicians for his lung cancer was delayed by Weir and use of homeopathy, but the potential for camistry to delay conventional care does concern current critics. When a lung operation was eventually agreed by the King, it was carried out at Buckingham Palace rather than in the conventional specialist hospital where the surgeons regularly worked.

In the first half of the twentieth century, the most eminent homeopaths were medically qualified, but more lay practitioners entered the field, favouring Kent's teaching and Tyler's emphasis on 'constitutional prescribing'. The homoeopath's objective is to identify an individual patient's *constitution*, and then the appropriate remedy is inferred. This has given rise to patients being described as a 'sulphur patient' or a 'thuja patient'. Homeopathy moved from what little science it had towards an ever more metaphysical practice and a faith. This has appealed to the growing number of lay practitioners.

Modern homeopaths have associated each specific constitution of a patient with a variety of symptoms which can be treated by homeopathic *polychrests* – remedies which are capable of curing many conditions (*poly*, many; *chrēstos*, useful). A homoeopathic consultation commonly takes at least an hour, during which the patient is questioned in depth on their health and emotions. Each homeopath conducts the consultation differently, and although the main headings of complaint, lifestyle and past history will be the same as in orthodox medicine, there will be additional emphasis on mental, emotional, psychological and spiritual matters. The consultation is highly individualised. That alone can make patients feel cared for and 'better'. Some homeopaths question the patient following an inquiry scheme akin to a decision tree and then apply their intuition. Some will use formal questionnaires, but there is no consensus as to which might be best, nor even audits as to what the outcomes are when using different schemes. As an example, the following questions are taken from a list of 176 employed by the Indian homeopath, Nancy Malik:

> Do you cry when thanked? Do you tend to sigh? Are you suspicious? Are you concerned with precision and accuracy? Are you vain? Are you are timid about public speaking? Do you like soft boiled eggs? Do you fear ghosts? Do you fear insanity? Are you uncomfortable wearing tight clothes? Do you have a chilly personality?

Such case history taking identifies a remedy based on the 'totality of the patient's personality and illness'. This has resulted in simplification, and most homeopaths nowadays use less than thirty remedies on any regular basis.[24] Hahnemann made preparations from a wide variety of substances including metals, minerals, vegetables, plants, herbs, and other chemicals, many of which were toxic in standard doses. *Natrum muriaticum* has been a popular homeopathic remedy – it is but common salt, diluted so the remedy contains no sodium chloride molecule. Today's homeopaths prepare their own remedies, or purchase them from commercial companies such as Nelson's, which also has a partnership arrangement with Prince Charles' Duchy Originals to produce 'herbal remedies'. Helios Pharmacy will provide the remedy *Luna* – prepared by exposing ethyl alcohol solution to moonlight, before being potentised by dilution and succussion. The same firm can provide remedies prepared from 'electrical hum'.[25, 26] The Centre for Bioliminal Homeopathy can provide Berlin

Wall 30C for 'those who feel a sense of separation from the world.' Ainsworth's will provide a combination of 'homeopathic tap water' (don't ask); rohypnol (yes, the 'date rape' anaesthetic drug, flunitrazepam); and *Tyrannosaurus rex* (I kid ye not). Ainsworth's have Royal Warrants from both HM The Queen and her eldest son, and meet the standards required by their Royal Highnesses. Those standards are covert, confidential and mysterious, but all patients should be informed what they are, as they may wish to apply them to their own healthcare decision making.[27]

Hahnemann's metaphysical approach appeals to many lay people in the UK, particularly those attracted to concepts of shamanism, vitalism, 'energy therapy', counter-cultures and New Age philosophies. Prominent among them were Thomas Lackenby Maughan (1901-1976) and John Da Monte (1916-1975). Maughan used the title 'Dr.' claiming a D.Sc.. Inquiries have not unearthed the university from which the doctorate was obtained. Both of these homeopaths had their own distinctive teaching styles and although the students in their rival schools did not mix, together the principals founded the Society of Homeopathy in 1970.

Gibraltan Da Monte had commenced a medical degree but never qualified. He also had interests in scientology, radionics, and energy philosophies. He claimed to have met Maughan whilst working in British intelligence in the war, and came to Britain to continue his studies of homeopathy and Druidism. He became a prominent member of the Radionic Association. In addition to an interest in eastern philosophies, Maughan became Chief Druid and held that homeopathy was more than a system of medicine and should incorporate concepts of chakras, karma, rebirth and the teachings of the Western Esoteric Orders. The homoeopathic higher potencies themselves were regarded as being highly spiritualised.

In Germany, Hahnemann's system of medicine developed as one of the 'natural therapies'. By the 1920s Germany was in crisis. In addition to the general economic predicament, health standards were low and not good enough for German industry to perform at optimum level. There was a widely perceived 'crisis in medicine'. Politicians criticised the mechanistic and sceptical approach of conventional medicine as doctors seemed to have become more and more detached from their patients. Quackery was a developing problem and orthodox doctors sought to prevent 'naturalistic' medically qualified homeopathic doctors and lay practitioners from receiving income from the social security system. There was a crisis of trust.
Others sought a different approach. Rudolph Virchow had developed his idea of the germ theory in a more holistic way as 'the theory of the human being and everything human.' In 1928 Georg Honigmann suggested 'unification in medicine.'[28] In 1937 medical specialities were redefined under a new system of Medical Regulation of the Reich, and a new policy, *Neue Deutsche Heilkunde* (New German Medicine) sought to integrate conventional medicine, natural therapies and homeopathy.
At the time, German 'natural therapies' were practised by lay people in a naturalistic movement comparable in size to that of conventional medicine. Additionally, some conventional university-trained doctors practised homeopathy. Not all were happy

to have the same professional status as lay practitioners whose practices were not science-based – but such policies were in accord with the ideology of National Socialism and hard to resist.[29]

New German Medicine policy integrated conventional medicine with German folk practices, and expected National Socialist attitudes. Doctors who adopted natural therapies and homeopathy were described as being 'biological doctors'. The term 'holism' had by now been coined by the South African politician Jan Smuts and was applied to this new synthesis between conventional and alternative medical systems, with their concepts of vitalism and natural therapy. At first, the control over all aspects of German life sought by the National Socialist Party was not apparent but became clearer with an article in 1933 in *Deutsches Äzteblatt* by Dr Gerhard Wagner, the Director of the German National Socialist Medical League and the Führer's Commissioner for National Health: 'I want to unite all doctors... I want to see them all together in one large and wide associative chain congregating all the biological doctors from all orientations. Only after this integration would it be possible for all therapeutic approaches to have the proof of recognition that they deserve, so they can offer training and improvement to doctors for the sake of the patients needing our help.'[30]

Lore Fortes has suggested 'the notion of integration, dictatorially instituted through the policy of the New German Medicine, had to be 'voluntarily' accepted by all doctors, homeopaths and lay naturalistic practitioners. In this way it was hoped that past conflict would be left behind and there would be no more controversy among all these professional categories.'[31]

The Rudolph Hess Hospital was founded in Dresden in 1934 for medical research in natural therapy and homeopathy. Diagnosis was carried out in the conventional way, but the treatment offered was 'naturalistic'. Dr Karl Kötschau, the Director of the Task Group of the Reich for a New German Medicine declared that natural medicine was successful, since official medicine had reached the boundaries of its wisdom.

When Rudolph Hess, Hitler's deputy, spoke to the General Assembly of the Central Association of German Homoeopathic Doctors later in 1937 he said 'it is for the sake of the people, that what seems to bring benefit must be integrated ... homeopathy is a therapy close to nature. It is always possible to intertwine opposites, which shows a parallel with National Socialism, that in its intertwining with socialism and nationalism it has attained the utmost political success of the State. Allopathy and homeopathy have nowadays in their joint work a great task to fill in many fields that have not yet been researched in medicine.'[32]

In 1939 a new profession of naturalistic practitioners was established under the term *heilpraktikern* (healers, therapy practitioners), but after 1940 the idea of integration and harmony between conventional medicine, homeopathy and natural therapies dissipated and today, whilst conventional doctors do practice homeopathy in order to placate their patients, conventional medicine regards homeopathy as an alternative system.

Edward Bach (1886-1936)

The 1920s saw other homeopaths develop even more idiosyncratic systems. Bach (pronounced *Batch)* qualified as a doctor from Birmingham University in 1912. He joined the staff of The London Homoeopathic Hospital as its pathologist in 1919, but three years later set up his own practice in Harley Street, specialising in the treatment of chronic diseases by diet and nutrition. He initially identified seven 'nosodes' in the bowel which were associated with different homoeopathic constitutional types (*nosode,* disease).

Bach manufactured a number of his own homoeopathic remedies but also utilised distance healing and radionics. He believed that diseases were triggered by negative emotions and could be treated by appropriate vibrations derived through God's gift of flowers. He investigated further by concentrating on one particular emotion at a time whist walking in the countryside, in all weathers, and sought to ascertain which plants had the appropriate energy vibrations to correct the emotion. By this means he identified twelve emotional types which could categorise all patients and which corresponded with specific flowers and plants which he was able to identify by his own intuition – not by scientific inquiry. It is said that 'Through his finely developed sense of touch he was able to feel the vibrations and power emitted by any plant he wished to test ...He drew on concepts used by the alchemist Paracelsus and developed remedies based on dewdrops and from flower petals which he floated in water exposed to sunlight for four hours – thus impregnating them with magnetic power.'[33]

Subsequently Bach added a further twenty six remedies. He claimed that by his own intuition he had identified a total of thirty eight wild flowers which possessed a soul or vital energy which could heal human diseases. '...early morning sunlight passing through dew-drops on flower petals transferred the healing power of the flower onto the water.' It was his psychic connection with the plants which enabled him to identify those which would treat different negative emotional problems. *Rescue Remedy* is probably the best known, and relies on Bach's view that 'Disease in is in essence the result of conflict between the Soul and Mind and will never be eradicated except by spiritual and mental effort.' *Rescue* comprises a mix of the other remedies – its timely use is held to prevent emotional imbalance developing. Bach moved away from the homeopathic 'Law of Similars', though preparation of his remedies involved homeopathic dilution and shaking techniques. This resulted in remedies containing little more than stream water. Taken as a tincture, often with brandy, the 'Flower Remedies' balance negative moods and energy blocking and restore harmony to the patient's soul. Systematic reviews have found no effects greater than those which can be achieved by placebos.[34] Bach's propensity to advertise his remedies led to him having a run in with the GMC. In Germany, Bach's remedies have to be sold as food supplements with no claim they can affect illness. In law, claims to be a 'medication' have to be substantiated by plausible evidence of efficacy – and for flower remedies there is no such proof.

Inevitably other camists have developed their own commercial remedies based on Bach's ideas – *Alaskan Flower Essences; Australian Bush Flower Essences; Native Indian Essences,* though none have been shown to contain any therapeutically effective active principle. Nora Weeks has described Bach himself as 'passing through terrible mental agonies accompanied by a physical malady in its most severe form ... a severe haemorrhage exhausted him and bleeding did not cease until the remedy for the mental state he was passing through was found. These might have included *Agrimony* for mental torture behind a cheerful face; *Crab Apple* for self hatred; *Cherry Plum* for fear of the mind giving way or *Sweet Chestnut* for extreme mental anguish and for when everything has been tried and there is no light left.' In 1936 Bach's Masonic lodge awarded him ten guineas in benevolence. Months later his death was certified as being due to 'cardiac failure, sarcoma'. He was fifty.

William Ernest Boyd (1891-1955)

Boyd qualified in medicine from Glasgow, became a homeopath and practised as a radiologist at the Scottish Homeopathic Hospital for Children.[35] Boyd invented an energy detection machine, the Emanometer, based on the 'Radionics' machine which had been developed in America by Albert Abrams. He claimed his device would help a homeopath find the appropriate remedy.[36] The American National Center for Alternative Medicine stated in 2008 'neither the external energy fields nor their therapeutic effects have been demonstrated convincingly by any biophysical means.' Scientologists today use similar E-meters, as proposed by science fiction writer L. Ron Hubbard as: 'A religious artefact used to measure the state of electrical characteristics of the "static field" surrounding the body.' There is no independent scientific evidence of such a field.

Current issues

To assist their diagnoses, homeopaths have also used charms, talismans, and pendulum swinging techniques. The latter take advantage of the ideomotor response and are well described in books on magic, as well as being basic to Applied Kinesiology.[37]

Today, Kentian homeopathy is described as 'classical'. Some modern homeopaths use lower potencies as 'isopathic homeopathy' and include acupuncture, herbalism, naturopathy, and other CAMs in their practice. Why these additional systems are needed if the homeopathic system is efficacious is not explained.

Any research on homeopathy has to bear in mind the diverse nature of homeopathy and associated philosophies. This has been acknowledged by the marketing director of Boots the Chemists when he gave evidence to the House of Commons Select Committee on Homeopathy (2010), yet pharmacists still sell such remedies on shelves identifying them as 'medicines'.

Because remedies are individualised and their effects are conflated with that of the consultation, the application of statistical methods of research such as randomised controlled trials are hard to apply. The consultation itself is highly dependent on the emotional rapport between homeopath and patient and the intuition of the homeopath to unearth deep personal emotional, psychological and spiritual determinants. Nevertheless, it is a matter of great regret that after more than two hundred years, proponents still do not differentiate properly between the practitioner and the product, the teacher and the tincture, the style and the substance. Homeopathic consultations are often described by patients as having 'worked' or been of 'benefit'. There does seem to be reasonable evidence that the experience of a consultation with a homeopath provides useful psychological and emotional support, which can then enable a patient to cope better with any fundamental and underlying stress or disease. The resultant emotional calm can have a physiological effect. There is no credible evidence that the remedies themselves have any effect on a specific disease, nor on emotional or psychological responses. Placebo effects are due to the patient-practitioner relationship.

By conflating the effects and experience of the constructive empathic therapeutic encounter between patient and homeopath, with the perceived effects of the pills or remedies themselves, it is not possible to quantify the effects of the latter. Francis Beauvais has proposed a methodology for avoiding problems using randomised controlled trials for research into the effects of homeopathy – by blinding the homeopath as to whether the patient received a homeopathic remedy or non-homeopathic sugar pill as a placebo. All other parameters should be the same. To date, no such research has been carried out.[38] There is no plausible evidence that homeopathic products and remedies have any discernible effect on disease or illness. They do however provide significant commercial benefit to Big Charma, (Complementary Health and Alternative Remedy Manufacturers), which has comparable vested interests in their products as does Big Pharma in pharmaceuticals.

The homeopathic remedy Oscillococcinum is prepared from a duck's liver, incubated for forty days and then filtered, freeze-dried, rehydrated and diluted in the ratio 1:100 on 200 occasions, accompanied by succussion. The resultant solution is then impregnated into sugar pills. At these dilutions the concentration of the duck's liver molecules would be 1 in 100^{200}. In the US a class action was filed on 4th August 2011 in the Superior Court of California for the County of San Diego, against Boiron USA Inc., a major homeopathic manufacturer. It was alleged that Boiron and its French parent company had violated consumer protection laws in falsely advertising and selling Oscillococcinum. The complaint charged that the product (a) is nothing more than a sugar pill, (85% sucrose, 15% lactose); (b) has no impact on influenza or accompanying symptoms, as is claimed; (c) contains no molecules of its allegedly active ingredient.[39] The suit claimed that the probability of getting one molecule of active ingredient of Oscillo in a regular dosage is approximately equivalent to winning the Powerball Lottery every week for an entire year.

In March 2012 it was announced that Boiron had set aside $5M to settle the claims, the company stating '…at the end of the day consumers need additional information that we're happy to provide.' Whether that additional information will in future include the fact that its products being marketed as Oscillo, Arnica pain reliever, Chestal cough remedy and Coldcalm do not work as claimed is unclear. It is estimated that re-labelling and explanation of the dilution process has cost $7M. Andy Lewis points out that 'over the past year, Boiron stock had been trading at over $30. After the suits were filed, their price dropped to below $20.' [40]

In 2014 The German Heel Group announced the cessation of its business activities in the United States and Canada. 'In the USA and Canada, manufacturers of over the counter homeopathic medicinal products have been confronted with accusations through class action lawsuits. Heel Inc. was also faced with two such attempts recently. Both cases have been settled without conceding the allegations. The financial burden however was substantial. In a subsequent risk-benefit analysis of its global activities, the Heel Group decided to focus on strengthening its excellent position in South America, Central Europe and Eastern Europe and to withdraw from business activities in the USA and Canada for the time being.'

Camees need to be aware of the concerns about Big Charma as well as Big Pharma. Contrary to statements made by some, BMA policy is not to oppose 'homeopathy' as such, but simply holds that homeopathic remedies should not be paid for by the tax-payer unless or until the National Institute for Health and Clinical Excellence (NICE) indicates that such remedies provide value for money. Past BMA President Prince Charles has been asked to make publically available the evidence he has that homeopathic remedies provide beneficial effects beyond the placebo. He declines to respond, yet continues to encourage 'evidence-based medicine'.

A major challenge for homeopaths is that instead of embracing the issues thrown up by the scientific method and moving on, they remain wedded to Hahnemann's original principles. 'A system for the cure of disease based on dogma set forth by its promulgator' is defined by Webster's dictionary as a cult. A sect is defined as 'a group adhering to a distinctive doctrine or leader.' Hahnemann set out his own principles of medicine which he called homeopathy. If ever homeopathy were to develop using the principles of scientific evidence-based medicine, chemistry, physics and pharmacology, Hahnemann's fundamental principles would have to be set aside – traditional homeopathy would be no more.

Those interested in how the 'repertory' of homeopathic remedies is created and the 'proving' trials of them are carried out should refer to www.nyhomeopathy.com/provings. Followed by the 'next' pages for *rubrics* and 'next' again for the 'words used' by the experimenter. Homeopathy should not be further contemplated until these web pages have been studied. Be prepared to be amazed.

Lionel Milgrom has offered some insight into the mindset of homeopaths in his paper *Toward Topological Descriptions of the Therapeutic Process: Two New Metaphors Based on Quantum Superposition, Wave Function Collapse, and Conic Sections:*

> Quantum theoretical discourse has previously illustrated the therapeutic process as three-way macro-entanglement (between patient, practitioner, and remedy), and depicted the Vital Force as a quantized spinning gyroscope. Combining the two via semiotic geometry leads to a topological description of the patient's journey to cure. In this article, two new metaphors for the homeopathic therapeutic encounter are described, based on a quantum mechanical model of adaptive mutation and the illuminated geometric patterns generated by a light source attached to a spinning gyroscope. [41]

It is impossible for conventional doctors or scientists to understand any of this. Patients must judge for themselves.

Homeopaths claim the process of progressive succussion and dilution imbues 'higher potency'. That is, the preparation is able to increase the healing energy in the remedy. This of course contradicts the Second Law of Thermodynamics which precisely precludes energy being created in this way. The Second Law states that everything in the universe runs down, wears out and decays. 'Entropy' describes on a probabilistic and statistical basis how mixed up things are (*en*, inside; *trope*, transformation). The higher the entropy of a system, the less it is able to do anything. Homeopathic remedies have such high entropy that they can do nothing. That is what the Second Law says. Hahnemann would not have known this physical fact. Albert Einstein said "The Second Law of Thermodynamics is the only physical theory of universal content which I am convinced will never be overthrown." Today's homeopaths either do not know or understand this, or do and are seeking to mislead and defraud.

Homeopathy is a cult – 'a faith based on novel beliefs in an authority and with a high degree of tension with surrounding society'. It was devised as an alternative to orthodox medicine and should continue to be considered as such. Its principles are shared with traditional magic. Those patients who want an alternative should have their right to choose respected – that respect need not extend to their choice. Attempts to integrate such alternatives with the orthodox are destined to fail, as the fundamental philosophies are so disparate. No one would expect Christianity to integrate with Islam, or monarchists with republicans. Patients must make their healthcare choices on that understanding and with guidance from *Real Secrets of Alternative Medicine.*

Additionally, some doctors, dentists, nurses, and other health professionals, who have no particular training in homeopathy, nevertheless like to recommend, and sell, homeopathic remedies to their patients on the grounds: 'I find many patients appreciate it.' No doubt some do. Such a service may well help marketing of practices and even give the practitioner/camist some vicarious satisfaction. For example, some like to prescribe patients homeopathic Arnica 30C 'to reduce bruising.' Several species of Arnica contain the toxin helenalin, a sesquiterpene lactone that is a major ingredient in anti-inflammatories (though proof of efficacy is sparse). Homeopathic preparations contain no Arnica whatsoever. Given the lack of evidence that homeopathic arnica 30C has any recognisable effect whatsoever on anything and the reliance of the practitioner on mere anecdotes, patients have to consider whether they are being quacked and even defrauded. The independent journal for evidence-based healthcare, *Bandolier,* points out:

> 'Clinical bottom line: There is no evidence to show that Arnica montana is more effective than placebo for a number of clinical conditions related to tissue trauma.'[42]

As in all these matters, the key is for patients to ignore anecdotes and demand to see the evidence on which the camist acts.

To protect the public from those who would prey on their trust, ignorance or vulnerability, the UK Advertising Standards Authority (ASA) requires that any claim made in an advertisement must be legal, decent, honest, truthful, based on reasonable evidence and capable of substantiation. Until October 2011 the home web page of the Society of Homeopaths claimed: 'Homeopathy is an evidence-based medicine which offers holistic, individual and integrated treatment with highly diluted substances with the aim of triggering the body's natural system of healing.' With the ASA's rules becoming more widely appreciated, the Society has changed its site to say 'Homeopathy is a form of holistic medicine in which treatment is tailored to the individual.' There is no longer a claim to be 'evidence-based', but patients will still have to decide for themselves whether they believe the sugar pills provide any effect beyond that to be expected of a placebo. The Society also claims 'Homeopathy can be used alongside conventional medicine when necessary to give an integrated approach to your healthcare.'[43] Obviously it can be used, given that it has no effect beyond the placebo – but how is the necessity determined? Is that claim designed to be misleading? The patient must be the judge.

In 2011 the UK Medicines and Healthcare products Regulatory Agency (MHRA) upheld a complaint against Boots Pharmacy Stores that point-of-sale advertising and 'indications for use' next to their displays of homoeopathic products contained information that was prohibited.[44] The MHRA ruled the homoeopathic products being advertised were not licensed to include indications for their use because they were registered under the MHRA's Simplified Rules Scheme for homoeopathic products, which prohibits indications. These rules are underpinned by the Medicines Act 1968, EU directive 92/73/EC and other regulations and directives. All are designed for the protection of the public and to avoid misleading advertising. Boots withdrew the point-of-sale information. Action against Canadian pharmacies which sell these products as 'remedies' are also in hand, and are reported by Canada's Center for Inquiry.[45]

In 2012 the UK Advertising Standards Authority issued 'advice to help marketers of homeopathic services comply with the Committee of Advertising Practice Code, and understand the ASA's current position regarding acceptable claims.' CAP represents the interests of the advertising industry and is recognised around the world for setting standards of honesty, fairness, truthfulness and integrity which protect consumers and provide a level playing field for advertisers.

> 'If you are making claims for a homeopathic product, or for a treatment based on a specific product, or combination of products, you may only make such claims as are permitted by the product licence. To date the ASA has not seen persuasive evidence to support claims that homeopathy can treat, cure or relieve specific conditions or symptoms. We understand this position is in line with other authoritative reviews of evidence.'[46]

If people want to sell sugar pills to patients they will be able to continue that practice. They simply have to be honest about it and not claim the pill is 'medicine' or can treat specific conditions.

There are large commercial interests involved in camistry which take significant steps to ensure their position in the market place is maintained. Andy Lewis has drawn attention to how some homeopathic remedy manufacturing companies pay Internet bloggers to challenge and smear any journalist or scientist who dares to reveal secrets of their products and subject their systems to critical analysis.[47] Notwithstanding that King Edgar established the Right to Petition in the 10th century (leading to modern rights to freedom of speech about matters of public interest) some camists resort to a SLAPP – a 'strategic lawsuit against public participation' – intended to intimidate and silence critics by burdening them with the cost of a legal defence until they abandon their criticism or opposition.[48] This practice may prevent us from being as fully informed as we should be when we make critical health care decisions. You must be the judge as to whether this is acceptable.

One might think universities are representative of a rational approach to scientific matters, but some endorse alternative systems of medicine. Exeter University offers a discount for its staff at its campus homoeopathic clinic. Its website suggests 'Examples of commonly treated ailments are: blood pressure, grief, depression, addictions, injuries and joint troubles, infections, asthma, hay fever, hormonal disturbances and pregnancy problems.'[49] Very ingenious – there is no claim that these conditions are treated successfully by homeopathy, or provide any benefit beyond the placebo – simply that they are 'treated'. Misleading? The patient must be the judge – the University should examine its conscience.

Hippocrates' system of Humourism has largely died out after two millennia and as a result of better scientific understanding. Present scientific consensus that Hahnemann's homeopathy has no value in treating any specific condition is not shared by believers. Many persist in promoting the idea that valid research has been done.

Sceptics point that not only are basic premises implausible, studies to date have been poorly designed, controls are rarely used, results have not been replicated by others, and there are serious methodological flaws.[50] NICE has declined to report on the value of remedies, possibly recognising none is likely. Apologists for homeopathy continue to press for homeopathy to be 'integrated' with 'standard care' but have failed to distinguish the undoubted benefits of a constructive therapeutic relationship from the remedies themselves. It may well be that homeopathy is popular, because patients have their anxieties assuaged, but those responsible for health systems have to consider that patients will desire many things, and rationing on the basis of need is necessary. Whims cannot always be satisfied. *Argumentum ad populum* is a logical fallacy. Claims that homeopathy 'reduces the use of potentially hazardous drugs including antimicrobials' are misleading.[51] If such agents can be safely set aside, they should have been – homeopathy is not a substitute. Reports of such effects prove homeopathy works as a placebo and simply provides psychological support.

In 1998 the German Medical Association's Drug Commission advised: 'Since over 140 years of existence of and experiences with homeopathy including the evaluation of its results with modern meta-analyses were not capable of making its efficacy probable ... it raises concern, if further costly studies are still required, instead of drawing consequences from present knowledge.' A further review (including other CAM modalities) was requested from the Association of the Scientific Medical Societies in Germany and published in 2015. It was recommended *inter alia*: 'Evidence of a clinically relevant efficacy as per the standards of evidence-based, science-oriented medicine, which could justify therapeutic use, is not generally available for CAM methods, and also not for placebo medication. Their effects are predominantly conditioned by treatment context. The patient needs to be informed about this.'[52]

At the beginning of the twenty first century doctors were becoming reluctant to refer their patients to the Royal London Homeopathic Hospital and the hospital rebranded, diluting 'homeopathic' to zero. In 2010 it changed its name, dropping 'Homeopathic' and creating confusion with the Royal London Hospital which already existed. In 2011 the Liverpool Homeopathic Hospital closed. Glasgow Homeopathic Hospital has closed its pharmacy and no longer offers attachments to medical students. Perhaps embarrassed by its homeopathic underpinnings, it has changed its name to 'Centre for Integrative Care'. Lothian Health Board no longer funds homeopathy. In 2012 the UK health insurer BUPA stated 'We no longer provide cover for homeopathic treatment.'[53]

In January 2013 Professor Dame Sally Davies, England's Chief Medical Officer, told the Commons Science and Technology committee that homeopathy 'is rubbish', and advised that there is no evidence to support the claim that homeopathic remedies have any medical impact beyond the placebo effect. Davies went on to condemn the public funding the controversial treatment receives, telling the committee: 'I am perpetually surprised that homeopathy is available on the NHS.' Professor Sir

John Beddington, speaking on his retirement as the Government's Chief Scientific Adviser in 2013 commented 'Homeopathy has no underpinning of scientific basis, it is mad.'[54] His successor, Sir Mark Walport said he would tell ministers there was no medical benefit to be had from homeopathy. 'My view scientifically is absolutely clear: homeopathy is nonsense. The most it can have is a placebo effect.'[55] The views of Conservative MP David Tredinnick, who endorsed homeopathy, were declared by fertility expert Professor Lord Winston as 'lunatic', though in 2010 Tredinnick had been elected by fellow MPs to the Commons Health Select Committee and with Jeremy Corbyn MP, (elected Leader of the Labour Party in 2015), he voted in 2010 in support of the provision of homeopathy on the NHS at taxpayers' expense. Corbyn tweeted: 'I believe that homeo-meds works for some ppl and that it compliments (sic) "convential" (sic) meds. they both come from organic matter.' Oh dear.

Reporting in March 2015 on more than 1800 papers on homeopathy, with 225 controlled studies, the Australian National Health and Medical Research Council concluded that 'Homeopathy is not an effective treatment for any health condition.'[56] In May 2015 the Royal Australian College of General Practitioners determined: 'GPs should not prescribe homeopathic remedies for their patients and pharmacists should not sell or recommend the use of homeopathic products. GPs practise evidence-based medicine and there was robust evidence homeopathy had no effect beyond a placebo as a treatment for various clinical conditions.'[57]

Writing in the Pharmaceutical Journal in 2015, Michael Marshall and Simon Singh emphasise:

> Advocates of evidence-based medicine are not dogmatic campaigners who are ideologically against homeopathy, or against alternative medicine as a whole, but instead call for scrutiny of any modality not supported by evidence, be they 'alternative', 'complementary' or indeed 'conventional'. Before a patient is subjected to any intervention, it is imperative first to have a good reason for believing it might be of benefit....Perhaps the most persistent criticism of our campaign to prevent the funding of ineffective homeopathic treatments on the NHS is that to do so would deny patients their right to choose a healthcare option. Of course, patients cannot have a completely free choice, otherwise the NHS would be forced to offer every therapy under the sun, from aura enhancements to chakra transplants. Moreover, fundamental to the notion of patient choice is informed consent: for a choice to be an informed choice, patients cannot be offered a treatment known to be no better than placebo, while being incorrectly told that it is effective. Such actions fundamentally undermine the nature of informed consent, and jeopardises the trust between a doctor and a patient.'[58]

And Professor Jayne Lawrence, the Royal Pharmaceutical Society's Chief Scientist asked: 'Surely it is now the time for pharmacists to cast homeopathy from the shelves and focus on scientifically based treatments backed by clear clinical evidence?'[59]A 'focused systematic review and meta-analysis of randomised controlled trials (RCTs) from Mathie et al (of the British Homeopathic Association and Faculty of

Homeopathy) in 2014 reviewed thirty two RCTs, of which only three met inclusion criteria. They concluded 'the overall quality of the evidence was low or unclear, preventing decisive conclusions'.[60]

As of 31st March 2015, NHS Lanarkshire ceased new referrals of Lanarkshire residents to the Centre for Integrative Care 'on the basis of the lack of clinical effectiveness evidence for homoeopathy, and other health interventions delivered by the CIC.' As of October 2015 the Bristol Homeopathic Hospital ceased to provide homeopathic remedies. Judgement is nigh.

Endnotes to Chapter 10

1. Oliver Wendell Holmes. *Homœopathy and Its Kindred Delusions.* Two lectures delivered before the Boston Society for the Diffusion of Useful Knowledge. 1842. https://ebooks. adelaide.edu.au/h/holmes/oliver_wendell/homeopathy. The traditional diphthong 'œ' is not generally used today.

2. Dan King. *Quackery Unmasked,* 1858. https://en.wikisource.org/wiki/Quackery_ Unmasked/Chapter_VI.

3. Martin Gumpert, L B Fischer Publ. Corp, New York, 1945, a translation into English of: *Hahnemann, die Abenteurlichen Schicksale eines Arztlichen Rebellen und seiner Lehre, der Homoöpathie.* S. Fischer, Berlin, 1934. Also, Richard Haehl, *Samuel Hahnemann – his life and works.* B. Jain Publishers. Delhi. 1922 & 1971.

4. Samuel Hahnemann. *Organon of Medicine.* (J. Künzli, A. Naudé, & P. Pendleton, Eds.) 6th ed. London: Gollancz. 1983. #54 p.50. Quoted by: Yu Hin Ng, D. (2011). *A discussion: the future role of homeopathy in the National Health Service* (NHS). Homeopathy, 100(3).

5. Samuel Hahnemann. *Indications of the Homoeopathic Employment of Medicines in ordinary Practice.* Hufeland's Journal. 1807. See Martin Gumpert, *Hahnemann: The Adventurous Career of a Medical Rebel.* Fischer, New York 1945.

6. Anthony Campbell. *Homeopathy in Perspective.* Lulu Publishing, 2008.

7. Samuel Hahnemann, *Materia Medica Pura,* vol. i.

8. Julian and Susan Scott. *Natural Remedies for Women.* Avon Books, 1991.

9. Christian Samuel Hahnemann. *Organon of Medicine.* Gollancz, 1986.

10. Ben Goldacre. *Bad Science,* Harper Perrenial, 2009.

11. Brien S, Lachance L, Prescott P, McDermott C, Lewith G. *Homeopathy has clinical benefits that are attributable to the consultation process but not the homeopathic remedy. A randomised controlled clinical trial.* Rheumatology. 2011;50:1070-82. First published online November 13, 2010.

12. www.wholehealthnow.com/homeopathy.

13. Samuel Hahnemann. *Organon*, 6th Edition, footnote to aphorism 270.

14. C.F.S. Hahnemann. *The Organon of Medicine*. 6th Edition. B. Jain Publishers. New Dehli 1978.

15. Trousseau A and Gourand H. *Repertoire clinique: experiences homoeopathetiques tentees a l'Hotel-Dieu de Paris*. Journal des Connaissances Medico Chirurgicales, 8, 338-41. 1834.

16. Jacques Benveniste. *Nature* 1988. 333:816.

17. Thomas Paine. *Age of Reason*, 1794, Part I, 14.

18. Wilson Sullivan, *New England Men of Letters*. New York Macmillan, 1972 , 233.

19. William Croswell Doane was the first Episcopal Bishop of New York, and author of *Ancient of Days*.

20. Oliver Wendell Holmes. *Homœopathy and Its Kindred Delusions*. www.ebooks.adelaide. edu.au/h/holmes, and www.quackwatch.org/01Quackeryrelatedtopics/holmes.

21. Samuel Hanhnemann. *Organon*, paragraph 110.

22. Anthony Campbell, *Homeopathy in Perspective*, Lulu Publishing 2008, revised Kindle edition 2014.

23. Mary Tyler's account of her practice, including her recognition of placebo effects and failure of homeopathy can be found at www.homeoint.org/cazalet/tyler/nottodoit.htm.

24. www.homeopathy-help.net/Remedies/polychrests.

25. www.homeovision.org/en/film offers a six minute film which demonstrates how the process of trituration, dilution and succusion is carried out.

26. Lawrence & King. *Luna – a Proving*. Phamflet, Helios Pharmacy 1993. Cited by Steven Ransom, *Alternative Medicine a Mind Blowing Magical Mystery Tour*. e-book from www. mindblowingdecisions.com.

27. Ainsworth's remedies: personal experience, and BMA Annual Representative Meeting Agenda 2015.

28. Georg Honigmann. *Tendencies to Unification in Contemporary Medicine*. Hippocrates, 1 1928/29.

29. Gerhard Wagner, Hippocrates 7, No 14 (1936). 'New German Medicine' is not connected with 'German New Medicine', *Germanische Neue Medizin* – a system of alternative medicine originated by Dr Ryke Geerd Hamer to cure cancer. His license to practice as a conventional doctor was revoked in 1986 and he was imprisoned on counts of fraud and illegal practice.

30. Gerhard Wagner, *'Anruf an alle Arzte'* , also *Hippocrates* 1933: 309; *Allgemeine*

Homöpathische Zeitung 181 (1993).

31. Lore Fortes. Dissertation for doctoral thesis, Universidade de Brasilia, 2000 and *Circumscribere* 8(2010):12-27.

32. Rudolph Hess. *Leipziger Populäre Zeitschrift für Homeöpathie* 68, No.10 (1937): 192.

33. Nora Weeks, *The Medical Discoveries of Edward Bach, Physician.* C W Daniel Co, 1973, and in *Alternative Medicine*, Steven Ransom, www.mindblowingdecisions.com.

34. Kylie Thaler et al, *Bach Flower Remedies for psychological problems and pain: a systematic review.* BMC Complement. Altern. Med. 9 (16).2009.

35. http://homeoint.org/morrell/glasgow/preface.htm. A useful review of homeopathy in Glasgow. Students should particularly note the section on *Homeopathic Consultation.*

36. William Boyd. *Electric field of the Human Body*, Brit J. Radiol., 1930, 1932.

37. H.J. Burlingame. *How to Read People's Minds,* 1907 and Paul Daniels. *Adult Magic,* Michael O'Mara Books, 1989.

38. Francis Beauvais. *A quantum-like model of homeopathy clinical trials: importance of in situ randomization and unblinding* . Homeopathy Volume 102, Issue 2, April 2013.

39. www.casewatch.org/civil/borion/oscillococcinum/complaint.shtml.

40. www.quackometer.net/blog/2012/03/borion-settles-for-12m.

41. Lionel Milgrom. *Toward Topological Descriptions of the Therapeutic Process: Two New Metaphors Based on Quantum Superposition, Wave Function 'Collapse,' and Conic Sections.* The Journal of Alternative and Complementary Medicine. June 2014.

42. http://www.medicine.ox.ac.uk/bandolier/booth/alternat/at012.html

43. Zeno's Blog 21.07.11 and 29.10.11.

44. www.MHRA.gov.uk/howweregulate/Medicines/Advertisingofmedicines/Advertisinginvestigations/CON134909.

45. http://www.youtube.com/watch?v=B_J7XFPFh4s&feature=youtube_gdata_player.

46. www.homeowatch.org/reg/cap-guidance-pdf.

47. www.quackometer.net/blog/2012/07/german-homeopathy-companies-pay-journalist-who-smears-UK-academic.

48. https://en.wikipedia.org/wiki/Strategic_lawsuit_against_public_participation

49. www.exeter.ac.uk/staffassociation/benefits/homeopathy.

50. Edzard Ernst. *Should doctors recommend homeopathy?* BMJ 2015; 351:h3735.

51. Peter Fisher. Ibid.

52. Haustein KO, Höffler D, Lasek R, Müller-Oerlinghausen B. Arzneimittelkommission der deutschen Ärzteschaft: Außerhalb der wissenschaftlichen Medizin stehende Methoden der Arzneitherapie. Dt Ärztebl. 1998; 95(14): A-800-5.

And: http://www.egms.de/static/en/journals/gms/2015-13/000209.shtml

53. www.quackometer.net. 18.11.2011 and 15.11.2011.

54. Sir John Beddington. *Daily Telegraph.* 10.04.13.

55. Professor Sir Mark Walport, Emeritus Professor of Medicine, Imperial College, London speaking at Cambridge University's Centre for Science and Policy Conference, 18th April 2013. Nick Collins: http://www.telegraph.co.uk/health/healthnews/10003680/Homeopathy-is-nonsense-says-new-chief-scientist.html.

56. Australian National Health and Medical Research Council. *Statement on homeopathy.* 2015. www.nhmrc.gov.au/_files_nhmrc/publications/attachments/cam02_nhmrc_statement_homeopathy.

57. http://www.racgp.org.au/yourracgp/news/media-releases/homeopathy

58. http://www.pharmaceutical-journal.com//opinion/comment/stop-funding-treatments-with-insufficient-of-evidence-of-efficacy.

59. http://blog.rpharms.com/england/2015/06/17/homeopathy-should-pharmacists-be-selling-homeopathic-products/?utm_source=Advisory+Panel&utm_campaign=de400

60. Mathie RT, Lloyd SM, Legg LA, Clausen J, Moss S, Davidson JRT, Ford I. *Randomised placebo-controlled trials of individualised homeopathic treatment: systematic review and meta-analysis.* Systematic Reviews 2014; 3: 142. Also see: http://edzardernst.com/2014/12/homeopaty-proof-of-concept-or-proof-of-misconduct.

Chapter 11

Beyond the Twinge:
From magnetism to manipulation –
Osteopathy and Chiropractic

*God is the Father of Osteopathy and I am not ashamed of the child of His mind.
Osteopathy is to me a very sacred science. It is sacred because it is a healing
power through all nature.*

*The work of the Osteopath is to adjust the body from the abnormal to the
normal; then the abnormal condition gives place to the normal and health is the
result of the normal condition.*

*The fundamental principles of osteopathy are different from those of any other
system.*

*The cause of disease is considered from one standpoint, viz.: disease is the
result of anatomical abnormalities followed by physiological discord. To cure
disease the abnormal parts must be adjusted to the normal; therefore other
methods that are entirely different in principle have no place in the osteopathic
system.*

*The rule of the artery is absolute, universal, and must be unobstructed or
disease will result.*
Andrew Taylor Still

*The philosophy of chiropractic is founded upon the knowledge of the manner in
which vital functions are performed by innate intelligence in health and disease.
When the controlling intelligence is able to transmit mental impulses to all parts of
the body, free and unobstructed – we have normal action which is health.*
Chiropractic is an outgrowth of magnetic healing.
Chiropractic is a science just so far as it is specific.
Chiropractic is founded upon different principles than those of medicine.
*Displacement, or 'subluxation,' of spinal vertebrae impedes the freedom of Innate
to flow from the universe through the human body. 'Adjustments' restore Innate's
ability to care for and direct the functions of the body.*
*That which I named innate (born with) is a segment of that Intelligence which fills
the universe, a 'part of the Creator.'*
Daniel David Palmer

We chiropractors work with the subtle substance of the soul. We release the prisoned impulses, a tiny rivulet of force that emanates from the mind and flows over the nerves to the cells and stirs them to life. We deal with the magic power that transforms common food into living, loving, thinking clay; that robes the earth with beauty, and hues and scents the flowers with the glory of the air.
Bartlett Joseph Palmer

The House of Lords classified those alternative systems of medicine which it regarded as being 'professionally organised' in Group One. This comprised five autonomous systems – homeopathy, acupuncture, herbalism and two others which originated with rival magnetic healers in America's Midwest of the late nineteenth century and are now styled as Osteopathy and Chiropractic. They are 'alternative' systems because their originators said they were.

In the seventeenth and eighteenth centuries some practitioners rejected orthodox medicine and genuinely felt they had a vocation as healers; some claimed to be divinely inspired; some tried but failed to train as orthodox physicians or surgeons; some took up alternative systems of medicine; some devised their own systems and sold training courses to other practitioners. For some, it was easy pickings to make a living selling secret remedies, nostrums, snake oil and convincing patients of their extraordinary powers to engage the very forces and spirits of nature. They knew perfectly well they had no plausible evidence their remedies and practices were effective but they sought to defraud the ignorant, gullible and vulnerable. They were quacks and charlatans. They were able to develop their practices because whilst many were downright crooks, they did offer care, compassion and hope and created the illusion of genuine clinical ability. Many conditions entered remission and many patients had worthwhile benefits from placebo effects.

Eighteenth-century Europe saw the introduction of Mesmer's techniques of 'animal magnetism' engaging the imagination of his patients, accessing their sub-conscious and introducing salutary suggestions. Although rejected by Louis XVI's Royal Commission of 1784, the methods nevertheless crossed the Atlantic and were taken up by a number of 'Magnetic Healers'. *Progressive Men of Iowa* tells of Paul Caster (born Custer) who claimed his ability to heal by animal magnetism was a divine gift. As such it could not be taught but he trained students who claimed similar abilities. 'Caster had a serious impediment in his speech, and some mental peculiarities which prevented him from receiving an education in the usual way and threw him entirely upon his own resources mentally.' He was clearly charismatic, and appropriating the title 'Doctor', he started his public career as a healer in 1866.

The 'can do' spirit drove the American Midwest where a number of people discovered they had the 'gift of healing' expressed by animal magnetism, gainsaying those who thought they were psychologically disturbed or were quacks. Caster's son Jacob continued the magnetic practice – other students went on to develop their own systems of unorthodox medicine and found schools to teach their idiosyncratic philosophies and practice. Two became particularly successful.

Osteopathy

Andrew Taylor Still (1828-1917) took exception to the orthodox and conventional American medicine of the late nineteenth century. As the son of a physician, Still was initially apprenticed to his father but was unable to qualify as a doctor. He went on to serve with the Union Army as a hospital steward. Like Hahnemann a hundred years earlier, he regarded the orthodox system as being hidebound by convention and morally corrupt. Conventional treatments by drugs and surgery too often did more harm than good. When three of his children died from spinal meningitis, Still became determined to find an alternative to conventional medicine.

After studying with 'magnetic practitioner' Paul Caster, Still set up practice as a 'Magnetic Bone Healer and Lightening Bonesetter' in Kirksville, Missouri. There he devised his own system of medicine which he called a 'rational medical therapy'. Acting on the principle that 'structure governs function', Still developed techniques for the mechanical manipulation of the spine and musculoskeletal system. Get that right, he advised, and all else would follow. He maintained that the cause of disease lay in dysfunction of bones and joints and particularly their blood supply:

> The bone is the starting point from which the practitioner may ascertain the causes of pathological conditions. Necessity is the mother of invention. It becomes necessary to have some method or system of the healing art based upon a philosophical foundation. This necessity is the mother of this invention or discovery, known as the mechanic's remedy for disease, and known as Osteopathy. Thus you see that the mechanical healer or Osteopath is the legitimate child of the mother of invention. Her name is necessity. My work for over thirty years has been confined to the study of man as a machine, designed and produced by the mind of the Architect of the Universe.[1]

Osteopathy is a belief (and having no rational basis, a faith) that diseases are caused by mechanical dysfunction of the skeletal system and can be remedied by manipulation. Still stated that necessity is the mother of invention.[2] Initially described as 'the mechanic's remedy', the term 'osteopathy' was first used in 1885 (*osteon*, bone; *pathos*, suffering). In 1892 Still founded the American School of Osteopathy in Kirksville. Lack of any real evidence of its efficacy, its religious underpinnings and its implausible rationale led the American medical profession to view osteopathy as a cult. Conventional doctors regarded it as being unethical for a physician to associate with an osteopath – or any other practitioner who was not regularly qualified. That proscription was how standards of professional practice were established and maintained. During the twentieth century osteopaths in the US came to use conventional pharmaceutical medicines and their training became more coherent with that of orthodox medical practitioners.

Although he never obtained the degree of MD from a recognised university, Still styled himself as a Doctor. His own School of Osteopathy 'awarded' the degree of Doctor of Osteopathy (DO). Students of osteopathy studied the same curriculum as students in conventional American medical schools and sought the same status as MDs but remained wedded to Still's philosophical and religious beliefs. In 1962 the American Medical Association in California allowed DO's to become members and in 1969 all US osteopathic physicians were allowed to participate in conventional postgraduate training programmes.

The AMA at one time hoped to merge the DO and MD professions. That has not happened fully and practice licences vary from state to state but the two professions now work closely together, albeit osteopaths retain Still's philosophy which is not shared by modern medical practitioners. If practitioners do not accept and endorse Still's philosophy, they can hardly be said to be osteopaths.

The value of osteopathic manipulative therapies remains contentious. Conventional doctors are concerned about the standards of educational achievement required for entry to osteopathic medical schools (the 'back door phenomenon') and the relative lack of research base for that profession, but in the US relationships are now more harmonious. In the UK, the gulf remains. There is only one standard to be expected of a doctor practising as a registered medical practitioner – that which is regulated by the General Medical Council.

Osteopathy is a system of medicine based on the principle that anatomical derangement of the blood supply to bones, muscles, tendons, ligaments and joints causes physiological dysfunction which leads to pathology – not only of the musculoskeletal system but also all other organs and systems including cardiac, digestive, respiratory, renal, neurological and immune. Osteopaths believe that these somatic diseases can be treated by spinal and joint manipulation. These are very bold claims and orthodox medical scientists have been quite unable to confirm any elements of them. Osteopathy remains an alternative system and its philosophy cannot be integrated with that of conventional medicine. Osteopathic techniques may have value as a method of physical therapy for specific parts of the musculo-skeletal system, but those techniques should be integrated with physiotherapy, not medicine.

The British School of Osteopathy web-site claims osteopathy to be 'a primary health care system' – a claim also made by chiropractic. Osteopathy is 'complementary to other medical practices. It is suitable for almost anyone and can contribute to the treatment and management of a wide range of conditions. A core principle behind osteopathy is that the body is an integrated and indivisible whole and contains self-healing mechanisms that can be utilised as part of the treatment. A wide range of gentle non-invasive manual techniques such as deep-tissue massage, joint articulation and manipulation are applied therapeutically.' This is of course what chiropractic and physiotherapy do. What these self-healing mechanisms are and how they work is not explained. Current promotional material studiously avoids mention of Andrew Still. More importantly, students contemplating studying osteopathy are offered no guidance as to how its practices or beliefs differ from chiropractic or physiotherapy, or why a student should choose to study osteopathy rather than physiotherapy, chiropractic or medicine.

Chiropractic

As with Osteopathy, Chiropractic claims it is 'a primary health system' and that its practitioners will diagnose and treat all manner of diseases and illness. Practitioners are not registered medical practitioners and should not give the impression they are. Chiropractic offers an alternative to conventional medicine based on the philosophy, practice and personal revelation of David Palmer, a grocer who became a magnetic healer in the American Midwest of the late nineteenth century. Chiropractors assert they are able to adjust 'subluxations' of spinal vertebrae, thereby releasing 'innate intelligence' and healing illness in distant organs and tissues. Regular sessions are frequently recommended for 'maintenance'.

Daniel David Palmer (1845-1913)

Generally known by his initials as D.D., Palmer was born near Toronto, Canada in 1845 and emigrated to the Mississippi in 1865. He moved to Iowa in his twenties and initially worked as a schoolteacher, farmer and grocer. After relocating to Burlington, near Ottumwa, he developed an interest in spiritualism, 'psychic healing' and 'magnetic healing'. Like Andrew Taylor Still, Palmer was taught the practice of 'magnetic healing' by Paul Caster. Some accounts suggest that Palmer was also Still's student for a time. Certainly Palmer said: 'Some years ago I took an expensive course in Electropathy, Cranial Diagnosis, Hydrotherapy, Facial Diagnosis. Later I took Osteopathy which gave me such a measure of confidence as to almost feel it unnecessary to seek other sciences for the mastery of curable disease, having been assured that the underlying philosophy of chiropractic is the same as that of osteopathy.' Palmer then went on to develop his own system of medicine, different from and in competition with Still's osteopathy. Any modern student contemplating studying one of these two alternative medical systems has to decide which one and rationalise why that system and not any other. Indeed, why an alternative system to conventional medicine and not medicine itself?

The essential difference between osteopathy and chiropractic is largely a matter of commercial branding for training courses and schools. Their originators were commercial rivals. Both systems manipulate. There is no scientific evidence for vital forces being relieved or balanced by either method and no evidence that, other than for local musculo-skeletal tissue, the health of somatic structures 'of the body' more generally can result from adjustment of abnormal anatomy by either method. Both systems were designed to be alternative to conventional medicine and practitioners have beliefs incompatible with scientific understanding. Quite on what basis or for what reason a student decides to enter either profession is unclear. Perhaps some think chiropractors earn more and because patients are more impressed by their claims. Many have excellent business acumen. Palmer's school paid particular attention to commercial aspects of practice – advertising, marketing, building a business and ensuring repeat custom as much as possible. That may be an attraction for some entrants to the profession. Using Google to ask 'What is the difference between osteopathy and chiropractic' necessitates passing through Lewis Carroll's Looking Glass into a world of fantasy. Studies of patients with low back pain having spinal manipulation by chiropractors, osteopaths or physiotherapists have not distinguished any difference in outcome. On his website, osteopath David Tio comments: 'When I was a student of osteopathy in the UK I used to attend meetings of complementary and alternative health practitioners and it was easy to tell who was who. The naturopaths would be wearing flowers and beads, while chiropractors would come with their suits and ties. Osteopaths were somewhere in between.'

After training with Caster, Palmer started his own healing career as a mesmerist and 'magnetic healer' in Burlington but being faced with competition for patients, moved to Davenport. Styling himself as 'Doctor' he opened the Palmer School for Magnetic Cure in 1886.[3] 'D.D. would draw his hands over the area of the pain and with the sweeping motions stand aside, shaking his hands and fingers vigorously, taking away the pain as if it were drops of water.' [4] This is not too dissimilar from the 'traction' offered by Perkins in the eighteenth century. By 1898 Palmer's annual income was $9276 – worth c. $1,780,000 today.

Palmer also had interests in mysticism, phrenology, 'natural philosophy of life' and spiritualism, claiming he was guided by the spirit of a dead physician.[5] 'For nine years previous to the discovery of adjusting vertebrae I was practising magnetic healing. I treated (as I supposed) the spleen for carcinoma of the breast, effecting a cure. Chiropractic is an outgrowth of magnetic healing, but is not magnetic healing.'[6]

Palmer's initial experience as a 'mesmerist and magnetizer' no doubt gave him considerable skill in harnessing patients' imaginations, reassuring them and giving them hope. There is no evidence that Palmer's hands generated a magnetic field, nor that magnetism had any effect on the pathology from which a patient might be suffering. He eventually gave up such claims – but his techniques were surely a variety of hypnosis and he continued in that vein.

In 1895 D. D. adjusted the spine of Harvey Lillard who had been deaf for seventeen years. After two treatments, he reported 'I could hear quite well.' Palmer did not appreciate that the auditory nerve, which conveys hearing, is a cranial nerve and does not pass through the spine. Palmer asserted he had been advised to try the method by Dr Jim Atkinson, a deceased doctor and 'intelligent spiritual being' who had communicated with Palmer 'from the other world' during a psychic séance.

D. D. moved from magnetic healing to hands-on vertebral adjustments. He felt the success he had with his new method was due to the effect of 'vital forces'. He was able to detect 'inflammations' which he claimed caused '...an obstruction to the blood circulation and injury to certain nerves. It is this combination which causes cancers. Having found the cause of cancer it is an easy thing to relieve the pressure upon the blood vessel and nerve... in curing Lillard's hearing I proved that disease does not originate outside the body – it is not the work of devils, for God created the universe. Drugs will not release pressure upon the spinal cord. It is the intelligence within – let us call it 'innate' – which transmits to every organ and cell the only real healing force. In other words, the power to heal is within us. Innate is an individualised portion of the All-Wise, usually known as the spirit.'[7]

Palmer went on to describe how the nervous system should have an optimal 'tone'

– any alteration of tone caused disease:

> Life is the expression of tone. Tone is the normal degree of nerve tension. Tone is expressed in functions by normal elasticity, activity, strength and excitability of the various organs. Consequently the cause of disease is any variation of tone – life is the expression of tone. In that sentence is the basic principle of chiropractic. Innate directs its vital energy through the nervous system to specialize the coordination and sensation and volition through the cumulative vegetative functions. That I named 'innate' is the segment of that intelligence which fills the universe. Chiropractors correct abnormalities of the intellect as well as those of the body. *Chiropractic is founded on different principles than those of medicine.*[8] (Italics for emphasis).

According to the Rock Island Union newspaper, in 1895 Palmer brought a lawsuit against a man who failed to pay: 'not so much for the collection of a bill as it was to establish Palmer's right to practice in Moline without a physician's certificate. During the course of the trial, D.D was questioned on the witness stand and testified his profession had nothing to do with medicine, that he healed by the laying on of hands and that he had a diploma from High Heaven.' Clearly, by Palmer's own declaration, Chiropractic is an alternative to evidence based medicine.

Palmer claimed that he occupied in chiropractic a similar position as did Mrs. Eddy in Christian Science. 'Mrs. Eddy claimed to receive her ideas from the other world and so do I. She founded a religion thereon, so may I. I am the only one in chiropractic who can do so. We must have a religious head, one who is the founder, as did Christ, Mohammed, Joseph Smith, Martin Luther and others who have founded religions.'[9]

Modern chiropractors and their patients need to appreciate that these are the principles under which chiropractic is conducted. They should also be aware that the *Davenport Leader* of 1894 reported: 'A crank on magnetism has a crazy notion that he can cure the sick and crippled by his magnetic hands. His victims are the weak-minded, ignorant and superstitious, those foolish people who had been sick for years and had become tired of the regular physician and want health by the short-cut method ... he has certainly profited by the ignorance of his victims, for his business has increased so that he now uses forty two rooms which are finely furnished... he inserts a wonderful magnetic power on his patients, making many of them believe they are well. His increase in business shows what can be done in Davenport, even by a quack.'[10] An article in the New Zealand Medical Journal has commented 'The intellectual standards of a nineteenth century Mid-Western provincial newspaper leader writer are rather better than the intellectual standards of the UK's Department of Health, and of several university vice-chancellors in 2007.'

Palmer was not the first to adjust the spine by manipulation; he acknowledged bone setters had been active since ancient times. He was not the first to identify the nervous system as being of importance in health; that was the basis of the 'magnetic healing' he had been practising along with Caster and Still. D.D. was the first to identify a problem with vertebrae being 'out of place' and seek to adjust them using adjacent vertebral spinous processes as levers, though how he did this was initially kept secret.

The term 'subluxation' as applied to the vertebral adjustment technique was introduced by chiropractor Solon Langworthy who, together with Oakley Smith, published the first book on chiropractic in 1906. This concept remains fundamental in chiropractic today and accounts for the difficulties the profession has in its dealings with evidence-based medical practice. Subluxations have never been identified by anyone other than chiropractors.

D. D.'s son B. J. Palmer was born in 1882 to one of D. D.'s five wives, and named Joseph Bartlett on his birth certificate. He recalled that D. D. had been harsh on his children:

> When each of our sisters reached eighteen they were driven out of home and onto the streets of Davenport to make their living any way they could. We were forced to sleep in dry goods boxes in alleys... all three of us got beatings with straps until we carried welts for which father was often arrested and spent nights in jail. Older sister was badly injured and has been sickly all her life. Our younger sister had a severe abscess caused by beatings. I have a fractured vertebra and bad curvature from the same source.[11]

In 1895 B. J. was expelled from his school for letting mice out in the schoolroom, became a juvenile delinquent, but was rehabilitated by 'Professor' Herbert Flint, a travelling hypnotist and showman. When D. D. was jailed for practising medicine without a licence in 1906, his school had financial difficulties and was taken over by his son. B. J. became a dynamic businessman, teacher and promoter of chiropractic and the school flourished. When he left prison, D. D., now styled 'Old Dad Chiro' became estranged from B. J. and opened a rival school. All who paid the fee were admitted.

D. D. Palmer died in 1913, three months after having been struck by a car driven by B. J. during a parade in Davenport. The cause of death was said to have been typhoid fever, but some have suggested the car accident was a deliberate act. [12] B. J. developed a business, not a profession: 'We manufacture chiropractors ...we teach them the idea and then we show them how to sell it ... we hold no entrance examinations ... the world is your cow – but you must do the milking ... early to bed and early to rise – work like hell and advertise.' [13]

After the First World War many veterans were unemployed and turned to healthcare to provide professional status and income. There was a ready supply of enthusiastic students. Many medical assistants who had served in the Army and had experience looking after soldiers' feet trained as chiropodists (*chiron,* hand; *pod,* foot). Others, keen to receive training which would offer some other form of qualification as a health professional found chiropractic ideal. Not unsurprisingly, confusion arose between chiropodists who treated foot problems and chiropractors and their subluxations.

In order to avoid the foot care profession being taken for a system of medicine that seemed to have no basis in science, in 1958 the name of the chiropodial profession in America was changed to 'podiatry'. Today in the UK 'chiropody' is gradually being supplanted by 'podiatry'. As for Chiropractic, many students remained faithful to D. D.'s original principles and techniques. Others developed their own, spawning a plethora of techniques and systems, many of which are well reviewed in *Technique Systems in Chiropractic.*[14]

B. J. Palmer refined his father's chiropractic system of medicine. He contended that diseases in all organs could be attributed to subluxations of the upper two cervical vertebrae (atlas and axis) and congestion of innate intelligence in the neck. Not all chiropractors agreed. There were various schisms and many new colleges were founded on a commercial and proprietorial basis, each emphasising their own approach. There were some amalgamations, but attempts to create a united profession failed. There simply was no adequate evidence base on which to make judgements and decisions. B. J. enthusiastically introduced x-ray techniques. He also insisted on the use of a 'neurocalometer' which purported to measure the heat produced in nerves during chiropractic adjustment. This device could only be hired from Palmer's School. It can be bought today for $799 from www.chirocity.com as a 'Nervoscope' and detects 'uneven distributions of heat along the spine which can be indicative of inflammation and pressure' (notwithstanding that the word *scope* means 'seeing' – temperatures are measured by 'thermometers'). Such instruments are not used by neurologists or spinal specialists practising orthodox medicine. There appears to be no scientific evidence that such minute temperature changes have clinical relevance, save to chiropractors.

John A. Howard qualified as a chiropractor but found B. J. Palmer overzealous and too wedded to the idea that all disease was due to subluxations of the vertebrae and could be treated by adjustment. Howard started his own school, the National College of Chiropractic in Davenport in 1906, moving to Chicago in 1908. Training in a variety of massage, hydrotherapy and other musculoskeletal techniques was offered. Howard's approach was regarded as that of a 'mixer' as he moved away from simply correcting subluxations. Those following B. J. Palmer's more traditional approach were referred to as 'straights' as they remained orthodox in terms of chiropractic theory and practice, although of course, 'alternative' to conventional, orthodox systems of medicine.

Some members of the osteopathic community harangued Palmer saying he was a thief who had appropriated Still's osteopathic concepts and repackaged them as chiropractic. D. D. left the osteopaths to their 'rule of the artery' and concentrated on the role of the nervous system itself. In 1907 a trial in Wisconsin acquitted a chiropractor of 'practicing osteopathy without a licence.' The defence averred osteopathy sought to release vital energy through the vasomotor system, whereas chiropractic concerned itself with inflammation and heat mediated through nerves.

Joseph Keating has studied the story of chiropractic and notes: 'Still manipulated any body part thought to obstruct the flow of endogenous healing substances from the brain, which were believed to reach the end organs through the circulation and through the nerves. Palmer on the other hand manipulated in order to reposition displaced anatomy and thereby relieve inflammation. Palmer's ideas were also unique in that he proposed repositioned anatomy would reform itself into better more functional shapes; in this he anticipated orthopaedic concepts that the stresses applied to osseous structures determine their form. Palmer thought he had the 'gift' of being able to detect inflammation with his hands, and to cool areas which had excess vital magnetic force. From this he developed the idea that cause of most dis-ease was displacement of anatomic parts, which gave rise to friction, and hence inflammation. By 1905 Palmer restricted his notion of the cause of disease to those anatomic displacements involving pinching of nerves, that is, "the subluxation". He always held that nervous innate intelligence was inhibited by such obstruction, and that adjustment of the subluxations could resolve diseases.' [15]

Today some chiropractors mix and match and describe their systems as using 'diversified techniques'. This implies that for some there is no such thing as a subluxation and any attempt to adjust one is irrelevant. Others maintain they can indeed adjust subluxations and thereby affect all parts of the human body and a multitude of diseases. Some chiropractors have claimed that adjustment of subluxations can treat all manner of children's health problems, including ear infections, eczema, asthma and bed-wetting. Most chiropractors derive the majority of their income from treating musculo-skeletal problems by manipulation although nowadays many seem to have need of other CAMs such as acupuncture, naturopathy and homeopathy. Each of these is based on entirely different principles and their use represents rejection of chiropractic. There is at least now a wider appreciation of the fact that no anatomical, pathological or surgical texts of orthodox medicine have ever identified the 'subluxation'.

Chiropractors also have a tendency to make diagnoses which would not sit comfortably with regular spinal specialists. 'Leg length discrepancy', 'spinal curvature', 'shoulder not level' are frequently identified – but are rarely the cause of genuine pathology needing treatment. Chiropractic adjustments may produce cracks sounding like a magician's gag cracker, but do not affect somatic structures.

For these reasons, students who are thinking of training in chiropractic will have to consider carefully just what they do believe about health and treatment and rationalise in what way learning chiropractic theory and practice will enable them to improve health and well-being. They will need to consider whether they might find greater professional satisfaction with osteopathy, another alternative medical system, or orthodox medicine, physiotherapy or a HPC regulated healthcare profession. If they do decide on chiropractic they will have to decide whether to train as a 'mixer' or 'straight'.

Equally, those who are thinking of visiting a chiropractor will have to think about why and how they think a chiropractor can help – rather than another camist whose primary qualification is in acupuncture, osteopathy, homeopathy, naprapathy, or any other CAM. And patients will have to decide whether they want the services of a 'straight' traditional chiropractor, a 'mixer' or, of course, conventional orthodox musculo-skeletal care such as that offered by physiotherapists. Nearly all chiropractors dip their toes deeply enough in the waters of rational science to give the impression their practice is well founded. Is this deceitful? You must be the judge.

In the United States there has long been controversy and disagreement between different groups of chiropractors. In 1996 the Association of Chiropractic Colleges declared that 'chiropractic is concerned with the preservation and restoration of health, and focuses particular attention on the subluxation.' In its 2012 Standards, the American Chiropractic Association used the term 'subluxation/neuro-biomechanical dysfunction'. Mirtz *et al* reported that 'no supportive evidence is found for chiropractic subluxation being associated with any disease process or of creating suboptimal health conditions requiring intervention.'[16] In which case, what is the point of chiropractic?

Doctor of Chiropractic Sam Homola suggests that 'patients who believe they have subluxations causing health problems may be subject to a powerful placebo effect when the spine is popped. Such popping does not mean a vertebra was out of place. Normal vertebrae can be popped when manipulated beyond the normal range of movement.' Homola goes on to suggest that the subluxation theory is becoming disregarded by many chiropractors, yet they are reluctant simply to give up the practice. They have invested too much time and money in their training and Colleges. Economists refer to this as the Sunk Cost Fallacy. The costs of training cannot be recovered, they have been sunk – but it is fallacious for decisions to be made for that reason. Decisions about career development should be made rationally on the merits of the graduate's situation. Nevertheless chiropractors may not always act rationally and when they feel they have passed the point of no return, continue to practise methods they may no longer believe in, enveloping themselves in the practices of other professions and stepping out on the path of quackery.

The Association of Chiropractic Colleges stated on its website (December 2011): 'chiropractic is associated with the field of complementary and alternative medicine.' Homola is concerned that 'alternative medicine may be a haven for unproven and implausible treatment methods.' He is concerned that many consumers are unaware of the great diversity in chiropractic.[17] He is not alone. Further cynicism about chiropractic has arisen from the ranks of manipulation therapists themselves. C.F. Nelson suggested how you can invent your own system in *Five steps to your own technique.* [18]

In 2010 The British Chiropractic Association was involved in a libel action against particle physicist and author Simon Singh. The BCA website had claimed that chiropractic can treat childhood problems such as eczema, bed-wetting and ear infections. As a result, Singh had written a newspaper article in the *Guardian* alleging that BCA members were 'happy to promote bogus therapies' and the BCA sued for defamation. Some McTimoney Chiropractic Association members had websites with similar claims but members were advised to remove them. This hardly helped the BCA case. The BCA eventually withdrew the case before trial. Singh has since successfully campaigned to reform UK libel laws so that commentators can freely and honestly discuss contentious scientific issues without fear of litigation.

Some techniques used by chiropractors may be of limited benefit. For neck pain, a Cochrane Review has compared randomised controlled trials of exercise regimes, neck manipulation and neck mobilisation (a rather more gentle technique used by physiotherapists who do not claim to adjust vertebrae). Outcomes were equivalent.[19] Chiropractic manipulation might also cause dissection of vertebral arteries and result in strokes. There are no satisfactory screening procedures to mitigate this risk.

Some patients want a metaphysical approach to their healthcare and want their innate intelligence unblocked by vertebral adjustment, others might prefer physiotherapy or exercise therapy. As ever, patients must be the judge but they must also be fully informed as to the metaphysical underpinning of osteopathy and chiropractic. They may not want their innate vital forces to be manipulated.

It is essential that camees, healthcare practitioners, managers and politicians give careful consideration to these important issues before committing any time, trouble or financial resources, especially that of tax-payers, to chiropractic. They would be assisted by reference to the Institute for Science in Medicine's White Paper of 2012, in which the point is made that: 'There is no scientific evidence that chiropractic subluxations exist or that their purported 'detection' or 'correction' confers any health benefit...Chiropractors cannot agree on what subluxations are, how they can be located, or how they should be treated. This has resulted in dozens of non-validated diagnostic and treatment modalities, inconsistent terminology, and a dearth of evidence-based practice guidelines...The public is largely unaware of the chiropractor's shortcomings. Government agencies are silent about this, while licensing and mandatory insurance laws lend an *imprimatur* of government approval.' [20]

The UK General Chiropractic Council has given guidance on 'claims made for the chiropractic vertebral subluxation complex.' They have now decided the complex 'is an historical concept but it remains a theoretical model. It is not supported by any clinical research evidence that would allow claims to be made that it is the cause of disease.' In which case, what is the point of chiropractic? Or the GCC?

The GCC emphasises that in advertising, claims for chiropractic care 'must be based on best research of the highest standard only.' [21] But that research shows there is no evidence that chiropractic has any more type II effect than physiotherapy. And if a chiropractor is not manipulating a subluxation to release 'innate intelligence', then exactly what are they doing? They are manipulating and massaging musculo-skeletal tissues. This is precisely what physiotherapists do. So why do potential students not join the physiotherapy profession? Or medicine? What is the Unique Selling Point of chiropractic if not the adjustment of subluxations?

In the UK there is now legislation for the statutory regulation of the professions of Osteopathy (Osteopaths Act 1993) and Chiropractic (Chiropractors Act 1994), but neither profession is under the aegis of the GMC nor the Health & Care Professions Council, and these systems of medicine provide 'alternatives' to otherwise regulated healthcare. The HPC, created in 2001, currently regulates fifteen healthcare professions including Physiotherapy. This concentrates, as its name suggests, on physical therapy including manipulation and mobilisation – but avoids the pseudoscientific philosophical and spiritual underpinnings of other systems of manipulative and musculoskeletal medicine.

In terms of their training, practice, scientific evidence for claims made and administration, neither the Osteopaths Act 1993 nor the Chiropractors Act 1994 identifies any significant difference between osteopaths and chiropractors. There is little difference between the two Acts themselves. Both the General Osteopathic Council and General Chiropractic Council have referred to a GCC funded report by chiropractors Gert Bronfort *et al* as the basis for the scientific evidence for manual therapies and for guidance to their registrants.[22] In fact none of the studies referenced by Bronfort were identified as being specifically of chiropractic or osteopathic manipulation – the report simply referred to 'non-specific spinal manipulation and mobilisation'. The Nightingale Collaboration contends that the continued existence of separate regulators of chiropractors and osteopaths in the UK cannot be justified. It recommends that if statutory regulation of chiropractors and osteopaths is to be continued, then they should be combined under one regulator.[23]

Such differences between chiropractic and osteopathy as there may be are matters of faith in the hand of God; the ability of massage or manipulation to affect the soul and release blockage of vasomotor constriction or innate intelligence; and the beneficial effects of such manual methods on pathological processes. As belief systems, neither chiropractic nor osteopathy needs to be regulated by governments – any more than Scientology, Mormonism, Christianity or Islam should be. Metaphysics should not be regulated by governments, for then there would be no freedom of faith. Those who suggest that health care philosophies need regulation because they might be harmful, must bear in mind the same concerns apply to religions. The techniques used by these practitioners might need regulating, but on a basis of scientific, not metaphysical, evaluation. Students interested in manipulative therapies should consider training as physiotherapists and only then specialise in such other techniques and for such philosophical reasons as they may have.

Osteopaths and chiropractors cannot, will not or do not comply with the regulation and registration arrangements for physiotherapy or medicine. They want to carve their own niche for philosophical and commercial reasons. Some even style themselves as 'Dr.' – even though they have no doctorate degree recognised by UK academic authorities and are not registered by the General Medical Council. This is allowable in a free society – but must be clearly explained to patients and the public. Why would such chiropractors use this title unless they intend misleading the public or their students? Ask them.

Some chiropractors now claim they do not believe there are subluxations and have switched the term to 'spinal dysfunction' or similar. Some claim that they have 'moved on' yet remain wedded to their traditional practices and belief systems and aspire to see chiropractic accepted by regular science based practitioners. We all have to accept that professional opinions will vary, but D.D. Palmer named his practice Chiropractic precisely to brand it, market it and distinguish it from Osteopathy and other medical and faith based healthcare systems in the American Midwest of his day – including 'orthodox medicine'. For whatever reason, chiropractic students want to learn how to offer an alternative to conventional medicine, and they avoid joining an orthodox profession.

Chiropractic is not just a technique – by its own claims it is a 'Primary Healthcare System'. This implies that anyone suffering from a health problem should in the first instance go to a chiropractor with the reasonable expectation they will be able to provide or initiate effective diagnosis and treatment. Intending patients should bear in mind that it was D.D. Palmer himself who said 'Chiropractic is founded upon different principles than those of medicine.' Check out these sites: 'As 97% of the world's Chiropractors accept and utilise the terms Vertebral Subluxation Complex and Subluxation, at this time we feel it is important information to be included on this site.'[24] 'The chiropractic subluxation complex is a functional biomechanical spinal lesion with purported altered neurological function that can result in neuromusculoskeletal and visceral disorders.'[25] 'These blockages are known as 'subluxations', and can affect any part of your body, preventing you from functioning to the best of your ability. Chiropractic is a highly skilled and developed approach to removing subluxations, allowing your body to fulfil its maximum potential.' [26]

Camees who buy into this will probably gain benefit from chiropractic ministrations but must beware the lure of Confirmation Bias – ascribing undue credit to anecdotal evidence which confirms their existing beliefs. As with all trials, any 'research' article or evidence should include not only details of the successes but also failures and how many patients were seen in total. Failure to provide this information renders any paper on a CAM in default of acceptable scientific standards – and demonstrates publication bias or 'file-drawer' effect if negative results are simply not reported. This is a serious problem which also affects conventional medicine and current campaigns to have 'All Trials Registered and All Results Reported' are addressing this issue.[27]

D.D. Palmer himself said: 'I believe, in fact know, that the universe consists of Intelligence and Matter. This intelligence is known to the Christian world as God. A correct understanding of these principles and the practice of them constitute the religion of chiropractic. Knowing that our physical health and the intellectual progress of Innate depend upon the proper alignment of the skeletal frame, we feel it our bounden duty to replace any displaced bones so that physical and spiritual health, happiness, and the full fruition of earthly life may be fully enjoyed.'[28, 29, 30.]

For a time, Palmer considered turning chiropractic into a religion (as Mary Baker Eddy had done with Christian Science). The metaphysical and religious underpinning of chiropractic is still prevalent – chiropractor Mike Reid recently elaborated on the spiritual meanings of Innate: 'We are spiritual beings who are a piece of an entire bigger picture with a purpose in life ... As chiropractors, we already know that the universal intelligence lies within us as innate intelligence, causes our heart to beat, digests our food, and allows us to think as free people ... Listen to your innate ... Sit in a lotus position with your palms opened up. See yourself as one and the same with the universe.'[31] If that were not the case, practitioners wishing to specialise in spinal manipulation would have trained as physiotherapists or if wishing to attend to diseases more generally, as doctors.

Manipulation may help musculo-skeletal problems, but that is not chiropractic. Chiropractors profess unique insights into and abilities to affect health and disease. Those claims are not supported by plausible evidence. A contemporary Cochrane Review concludes: 'Spinal Manipulative Therapy is no more effective in participants with acute low-back pain than inert interventions, sham SMT, or when added to another intervention. SMT also appears to be no better than other recommended therapies.'[32]

Camees and camists interested in chiropractic and osteopathy must be aware of these issues and must judge. May the forces be with you – whether of high amplitude, low impact, or imaginary.

Endnotes to Chapter 11

1. A.T. Still. *Autobiography.* Kirksville Missouri, 1908.

2. The aphorism is sometimes ascribed to Plato. It appeared in a book of aphorisms in 1519 – sometime before Frank Zappa's 1960s band *The Mothers of Invention.*

3. Joseph C. Keating. *B.J. of Davenport: the early years of Chiropractic.* The Association for the History of Chiropractic. Davenport. 1997.
B.J Palmer, quoted on website of World Chiropractic Alliance. 2014.

4. J. White to R.B. Jackson, correspondence c. 1995.

5. Vernon Gielow . *Old Dad Chiro,* Davenport, Bawden Bros. 59, 1981.

6. D.D. Palmer, *The Chiropractor's Adjuster: Text-book of the Science, Art and Philosophy of Chiropractic for Students and Practitioners* .111. Portland Printing House, 1910.

7. Ibid.

8. Google: *D. D. Palmer quotes*. Identified by Kurt Youngman.

9. D. D. Palmer, letter to PW Johnson, archives of David D. Palmer, Health Sciences Library, Davenport, Iowa, 1910.

10. *Davenport Leader*, 1894, quoted in Vernon Gielow, *Old Dad Chiro: A Biography of D. D. Palmer*, Bawden Brothers, 1981.

11. B. J. Palmer. *Fight to Climb*. Palmer School of Chiropody, Davenport. 1950.

12. David Daniel Palmer (son of B. J.) *The Palmers*. Bawden Bros. Davenport.

13. Ralph Lee Smith. *At your own risk: the case against chiropractic*, Simon and Schuster, 1969.

14. Robert Cooperstein and Brian J. Gleberzon. *Technique Systems in Chiropractic*. Elsevier Ltd. 2004.

15. Joseph Keating PhD. http://en.citizendium.org/wiki/Chiropractic/Timelines

16. Mirtz, *et al*. *An epidemiological examination of the subluxation construct*. Chiropractic and Manual Therapies. 2009; 17:13.

17. Sam Homola: *Subluxation Theory: a belief system that continues to define the practice of chiropractic*. www.sciencebasedmedicine.org. December 30th 2011.

18. Nelson C.F. 1993. *Five steps to your own technique*. Journal of Manipulative and Physiological Therapeutics 16 (2). Similar proposals are made in *How to be a Charlatan and Make Millions*, Jim Williams, www.authorsonline.co.uk.

19. Gross A., et al. *Manipulation or Mobilisation for neck pain*. Cochrane Database Syst. Rev. 2010; 1:CD004249.

20. Jann Bellamy JD. *White Paper: Chiropractic*. Institute for Science in Medicine. Ed. Stephen Barrett. August 2012. www.scienceinmedicine.org/policy/papers/Chiropractic.

21. *Guidance*, General Chiropractic Council, London. 18th August 2012.

22. Gert Bronfort et al, *Effectiveness of Manual Therapies: The UK Evidence Report*. *Chiropractic & Manual Therapies*, www.chiromt.com/content/18/1/3.

23. www.nightingalecollaboration.

24. http://www.wightchiropracticclinic.co.uk/history.html

25. http://www.chiropractic-uk.com/subluxations.htm

26. http://arrowbankchiropracticclinic.co.uk/

27. See Dr Ben Goldacre's *Bad Pharma* and the AllTrials campaign supported by over 250 organisations including the BMJ, BMA and many politicians such as MP Dr Sarah Wollaston. The Public Accounts Committee placed the issue on the public agenda in 2014. Watch this space: http://www.alltrials.net.

28. D.D. Palmer. *The Chiropractor*. Los Angeles: Beacon Light Publishing Co.; 1914.

29. Kenneth John Young. *Gimme that old time religion: the influence of the healthcare belief system of chiropractic's early leaders on the development of x-ray imaging in the profession.* Chiropr. Man. Therap. 2014; 22(1): 36. Published online Oct 28, 2014. doi: 10.1186/s12998-014-0036-5;

30. Edzard Ernst. http://edzardernst.com/2014/12/chiropractic-education-seems-to-be-a-form-of-religious-indoctrination.

31. Mike Read. *The Seven Laws of the Power of Attraction,* Chiropractic Journal: A Publication of the World Chiropractic Alliance. 2007. WCA Mission Statement on website: 'We promote chiropractic as a drug-free, subluxation-based health care approach providing lifetime, family wellness care. It should be available to all people, from infancy to old age, regardless of the presence or absence of symptoms. We work constantly and vigorously to ensure that chiropractic does not deteriorate into a medical therapy or incorporate drugs, surgery or other medical techniques.' Chiropractic's alternative nature is clear and unequivocal. Integration with conventional orthodox medicine is impossible.

32. Cochrane Review: http://www.ncbi.nlm.nih.gov/pubmed/22972127.

Chapter 12

House of Lords CAM Group One, Part Three:
Herbalism
Also styled as Herbal Medicine, Botanicals, Phytotherapy[1]

The art of medicine consists in amusing the patient while nature cures the disease.
Voltaire

Ah me! Love cannot be cured by herbs.
Ovid

Herbalism involves giving patients unknown doses of ill-defined drugs of unknown effectiveness and unknown safety.
David Colquhoun
Professor of Pharmacology, UCL

Plants have been used to treat diseases since time immemorial and are the origin of many modern therapeutic drugs, usually dried out and ground down (Old Saxon: *drōgi*, dry). In evolving defences against animals and fungi, some chemical compounds made by plants undoubtedly have a beneficial effect on human disease. Some are extremely toxic, poisonous and dangerous. All the chemicals in plants are made of the atoms and molecules which originated from the same place as all others – stardust. Alchemists tried to change one element into another, usually base metal into gold – they failed. As alchemy gave way to chemistry, so apothecaries developed ever more refined, sophisticated and efficient techniques for extracting active compounds to be found within spices and plants and for excluding the more harmful and dangerous metabolites. Lists of useful plants were drawn up in *Herbals.* The first in English was the anonymous *Grete Herbal* of 1526. Nicolas Culpeper's *The English Physician Enlarged* (1653) became a classic, in spite of being plagiarised and promoting astrology, magic, witchcraft and folk remedies. The Worshipful Society of Apothecaries of London had its own elaboratory for manufacturing drugs from 1672 until the twentieth century. To provide medicinal plants, the Society's Physic Garden was established in Chelsea 1673 and visitors are still welcome.

The use of chemical methods in the manufacture of drugs is *pharmacy*. Given the possibility of seriously harmful effects, inappropriate formulation, adulteration with toxic minerals, drug interaction and potentially lethal consequences – stringent regulations have been developed for the manufacture of modern drugs – and for their sale and promotion as 'medicines'. Compounds not meeting those standards should not be described as medicines. The US National Institutes of Health describes therapeutic herbs as 'dietary supplements'.

Pharmaceuticals are expensive. Intensive research is followed by a multitude of animal and human clinical trials with an emphasis on safety. Even then, when a pharmaceutical drug is brought to the market the manufacturer only has exclusive marketing rights for a limited period. Herbal remedies are very much more easily grown from seed and do not have to meet the demands of pharmaceutical regulation. More pertinently – there is no requirement to demonstrate effectiveness or safety. These features may have particular attraction for practitioners who feel they have special gifts or powers which they can combine with herbs in a variety of magical, thaumaturgical and shamanic medical practices. Many practitioners remain wedded to the principles of humours promoted by Hippocrates and Galen. Given ancient concepts that diseases are hot, cold, wet or dry, the herbalist uses a plant to balance a patient's temperament or clinical status. For hot: peppers; bitter: dandelion, angostura, cinchona or opium; cool: Echinacea, cucumber (containing salicylates); sweet: agave, flower nectar. Other practitioners believe plants and flowers can release 'energies' which can affect the soul, or that plants should be used as a whole, 'holistically', with their multitude of component molecules acting in synergy.

Pharmacists and physicians expect plant extracts to be refined and doses standardised before being marketed as medicines. What is left over after extracting the useful compounds can be used as pot-pourri or to garnish a salad. Given the paucity of evidence for efficacy, dosage, safety, and identification of side-effects of unrefined plant material, herbalism remains an alternative medical system and is listed as such by the House of Lords Committee.

The National Institute of Medical Herbalists states its members are 'health care providers trained in Western orthodox medical diagnosis who use plant based medicines to treat their patients. In the UK, medical herbalists have the right to primary diagnosis. For many patients, their first visit to a medical herbalist can be a life changing experience and a chance to experience true healthcare. Your medical herbalist is a genuine, caring partner in health from the cradle to the third age. Many people come to appreciate the power of correctly prescribed, natural herbal medicines dispensed by a highly trained medical professional.'

In other words, they are practicing medicine, but without a licence from the GMC. Why they have not trained and registered as doctors is not explained. The Institute's members must affirm 'With purity and holiness will I pass my life and practise my art.' The origin of that holiness is not explained. In the UK there is no bar to anybody offering a 'primary diagnosis' – all that phrase means is that nature of a disease or condition is discerned. There is no 'right' to do this which can be conferred. As to whether patients might be confused and misled by the claims of being 'medical' – you must be the judge.

The sugars and fats extracted from plants are likely to provide evidence-based medicines for the regulated conventional pharmacopoeia for years to come. Plant and herb chemicals can be scientifically analysed, their properties established, their value and danger assessed – and regulated. That is what pharmacists do, as part of the regulated conventional, orthodox, medical system. Problems arise with camists who wish to ascribe esoteric, metaphysical and supernatural qualities to otherwise perfectly normal natural chemicals. In the West, herbalists who wish to practice conventionally, and be accepted by the conventional medical community, can qualify as pharmacists, pharmacologists or doctors and then develop their interests in plants as they may.

Herbalists even claim they can use herbals 'in tandem with modern medicine.' In parts of the world, modern medicine is hard to come by. The Bhumi Vardaan Foundation was launched by the Prince of Wales in 2006 to support Indian rural lifestyles, but also to support the production of herbal medicines and beauty products 'within the tradition of Ayurvedic medicine'. Ayurveda is a system based on religious texts of the Hindus and the Vedic belief in a pantheon of deities. The Foundation accepted that 'Published information about the efficacy and safety of traditional medicines in the scientific literature is scanty... quality of production is not always assured.' As always, the patient must be the judge. *Caveat emptor, caveat imperator.*[2]

Herbs are often promoted as being 'natural' with the implication they are safe – but they may not be. Toxins and the herbs tobacco and opium are 'natural'. Preparations containing extracts from *Aristolochia* plants are banned in Europe and mainland China. They are held to be highly dangerous and 'an international public health problem of considerable magnitude' as they may be the cause of high incidence of upper urinary tract cancer seen in Taiwan and other Asian countries.[3] They continue to be an ingredient of some 'Traditional Chinese Medicines'.[4]

Use of DNA analysis has also shown that some traditional herbal preparations contain ingredients derived from endangered animal species such as black bear, rhinoceros, saiga antelope and toxic plants. Most have not been proved to be effective. An active component of many preparations, *aristocholic acid* has been shown to damage human DNA. This information is absent from package labelling – a practice which has been regarded as dishonest.[5] The popular bruise remedy *Arnica* contains the sesquiterpene lactone *helenalin* which is toxic and causes gastroenteritis.

There is little help from the UK Government, which permits the Medicines and Healthcare products Regulatory Agency (MHRA) to regulate herbal preparations. This can give the impression to the unwary that herbal products are comparable to pharmaceutical medicines – although they do not meet the same high standards. Not every patient, nor policy maker, appreciates that though herbals may be regulated by MHRA, they are under the Traditional Herbal Medicines Registration Scheme – a totally separate regulation from pharmaceutical medicines. Quite what advantage 'tradition' provides is obscure, other than as a sop to traditionalists. Slavery was once 'traditional'. We have moved on. So has conventional orthodox medicine.

The term 'herbal medicine' is usually applied to remedies that are used in the same way as prescription drugs. There is no reason why these products could not be described as 'medicinal herbs' but for some reason many herbalists prefer 'herbal medicine.' The camee must judge if the intention is to deceive them into thinking the herbal product is a regulated medicine. 'Herbalism' is a belief system combining metaphysical concepts of holistic 'natural' care with plant preparations. Some of these decoctions may be extracted by distillation as was the case with alchemy; some are extracted into alcohol and termed 'tinctures'. Herbs are chosen by how they are believed to affect the harmony of internal vital forces – but different cultures, and certainly different herbalists, will choose different herbs.

Many traditional drugs sold in the Orient owe their alleged properties to the 'Doctrine of Signatures' – the ancient wisdom that the form and shape of a drug source determines its therapeutic virtue. To some it seems obvious that ginseng roots and rhinoceros horns are aphrodisiacs.

In an attempt to 'move forward' some herbalists now style themselves as 'phytotherapists' (*phyton*, a plant) – although herbalism remains an imaginative magical system which conveniently overlooks the fact that the active principles are just chemicals – and unrefined chemicals at that. Herbalists deny they are trying to be deceptive. Some commentators have recommended all herbals should be regulated

– but this ignores the fundamental philosophy, which is that they are 'natural' and 'traditional': – and which 'tradition' varies enormously. All that regulation of herbal products achieves is spurious and misleading endorsement that they can be regarded in some way as being equivalent to pharmaceutical preparations.

Some herbalists want their 'profession' to be regulated by the Health & Care Professions Council. Dr Michael Dixon, Chairman of the 'College of Medicine' claims 'stricter controls are needed so that the public has a real choice about treatment and is properly protected.' He appears to discount the extensive protection against false claims and harmful products and practices already afforded by existing regulations. The Prince of Wales has opined 'regulation would build confidence in making choices.' There already is regulation of healthcare practitioners – by the GMC and HPC. What we are seeing here is an attempt to have un-scientific precepts recognised as having the same validity as scientific medicine. This is promoting a faith. Commentators note the HPC does not regulate other belief systems, yet seems prepared to consider regulating herbalists and their faith in a metaphysical but unidentified 'vital force of nature.' The HPC has stated it 'will work with the Government and other stakeholders on the proposals to enhance public protection.' Protection from what – a faith? The GMC already forbids registered medical practitioners from proselytising any faith they may have to their patients.

In March 2015 health officials concluded there is insufficient evidence that herbalism works. The Chief Medical Officer Professor Dame Sally Davies told the House of Commons Select Committee on Anti-microbial Resistance that 'plants/herbs have long been appreciated as sources of efficacious medicines, but they require substantial work to precisely determine the testable active ingredient, rather than the haphazard administering of soups of chemicals.' Professor David Walker, Deputy CMO, said the government will not regulate herbalism.
Patients should guard against being misled as to the true status of this belief system and its practitioners. The buyer must beware, and not be taken in by pseudoscience, wishful thinking, false promises, misleading legislation, personal whim and political ambition.

Those interested in herbal medicines should ponder Maurizio Pandolfi's advice:

> They are real, albeit impure, drugs and therefore fully capable of producing undesirable consequences if misused. Why should un-purified or partially purified vegetable material be prescribed to a patient instead of their isolated therapeutically active ingredients? Herbalists are vague in this respect and postulate a favourable synergy among the active ingredients present in plants....the main rationale of herbal medicine is more cultural than scientific and consists in the ancient belief that nature is particularly friendly to humans who are considered the purpose of creation...And as Karl Popper made clear, what cannot be tested is not experimental science, and therefore not acceptable medicine, since medicine is just experimental science.[6]

To help protect patients in the European Union, since December 2012 health claims which suggest that foods, supplements and natural health products have disease specific beneficial properties are no longer permitted on labels unless there is good scientific evidence to back up the claims. Practitioners may speak and write in generic terms about the health benefits of food but risk breaking the law if they refer to specific commercial products whilst making such claims or claim their products are medicines – unless they are licensed as such. That should offer protection enough for all but the most gullible.

The National Institute of Health has a comprehensive web-based guide to the use of unrefined plant chemicals for healthcare.[7]

Endnotes to Chapter 12

1. Not *Phidotherapy,* that is treatment by dogs.

2. www.plant-medicine.com.

3. Chung-Hsin Chen et al. *Proceedings of the National Academy of Sciences* (doi/10.1073/pnas.1119920109).

4. Nigel Hawkes, *BMJ* 2012; 344:e2644.

5. Coghlan, Megan L. et al, *Deep Sequencing of Plant and Animal DNA Contained within Traditional Chinese Medicines reveals Legality Issues and health Safety Concerns.* PLoS Genet. 8 e1002657 (2012).

6. Maurizio Pandolfi, Lucilla Zilletti. *Herbal Medicine, Chaplin, and 'The Kid'.* European Journal of Internal medicine. Vol 23, Issue 4, June 2012.

7. http://www.nlm.nih.gov/medlineplus/druginfo/herb_All.html

Chapter 13

House of Lords CAM Group One, Part Three:
Acupuncture

Latin: *acus,* a needle.

Greek: *belone,* a surgeon's needle.

Acupuncture is no better than a theatrical placebo.
David Colquhoun and Steve Novella[1]

As with other CAM systems, Acupuncture conflates two constituents – the physical and metaphysical. Stone Age man used sharp flints or bones for many purposes – records suggest that skin puncturing, presumably for health, was being used in the first millennium BC. In time the principle extended and the practice of bloodletting developed. Chinese techniques used sharp thin solid needles to encourage the flow of 'vital energy'.

The first medical textbook, *The Yellow Emperor's Inner Canon* of about 250 BC described acupuncture with needles and blistering of the skin with a burning moxa herb in the practice of moxibustion. Traditionally the needles were placed randomly, but over time practitioners determined principal points where they felt the stimulus of the needle would affect the disease of the patient and balance the esoteric forces of *yin* and *yang*. These points were described as lying on specific lines described as 'meridians'. The number of meridians described in different texts varies enormously from four, to one for every day of the year – conveniently fitting in with astrological precepts. Twelve is classic, there being twelve great rivers in China. Additionally, there are many acupuncture points along or near each. How any particular point is chosen is a mystery and akin to magic.

Dutch doctor Willem ten Rhijne published the first Western text on the art in 1683 but in China, the system went into decline and in 1822 the Emperor banned it. At the time of the Cultural Revolution, Mao Zedong was keen to advance modern scientific medicine but he came to realise that it was simply not possible to provide the vast population with anything other than 'barefoot doctors'. In these circumstances, traditional medical systems including herbalism, moxibustion and acupuncture were once more encouraged. Better to have some care than none. That policy may be reflected in the contemporary support CAM receives from a number of governments. When Richard Nixon witnessed major surgery on conscious patients under acupuncture during his 1972 China visit, wider interest was aroused. We now know the patients that Nixon saw were sedated, received analgesia and were hypnotised – however, acupuncture got the credit. Today in China, if acupuncture is used at all for analgesia, it is usually in conjunction with conventional techniques.

In 2010 Professor John McLachlan of Durham University submitted a paper for presentation at the Jerusalem International Conference on Integrative Medicine, in which he described his discovery of a homunculus represented on the human buttocks. The 'map' responds, so he said, to needling and cupping as in acupuncture. His subsequent paper in the BMJ explained 'So called integrative medicine should not be used as a way of smuggling alternative practices into rational medicine by way of lowered standards of critical thinking. Failure to detect an obvious hoax is not an encouraging sign.'[2]

Investigation into the effectiveness of acupuncture continues and proponents inevitably identify conditions where some benefit is perceived. Irritable Bowel Syndrome is said to affect up to one in five people at some point in their lives. Oft quoted is a meta-analysis of seventeen studies showing that acupuncture seemed to be superior to drugs in several randomised controlled trials in China. More careful analysis showed any benefit to have been no better than sham controls, and therefore any reported benefits may have been due to the patients' expectations – that is, there were strong placebo effects.[3]

There is no plausible evidence that acupuncture needling has an effect greater than might be expected from a placebo. Many journalists report that 'acupuncture works' but fail to distinguish between the beneficial effects of a therapeutic relationship with an empathic practitioner and the actual needling. Indeed, in most studies, controls have not been used. The best trials have been controlled with sham needling – fakes designed on the same principle as retractable stage daggers. For all practical purposes, acupuncture is a placebo, and should be accepted as such. Camees who express delight their IBS, hay fever, psoriasis, aches and pains have gone since having acupuncture need to consider very carefully that these are all self-limiting diseases, which would have improved in any event, and which may even yet return. Correlation of perceived benefit with treatment does not imply causation.[4]

The Royal London Hospital 'for Integrated Medicine' has advertised that in addition to homeopathy it provides acupuncture for a wide variety of conditions. A complaint about the advertising led to a two-year review by the Advertising Standards Authority that adjudicated in June 2013. The Nightingale Collaboration Newsletter number 44 reports: 'The adjudication is lengthy, running to some nine pages and four-and-a-half thousand words. In it, the ASA carefully consider each of the claims made and whether the evidence provided was sufficient to substantiate them. It was not. The advertisements breached CAP Code rules 3.1 (Misleading advertising), 3.7 (Substantiation) and 12.1 (Medicines, medical devices, health-related products and beauty therapies). The ASA concluded: (The leaflets) must not appear again in their current form. We told RLHIM they should not state or imply that acupuncture was efficacious for conditions for which they did not hold adequate evidence. The ASA's rules are there to protect the public from misleading claims. We hope all acupuncturists now get the point.'

A recent systematic review of twenty nine randomised controlled trials on acupuncture in *Archives of Internal Medicine* suggested 'acupuncture is effective in the treatment of chronic pain and is therefore a reasonable referral option.'[5] A significant problem has arisen because some media reports took that extract at face value and as a result have seriously misled their readers. The study showed that real acupuncture is better than sham, but did not show there was any substantive genuine physiological effect. As there was no comparison with placebo procedures in which the practitioners were also blinded, this allowed subjective bias. The analysis simply showed there are no specific effects of acupuncture beyond placebo. The *Archives* also published an independent commentary on the paper suggesting the assertions were 'difficult to substantiate' and of 'dubious clinical relevance' – but the media failed to report this. The result is that the public are left with the impression acupuncture has a value – which was not in fact shown by the review in question.

In his own commentary on this issue, Andy Lewis notes placebo effects 'may indeed lead to genuine subjective improvements in the experience of pain and so lead to a better quality of life. However, placebo effects can also be little more than measurement artefacts. Patients may be inclined to report their pain less in order to reciprocate goodwill toward their acupuncturist. The expectations of improvement and natural desire to please may introduce bias in score results towards positive effects.'[6] Poor media reporting may introduce bias and has to be guarded against, as deliberate mis-representation might be involved.[7]

To date, much research on acupuncture is inconclusive – studies have not been placebo controlled and subjective bias could not be excluded.[8] Acupuncture has to be classified as an alternative medical system because of the fundamental belief of practitioners in meridians and in the manipulation of *ch'i* by needles. Neither meridians, *yin*, *yang*, nor the energy of *ch'i* have ever been identified or observed. They are entirely speculative and theories based on them are pseudo-scientific. They remain metaphysical concepts. Contrary to the claims of its proponents, acupuncture is not devoid of risks – there are reports of lung puncture and even death. Wheway and Ernst have identified 86 acupuncture related deaths between 1965 and 2009.[9] 'Although the risks are small – they could well outweigh the benefit, which is next to non-existent.'[10]

The patient advisory web site NHS Choices reviews the evidence for the usefulness of acupuncture and advises: 'In many conditions where acupuncture is used, there is not enough good quality evidence to draw any clear conclusions over its relative effectiveness compared with other treatments.'[11] So, the conclusion has to be that acupuncture has no worthwhile effect – application of the null hypothesis is how science works. Those less enamoured of the scientific method will disregard these conclusions.

The Oxford Centre for Evidence Based Medicine has updated its analysis of acupuncture for back pain – their verdict was: 'Clinical bottom line: Acupuncture is no better than a toothpick for treating back pain.'[12] The National Institute for Health and Clinical Evidence (NICE) advises acupuncture should not be used for nine stated conditions, including osteoarthritis, and that for chronic non-specific low back pain it can be 'considered'. As no evidence was offered that needling has a meaningful effect on such pain, such 'consideration' is simply to assuage patients' concerns and enhance placebo effects.

Belonetherapy
In order to distinguish 'acupuncture' with its esoteric and metaphysical connotations from techniques which really do cause the release of identifiable chemical mediators and initiate type II effects on disease, practitioners should style their practice in this domain not as 'acupuncture' but as 'belonetherapy', from *belone*, a surgeon's needle.[13]

Needling may generate beneficial neuro-chemicals, but the effects are not significantly greater than can be achieved by other placebos. Acupuncture and its mythical mystical *ch'i* generate placebo effects. Belonetherapy may produce type II effects but it will be scientists and belonetherapists who will fill the gaps in knowledge – not metaphysicians.

Endnotes to Chapter 13

1. Profs. David Colquhoun and Steve Novella. *Acupuncture is a Theatrical Placebo.* http://www.dcscience.net/Colquhoun-Novella-A&A-2013.pdf. and Journal of International Anaesthesia Research Society, June 2013 Vol. 116 No. 6.

2. John McLachlan. *Integrative medicine and the point of credulity.* BMJ 2010; 341:c6979.

3. Alexander C Ford, Nicholas J Talley, *Irritable Bowel Syndrome.* BMJ 2012;345:e5836. 8 September 2012.

4. In December 2012 the Royal College of Veterinary Surgeons found a member guilty of disgraceful conduct because she had performed acupuncture on a dog with renal failure. It seems animals have better protection from un-scientific practice than humans. Daily Telegraph, 29th November 2012.

5. Vickers A J, Cronin AM et al. *Acupuncture for Chronic Pain: Individual Patient Data Meta-Analysis.* Archives of Internal Medicine. Online September 10, 2012: doi:10.1001/archintermed.2012.3654.

6. Andy Lewis. www.Quackometer.net/blog/2012/09/spinning-acupuncture.

7. Yavchitz A, Boutron I, Bafeta A, Marroun I, Charles P, et al. (2012) *Misrepresentation of Randomized Controlled Trials in Press Releases and News Coverage: A Cohort Study.* PLoS Med 9(9): e1001308. doi:10.1371/journal.pmed.1001308.

8. Abi Tilu et al. *Effect of Acupuncture on Treatment of Heel Pain.* Acupuncture in Medicine 1998, Vol. 16, No.2. Includes studies on patients from the author's clinic.

9. Jayne Wheway, Ezard Ernst, *Patient Safety Incidents. Report to National Patient Safety Agency.* International Journal of Risk & Safety in Medicine, Vol. 24, No.3 2012. DOI:10.3233/JRS-2012-0569.

10. www.newscientist.co./article/dn22247-acupuncture-treatment-is-not-as-safe-as-advertised.

11. http://www.nhs.uk/conditions/Acupuncture/pages/evidence.aspx.

12. *Acupuncture for back pain*: http://www.medicine.ox.ac.uk/bandolier/booth/painpag/Chronrev/Other/acuback.html.

13. *Belone* is the word used by St. Luke the physician in the original gospel as written in Greek – when referring to the difficulty a camel might have passing through the eye of a

needle. Luke 18:25. Galen (130 AD) also used *belone.*

Chapter 14

House of Lords CAMs Groups Two and Three
Other Alternative Systems
Reiki, Johrei and 'Energy Therapies'

Love one another and help others to rise to the higher levels, simply by pouring out love. Love is infectious and the greatest healing energy.
Guru Sai Baba

The House of Lords identified a number of CAM systems as 'alternative disciplines and complementary therapies other than those professionally recognised.' Techniques range from manipulative therapy and 'bodywork' to energy medicine with emphasis on the mind/body/spirit triad. Examples of the more commonly encountered are considered in the next chapter. Here, some non-touch 'energy' therapies are reviewed. The scientific basis of the energies these practices employ is not explained, no such energies have been identified by reputable scientists, and claims for their use raises issues of quackery and fraud.

Reiki.

Mikao Usui (1865-1926)
Usui was a Japanese businessman and a Buddhist who also practised Shintoism. This spiritual system recognises *kami* – the spirits and deities of animals, trees and mountains. With historical records dating from the seventh century, Shinto folklore and mythology has led to a range of religious practices associated with nature and today is often combined with Buddhist ancestor worship (Japanese: *Shinto;* Way of the Gods from Chinese: *shin,* kami, spirits or deities + *dō (Tao)*, philosophical path, way, or study).
The details of the origin of Reiki are shrouded in mystery and have resulted in some dispute. In 1922 Usui encountered financial problems with his businesses, stepped back, and took a twenty one day Buddhist training course at a mountain retreat involving prayer, fasting and meditation. Usui had a mystical revelation which empowered him with energy and enabled him to develop his *Reiki Ryoho Gakkai* ('Spiritual Energy Therapy Society'). 'Reiki' is pronounced 'ray-kee'. Japanese: *rei,* soul, spirit + *ki* , vital energy. Chinese: *ch'i* or *qi*).

In 1923 an earthquake devastated the Kanto region of Japan including Tokyo and Yokohama. Up to 145,000 people were killed. There was a great demand for medical attention and for emotional and psychological support. Fully qualified medical practitioners were in short supply and given the demand for care, Usui quickly trained students in his methods of transmitting 'spiritual energy' to patients.

Two conventions have emerged – one based on the traditional Japanese practices and the other referred to as 'Western Reiki'. Many traditional Japanese practices reflect the spiritual development of its culture and the influence of Chinese and other Asian civilisations – *Chado,* the 'way of the Japanese Tea Ceremony' is underpinned by Buddhism. Some suggest that Usui's inner teachings are secret, hermetic, and known only to selected initiates. The principles however, are clear: the practitioner's hands are held on or near the patient in a variety of different positions and energy is channelled from practitioner to patient, activating natural healing processes at physical, mental, emotional and spiritual levels.

The nature of this energy has never been determined but it is obviously very powerful if it can affect diseased cells. There is concern that a slight malposition of the hands might cause damage. Institutions offering Reiki must have good health and safety procedures to ensure patients are not harmed by these powerful energies as there is no explanation as to how practitioners can switch them off. Interested camees must inquire further. So should health authorities and politicians who are concerned about healthcare safety.

Hawaiian born Madam Hawayo Takata (1990-1980) trained with Usui and then developed a different set of hand positions and a system which better suited Western patients and practitioners. *Usui Reiki Shiki Ryoho*, Usui's Spiritual Energy Style of Medical Treatment, was initially set up by Takata in the 1970s. Her fee for a course of study leading to the degree of Master and to 'call out a student's commitment and lead the student into a deeper understanding of the energy of money' was $10,000.

Reiki practitioners advance through three or four degrees of training before becoming a Master. In the first degree, most systems teach students to channel the 'energy' with hands placed on, or merely near, the patient, employing a series of up to fifteen positions over the course of an hour. In the second degree, the student learns to attune and send the Reiki energy to patients over significant distances in a process referred to as 'distant healing'. Some claim international distances can be covered. This may take twenty years of study. On passing the third degree (or fourth degree in some systems) the practitioner will be referred to as a 'Master' – as a teacher of other students (Old English: *magester,* from Latin: chief, head, teacher). At each level the student is given different symbols or talismans which assist the flow of energy. These are supposed to remain secret and only made available to students who have purchased appropriate courses. The Internet offers a number of websites which explain the various symbols, their meanings and their effects. None offer any evidence of how Reiki energy is activated by these symbols, or evidence of any activation. Reiki has been likened to extra-sensory perception or mindreading, with both the practitioner and patient becoming 'psychically attuned'.[1]

Some hold that Reiki energy itself is not a psychic force, others suggest that is precisely what it is. Some declare Reiki is not a religion – others, that sacred energy is released. Given there is no evidence for ESP or other such energies or forces, further consideration will not be given here, save to say the talismanic symbols appear to act as a 'trigger' in some subjects or students, in much the same way that some hypnotherapists use bright objects to aid concentration and focus imagination during hypnotic induction.[2]

Currently, Western Reiki teaches that the hand positions align the Reiki energy with the major 'meridian energy lines' as described in Chinese acupuncture or the seven 'chakras', described as vortices of energy in the early Hindu philosophical texts. These systems of energy have never been identified by scientific inquiry and there is no evidence they can be manipulated nor that they have any bearing on human health.[3] These energies appear to have no basis in reality and must therefore be regarded as speculative, imaginative and metaphysical. This is why systems of medicine based on them have to be termed 'alternative'. Either Reiki practitioners are using a form of energy quite unknown to science; or they are not, but not knowing this are deluded; or they are not, and knowing this, are quacks and charlatans and may be frauds and scamists. How are we to know which?

University College Hospital London has advertised for a practitioner who holds a 'Reiki Masters Certificate via the Usui system...salary up to £29,764.' The Royal London Hospital for Integrated Medicine also lists Reiki amongst the 'treatments' it offers. The RLHIM was formerly the Royal London Homeopathic Hospital, based on the UCH site. It should not to be confused with the Royal London Hospital itself. [4, 5]

Johrei /Jyorei

Mokichi Okada (1882–1955)

Initially Okada followed a Shinto sect Oomoto, a new Japanese religion founded in 1892. Okada made his fortune in the jewellery business, but after a divine revelation in 1926, founded his own Church of World Messianity in 1935. He went on to develop *Johrei* (Japanese: purification of the spirit/God's healing light): 'A healing ritual that channels divine light to dissolve the spiritual impurities that are the source of all physical, emotional, and personal problems...Johrei's blessings are even greater for the giver.'[6] The Mokichi Okada Association (MOA) was established in 1980 to continue his work 'toward the creation of a new civilization.' Okada's considerable art collection was left to MOA, now a wealthy organisation capable of funding travel expenses for supporters to attend its conferences.[7]

Ernst and colleagues have carried out a pilot trial aimed to identify any potential benefits of family-based Johrei practice in childhood eczema and for general health. 'There were no improvements on other outcomes measuring general health and psychological wellbeing of family members.'[8]

A recent Cochrane review found no evidence that Reiki has any effect on anxiety or depression.[9] If it is the case that Reiki, Johrei and other 'energy therapies' are capable of transferring energy from practitioner to patient, powerful enough to activate healing at physical as well as psychological levels, then the practices should comply with the full panoply of health and safety and other regulations designed to protect the patient against harm from advancing medical technology. If the energies are simply 'psychological', then treatment should be regarded as a form of psychotherapy and patients should be given this information clearly and in a manner they can comprehend, otherwise they are unable to give fully informed consent to have the treatment. The relevant health service authorities need to consider how they distinguish between a well-meaning, albeit deluded, practitioner – and a quack who is seeking to gain advantage and defraud. Patients, politicians and tax payers need assurance that health authorities are not complicit in deception, quackery or fraud.

Endnotes to Chapter 14

1. www.reikiann.com.
2. www.cedarseed.com/air/reiki.html and www.reiki-evolution.co.uk.

3. From Bronwen and Frans Stieine, *The Japanese Art of Reiki: A Practical Guide to Self-Healing.* O Books, Hampshire, UK, 2005, and William Rand, *Reiki, The Healing Touch.* Southfield, MI: Vision Publications, 1991. Also refer to: www.reikiassociation.org.uk and Sandi Leir-Shuffrey. *Get Started in Reiki.* McGraw Hill. 2010.

4.UCH Cancer Unit, advertisement, www. nfsh.org.uk, 2007, and Rose Shapiro, *Suckers,* Vintage Books 2009.

5.Why would the name of the Royal London Homeopathic Hospital be changed to one so closely similar to the other long standing and respected Royal London Hospital in Whitechapel unless it was intended that patients, practitioners and politicians would be misled?

6. http://www.jyorei.org

7. The sponsors of research into Johrei healing have provided business class flights to Japan for Dr Michael Dixon of the College of Medicine, his wife and three children. http://edzardernst.com/2015/05/johrei-healing-and-the-amazing-dr-dixon-presidential-candidate-for-the-rcgp/

8. Canter PH, Brown LB, Greaves C, Ernst E. *Johrei family healing: a pilot study.* Evidence Based Complementary & Alternative Medicine. 2006 Dec;3(4):533-40. E-pub 2006 Jul 21.

9. http://www.ncbi.nlm.nih.gov/pubmed/25835541

Chapter 15

Other Alternative Systems

A merry heart doeth good like medicine.
King Solomon

Of several remedies, the physician should choose the least sensational.
Hippocrates

In 2000 the House of Lords Select Committee on Science and Technology reported on Supplementary, Complementary, and Alternative Medicine. Three groups of CAM systems were identified. Those 'energy therapies' in group one and group two are considered in earlier chapters. This chapter reviews other CAMs classified as 'alternative disciplines and complementary therapies other than those professionally recognised', together with some disciplines from the Foundation for Integrated Health's former web site. Some have developed as distinct medical systems and as alternatives to evidence-based scientific medicine. Techniques range from manipulative therapy, to breath work and energy medicine, commonly with emphasis on the mind/body/spirit triad. Many camists claim to be able to manipulate energy fields that affect the health of their patients. There is no plausible explanation for the basis of the energies these practices employ.

Many patients are satisfied that camists provide benefit. 'I saw conventional doctors for many years and also tried many alternative therapies until I discovered z-therapy. I have been better ever since.' Fair enough, we can be delighted for such patients – but there is no evidence z-therapy works any better than placebos and even intractable conditions may enter spontaneous remission eventually. Those patients who have been treated but not benefited from z-therapy are conveniently overlooked and not reported on. One patient's anecdote does not constitute sufficient evidence to direct treatment for others. Z-therapy works for a given patient because the neurochemicals released during the therapeutic relationship and by the treatment create brain patterns particular to that individual patient. Those are insufficient grounds on which to move z-therapy from the category of 'complementary and alternative'.

Examples of the House of Lords
CAM Groups Two and Three and 'other disciplines'

Thomsonism
Samuel Thomson (1769-1843) was born into a farming family in New Hampshire. As a boy he gave wild Lobelia to his playmates 'merely by way of sport to see them vomit.' In 1790 his wife became seriously ill and local doctors were unable to help. Two herbalists had more success, and Thompson became disenchanted with orthodox medicine.

Receiving further instruction from a local wise woman, Thomson developed his own medical system based on herbs and the principle that 'toxins' (which he did not define) should be removed by herbal emetics and purgatives. Orthodox practice was comparable but used relatively large doses which had significant effects. Thomson's herbs were less toxic and more gentle. He subsequently claimed a patent for 'the exclusive right of using lobelia for medical purposes.' At that time there was no effective system for licensing doctors to practice, and although Thomson was not qualified by having an education and degree in medicine, his ministrations became widely sought, evolving into a crusade. He avoided bloodletting, which was then the staple of the orthodox armamentarium although he based his theories of disease and therapies on Galen's humoral principles. Diseases caused a patient to be 'hot' or 'cold' and appropriate herbs and spices such as peppers and bitters would enable a balance. Unlike apothecaries, he did not actually analyse what the therapeutically active components of the herbs were. Pharmaceutical manufacturers now know the formulae of capsaicin, opium and other plants and offer the active chemicals in refined form.

In the pioneer spirit of egalitarianism and freedom of expression which underpinned the new United States, many Americans, particularly in rural areas, were content to turn to practitioners such as Thompson as an alternative to the orthodox. Frequently they had no choice.

Thomson set out his *New Guide to Health; or Botanic Family Physician* in 1822, and developed a large business selling his patented remedies. He trained other practitioners in his system, but would have nothing to do with orthodox doctors whom he regarded with contempt. Eventually this arrogance led to a parting of company with many of his own students who founded the Independent Thomsonian Medical Society which evolved as Eclectic Medicine. After a few years of illness Thompson 'passed from life heroically partaking of lobelia, enemas, and the recognised Thomsonian syrups and teas.'[1]

Eclectic Medicine

Based on Thompson's methods, this development also included an understanding of medicinal plants used by the Native Americans. The Eclectics themselves were qualified doctors who chose whichever medical system might best suit the patient, but with emphasis on nature and herbal remedies (Greek: *eklektos*, selected – hence physicians who choose from diverse sources). The Eclectic Medical Institute was established in Ohio in 1830.

Eclectics tended to avoid expensive and powerful purgatives, often mercury-based, and they rarely used bloodletting. Eclectic Medicine became more popular as the authority of orthodox doctors waned. Unlike Thomson, the Eclectics studied physiology and pharmacology. The Flexner report of 1918 reviewed all medical schools in the United States, but the Eclectic schools were not accredited. There has been criticism that this was largely because the American Medical Association supported medical schools which supported pharmaceutical medicine and by inference, were supported in turn by the pharmaceutical industry. The Eclectics' vitalist philosophy and herbalism was not regarded as orthodox.

In 1934 the president of the Eclectic Medical Association expressed concern at the challenges facing that system of medicine. 'We must choose between being absorbed by the dominant section, subject to the approval of an unfriendly, prejudiced, self constituted authority ... or adapt ourselves to the general social change and retain the old eclectic values of individual freedom of thought and action, independence of practice and the right to use that which has stood the test of experience in our service to mankind.'² The last Eclectic medical school closed in 1939. Eclectic Medicine is still practised – by herbalists rather than doctors.

Spondylotherapy

Dr Albert Abrams (c.1863-1924) wrote *Spondylotherapy: Spinal Concussion and the Application of Other methods to the Spine in the Treatment of Disease* in 1910. (Greek: *spondulos,* vertebra of the spinal column). The American Journal of Medical Sciences offered a review suggesting: 'This is rather a curious book which has not altogether repaid the time spent in its perusal.'

Being inspired by chiropractic, Abrams described how, by placing a block of wood against the vertebral spinous processes and then pounding it with a hammer, the subluxations described by D.D. Palmer could be adjusted. For a time these methods were enthusiastically taken up by many chiropractors.

Radionics

Albert Abrams then moved away from the mechanical into the realm of electronics and 'energy medicine' and invented a number of machines for diagnosis and cure. No plausible evidence of benefit could be identified and many doctors alleged Abrams was being intentionally deceptive. That is, he was a quack and fraud.

Abrams claimed to have registered as a student of the Cooper Medical College, San Francisco, in 1881, being awarded an MD in 1883, although his regular attendance seems doubtful. He was on the staff at the college between 1885 and 1898 when 'Dr Abrams submitted his resignation and it was accepted without the usual expression of appreciation for prior services. The records of the College contain no information as to the reasons for the resignation. However, considering the nature of Dr Abrams' practice, it can be assumed that he was requested to resign. Cooper College was subsequently taken over by Stanford Medical School.'³ His claim to have qualified in medicine at the University of Heidelberg was simply false. Dr Ray Wilbur recalled:

> It was during my student days at Cooper I made my first personal acquaintance with a quack, Albert Abrams, then (unfortunately) Professor of Pathology, until his connection with the college was severed. Abrams became one of the most sensational medical characters of the early 1900's. He had an electrical machine with which he claimed to diagnose almost every ailment. It was known as the Magic or Black Box. He was so plausible and those interested in him so guileless and gullible that he made quite a stir. He was a complete and total fraud.

Adams' ridiculous paraphernalia and preposterous claims were exposed by the *Journal of the American Medical Association* and the *Scientific American:*

> Dr Albert Abrams is the latest rocket to blaze a somewhat polychromatic course across the firmament of pseudo-medicine. He claims to have evolved a system of abdominal percussion from which he derives what he is pleased to term the "Electronic Reactions of Abrams". By means of this system Abrams claims he can

diagnose the sex, race and disease of a patient that he has never seen and who does not need to be present. All Abrams needs is a sample of blood from the patient.... the mysterious energy sets up a mysterious electronic emanation which may be detected by percussing the subjects abdomen.[4]

The black boxes were not for sale but could be leased – the contract confirming it would never be opened. Opening any of Abram's boxes damaged the sensitive internal electronics and they ceased to work. Or so he claimed. The History of Stanford Medical School reports:

> By 1923, thousands of American doctors and imposters were dabbling in "electronic medicine" which had many manifestations; chief among them was the Abrams cult. The mystique of the bogus technology made it a simple matter for the unscrupulous practitioners of this thriving fad to dupe and defraud the credulous public. The extravagant aura of science and progress at the time gave free range to idiotic ideas...Medical imposters have always victimised the public, and "other than science-based systems of medicine" will always persist because of their peculiar emotional appeal, and in spite of their nonsensical basis. Abrams phenomenal success over a period of twenty years was based on his ability to convince his followers and hordes of patients that his pseudoscience was at the forefront of the medical renaissance then clearly in progress. Scientific American found: "The claims are not substantiated and have no basis in fact. They are merely products of the Abrams practitioner's mind. At best, it is all an illusion. At worst it is a colossal fraud." [5]

More than fifty different devices and hyperbolic names were developed on Abrams' themes. 'Radionics' became a style used by many. Practitioners sometimes used a pendulum held over a sample of hair, termed a 'witness', and watched for different movements indicating 'yes' or 'no' to questions asked – an example of the ideomotor effect used in pendulum dowsing by many camists, and magicians. The box was not connected to a source of electricity, but relied on the 'universal energy grid'.[6] The Radionics box was banned by the US Federal Drugs Administration in 1958, and criminal charges were laid against the Electronic Medical Foundation in 1961.

The principle of a 'black box' was taken up by others. Dr William Ernest Boyd qualified conventionally from Glasgow, practiced as a homeopath, and devised a box to diagnose and proscribe which homeopathic remedy should be used. Naturopath and chiropractor Ruth Drown invented a device claimed to be capable of transmitting healing energy across vast distances. British radionics enthusiast George De La Warr used a form of Drown's box which certainly looked impressive, but its many dials and rubbing plates served no useful function.

American chiropractor Irwing N. Toftness, developed his version of the Black Box in 1936. In 1982 the US District Court of Wisconsin prohibited any use of the Toftness Radiation Detector as such devices were deemed 'in violation of the Food, Drug, and Cosmetic Act.' A permanent nationwide injunction against use of any TRD or similar device was issued, although some chiropractors developed alternatives. In

1984 the US Supreme Court denied an appeal to hear the case and all chiropractors using the detector were instructed to return the devices.[7] The Toftness School of Chiropractic was inherited by his nephew and as recently as August 2013 was fined $50,000 for shipping unlicensed medical equipment in interstate commerce.[8]

Chiropractor and psychotherapist Volney Mathison invented the 'The Mathison Model B Electropsychometer' or 'E-meter'. The measurement of small voltages passing through the hands of a subject holding two terminals was claimed to indicate aspects of their personality. Subsequently taken up by science fiction writer L. Ron Hubbard, who developed the psychological healing modality of *Dianetics* in the 1940's, E-Meters currently cost about $4000.[9]

The Radionic Association (UK) currently describes Radionics as: 'A healing technique in which our natural intuitive faculties are used both to discover the energetic disturbances underlying illness and to encourage return of a normal energetic field that supports health. It is independent of the distance between practitioner and patient. Radionics can be used to help humans and animals in agriculture....the name reflects the view of early practitioners that they were "broadcasting" healing, but we now believe that radionics treatment occurs at a level of reality where there is no distance between us. This is a challenging concept, but it is entirely compatible with modern physics and also with the ancient mystic teaching that at some level we are all one, and that at this level, exchanges of healing energy can occur.'

Naturopathy
A wide variety of different systems of medicine, remedy and cure were available in Europe during the 19th century. Many set aside the heroic treatments of conventional physicians, and identified natural ways to achieve and maintain good health. Those orthodox heroic treatments had involved bloodletting and purging which we would today regard as quite negligent. Nevertheless, slowly and with the application of the scientific method, those practices were abandoned. Meanwhile many other systems developed, promoted by practitioners without regular formal qualifications. Most sought to treat the whole person as mind, body and spirit – emphasising how in various ways an innate natural 'vital force' could enable patients to heal themselves. Proponents adopted a decidedly commercial approach.

Many patients wanted a more 'natural' approach, though they could not always clearly articulate why – it just seemed like a good idea.

Amongst the purest of natural resources is water – used as a component in the care and treatment of patients since time immemorial. Hippocrates recommended the 'qualities of the waters' both internally and for therapeutic baths. Various techniques have been formalised and promoted down the centuries, though without scientifically derived evidence for effect on specific diseases. No doubt pampering and attention was pleasurable and patients felt benefit. Diverse cures involving water together with natural herbs, diet, good nutrition, clean air, light and hygiene evolved. Practices included cold baths, hot tubs, saunas, showers, wraps, and colonic irrigation.

Siegmund Hahn (1696-1773) and his son Johann were physicians and pioneers of 'nature care' in Germany. Johann's book *'Lessons of the Power and Effects of fresh water in the bodies of the people'* (1738) laid down the principles of 'hydrotherapy'. Vincent Priessnitz (1799-1852), a farmer in Gräfenberg, Austrian Silesia, developed similar treatments to the Hahns' using nothing except cold water, a simple diet and exercise – a system of medicine alternative to the mainstream that became known as the 'Nature Cure'. Priessnitz became famous throughout Europe and his ideas were taken up by many spas and health resorts. In the UK twenty 'hydropathic' facilities were eventually constructed. There are now just two. Priessnitz died at the age of 52, exhausted from his own water cures.

Arnold Riki (1824-1897) added sun baths to the regime. Adolf Just published *Return to Nature in* 1896 and opened a retreat in the Hartz Mountains, the better to enable clients to commune with nature. Louis Kuhne of Leipzig published *The New Science of Healing* in 1899. He was a strict vegetarian who also forbid salt and sugar, believing that the cause of disease was a surfeit of 'toxins'. The term *Lebensreform* (life-reform) appeared in1896 to describe these various developments, which amounted to a rebellion against scientific-based medical practice. Richard Ungewitter's 1904 book *Nakedness* added naturalism to the naturopathic mix. In 1944 Mahatma Gandhi opened his Nature Cure Sanitarium in Poona, based on Just's retreat.

Father Sebastian Kneipp (1824-1897), emphasised the importance of achieving a balance between work and leisure and considered the effects of stress, social circumstances and emotions on health. This is not so different from today's emphasis on 'person centred medicine', though PCM tries to base its principles and practice on the scientific method, and expects some scientifically credible evidence of beneficial outcomes – not simply anecdotes. Kneipp developed a number of healthcare products, herbal remedies, calisthenics and methods of hydrotherapy. The holistic 'Kneipp Kur' is now recognised for health reimbursement in Germany. Kneipp Bread is still very popular in Norway and today's Kneipp Group sells more than two hundred different phytomedicines, nutritional supplements, body care and bath products.[10]

Benedict Lust, born in Baden, emigrated to the United States in 1892. He returned to Germany severely affected by tuberculosis and sought the water cure from Father Kneipp. He recovered, and Kneipp persuaded him to settle in the United States to promote his merchandise, along with hydrotherapy. Lust established a health food store in New York to sell Kneipp products and the books of Kuhne and Just. There he met John Scheel, a homoeopath who was also using hydrotherapy, and who had trademarked the term *'Naturopathy'* in 1895. Lust qualified as a homoeopath from the New York Homoeopathic Medical College in 1901, though it is said he was ridiculed for his beliefs in 'natural medicine'. He went on to qualify as an osteopath and then purchased the rights to the name 'Naturopathy' in 1902, opening the American School of Naturopathy to train other homeopaths, osteopaths and chiropractors in these new principles of nature cure. This included a Department of Astroscopy to explore the effects of astrological determinants on disease.

Lust published the *Universal Naturopathic Encyclopaedia for Drugless Therapy* and the magazine *Nature's Path*. Apart from healthcare methods originating in Europe, he introduced Ayurvedic medicine and Yoga to America and established health resorts in New Jersey and Florida. Lust thought of Naturopathy as a way of life, a belief system, philosophy and a system of healing alternative to conventional medicine. He emphasised the importance of prevention of disease and promotion of health: 'We plead for the renouncing of poisons from the coffee, white flour, glucose, lard, and like venom of the American table, and of patent medicines, tobacco, liquor and the other inevitable recourse of perverted appetite. Naturopathy stands for the reconciling, harmonizing and unifying of nature, humanity, and God.'[11]

As the 20th century moved on, scientific evidence-based conventional medicine developed better and more clearly effective therapies for many problems. The best principles of Naturopathy became incorporated into the orthodox practice of doctors and nurses. The medical profession expects those who wish to practice medicine and become 'doctors' to train and qualify as such. Some Naturopaths have a college education, but many do not. Many exhibit a lack of scientific rigour and appear unable to critically analyse the wide variety of treatments and therapies practised under the banner of 'Naturopathy'.

Naturopathy remains wedded to the principles that 'the body can heal itself due to a vital life force'. The body can heal, but not due to any 'vital force' for which there is no evidence. A naturopath's task is to enhance healing by using natural non-toxic therapies. 'Harmony', 'balance', 'energy', 'detoxification' are prevalent. Many naturopaths believe that diseases, including cancer, are caused by faulty immune systems. Many naturopaths oppose vaccination and recommend avoidance of pharmaceuticals. Some prescribe and sell unnecessary supplements as remedies.

Today, 'Naturopathy' covers a wide range of alternative therapies and is described by the UK General Naturopathic Council:

> The Naturopathic Practitioner makes use of supportive physical forces and agents such as: light, water, air, thermal effects, magnetism, Earth, electricity or vibration; and seeks to harness the patient's own life force more directly with massage, through rest, by exercise, by stimulating reflexes, by making dietary prescriptions, by psychotherapeutic interventions or by employing the patient's own heterostatic capacity. The Naturopathic Practitioner may achieve alternative effects by a number of therapeutic approaches, for example: acupressure, acupuncture, colonic hydrotherapy, homeopathy, hydrotherapy, iridology, kinesiology, massage therapy, nutritional therapy, osseous manipulative therapy, phytotherapy (herbal medicine).[12]

The University of Maryland Medical Center escribes naturopathy, or naturopathic medicine as: 'A system of medicine based on the healing power of nature. Naturopathy is a holistic system, meaning that naturopathic doctors strive to find

221

the cause of disease by understanding the body, mind, and spirit of the person.' If that doesn't sound very scientific, naturopaths agree. In one revealing interview, naturopathic oncologist Daniel Rubin states: 'One of the greatest challenges we face as naturopaths is the widespread public belief in the scientific method.'

In 2013 the UK College of Naturopathic Medicine claimed on its website that 'By using natural therapies (a naturopath) is able to treat both acute and chronic ailments successfully.' Additionally the website implied that practitioners were physicians. In the UK, only doctors registered with the GMC can claim that status. The Advertising Standards Authority found no evidence to support the contention that naturopathy could treat medical conditions nor that naturopaths 'were medical professionals suitably qualified to diagnose and treat disease'. The ASA upheld complaints that these claims were misleading and required them to be removed.

Naturopathy remains an alternative health system to medicine, though given the 'freedoms' offered in the US, some states licence naturopaths as 'doctors'. Naturopaths who seriously wish to become doctors should be encouraged to qualify in the conventional manner, and then take every advantage of those elements of naturopathy which have a credible evidence base such as promotion of a healthy diet and exercise. Conventional doctors could do more to use techniques of support and provide consolation, hope and love, but they do not need to integrate COM with metaphysical CAM belief systems. If regular doctors do wish to employ alternative methods for which there is no evidence of benefit (other than anecdotal and that due to placebo) they must expect to have obtained fully informed consent and to be accountable.

Naprapathy

'Dr' Oakley Smith, started out as a student of orthodox medicine and then considered osteopathy before qualifying as a chiropractor. Like many chiropractors he sought to develop wholly new concepts of healing. He rejected Palmer's notion of vertebral subluxation, laying emphasis instead on his own doctrine of disease based on 'connective tissue.' He claimed 'ligatite' causes tension in connective tissue and therefore structural imbalance. Whilst travelling in Czechoslovakia he studied a system of manual connective tissue techniques which were similar to his own. Smith styled his system as *Naprapathy,* founding the American Naprapathic Association in 1907 (Czech: *náprava,* correction). Naprapaths claim to remove blockages to the natural flow of blood, lymph and nervous transmission and thence to improve health. Scientific evidence supporting these claims is awaited. Naprapaths are licensed to practice as 'doctors' in Iowa. Some who value the influence of the Orient now refer to Naprapathy as *Tui Na* (Chinese: push and grasp), a form of massage which seeks balance by acting on 'eight gates', *meridians* and *chi* [13]

'Dr' Harlan Tarbell (1890-1960) who is best known for having created the classic *Tarbell Course in Magic* in the 1930's, originally qualified as a naprapath. Hence his title of Doctor of Naprapathy. Ever the illusionist. When teaching magic he emphasised 'there is a big difference between a magician and a man who does tricks

... fundamentally the making of a magician is no different than the making of other professional people. One must be trained in the mechanics, the alternate methods and be skilled in the presentation in order to meet any conditions which may arise.' These considerations very much apply in medicine, both orthodox and alternative. No doubt Tarbell's experience in dealing with patients as a naprapath contributed to his undoubted skills in reading body language, using sleight of hand and sleight of tongue for deception and misdirection in his career as a magician.[14]

McTimoney Chiropractic
John McTimoney (1914-1980) was born in Birmingham, UK, and trained at the Birmingham School of Art. McTimoney became a jeweller and technical illustrator, though he often said he would love to have been a doctor. [15]

In 1942 McTimoney was treated by a chiropractor who had trained with D.D. Palmer. Being impressed by that system, McTimoney trained for three years with another of Palmer's students and after examination by two 'doctors of chiropractic', was granted a qualification by the Palmer College in 1950. He developed Palmer's system and went on to found the McTimoney College of Chiropractic near Oxford in 1972. The College is in competition for students in the UK with the Anglo-European College of Chiropractic based in Bournemouth. The McTimoney Chiropractic Association was founded in 1979 rivalling the British Chiropractic Association. When the UK Register of Chiropractors was created in 1999, many McTimoney practitioners declined to join. Those who are not registered are no longer legally allowed to style and market themselves as 'chiropractor' and instead now use 'spinal therapist' or similar designations. One wonders why John McTimoney's name is to be seen on the 'Wall of Honour' at the Royal Society of Medicine.

Cranial Osteopathy and Craniosacral Therapy
Many osteopaths and chiropractors have developed their own manual therapy techniques, and schools to teach their idiosyncratic methods. Parallels can be seen with a wide range of 'body work' techniques including reflexology, reiki, therapeutic touch.

William Garner Sutherland (1873-1954) developed 'Osteopathy in the Cranial Field' (OCF) in 1899. Sutherland honed his sense of touch – his 'thinking fingers' – to such an extent he claimed he could feel changes in the shape of the bones of the skull, and later, other soft tissues. After compressing his own head he had severe psychological and physical reactions, but he was able to identify an 'involuntary mechanism' represented by a deep pulse through the body. He determined that this 'Primary Respiratory Mechanism' was the cause of dysfunction and disease and devised methods of massage to effect correction by freeing up passages through which the cerebrospinal fluid bathes the brain and spinal cord. These ideas reflected Swedenborg's (inaccurate) accounts of brain physiology.[16] The American School of Osteopathy created a course to teach OCF and the practice became known as 'cranial osteopathy'.

223

John Upledger (1932-2012), also an osteopath, studied Sutherland's theories, and carried out research to demonstrate cranial bone movement and pulse. He then claimed to have discovered a 'dural pulse' and established a practice he coined as 'Cranio-Sacral Therapy.' He also developed Somato-Emotional Release.

That work has not been regarded as being of sufficient quality to be accepted by mainstream neurologists, neuro-surgeons, orthopaedic surgeons, cranial anatomists or pathologists. The joints between cranial bones (sutures) are fused and immobile in adults, and take considerable force to move in children. Though why anyone would want to move bones of the skull, unless treating a case of trauma is beyond comprehension.

CST is based on the notion that there is a rhythmic impulse in the flow of the fluid that surrounds the brain and spinal cord, that diseases can be diagnosed by detecting aberrations in this rhythm and can be corrected by manipulating or lightly touching the skull. There is no plausible evidence that 'the gentle application of manual force' on the skull influences the course of somatic diseases in distant body systems. In 1999, after a meta-analysis of published studies, the British Columbia Office of Health Technology Assessment concluded that CST's theory is invalid and that practitioners cannot reliably measure what they claim to be modifying. There was 'insufficient scientific evidence to recommend Cranio-Sacral Therapy to patients, practitioners, or third party payers for any clinical condition. CST may induce a sense of deep relaxation or feeling light headed, as if they have been hypnotised – probably as a result of activation of the endocannabinoids system.' [17] Why 'as if hypnotised'? The mechanism is surely that of hypnosis. Just as occurs with any type I placebo effect resulting from a constructive therapeutic encounter with an empathic practitioner.

Today, Cranio-Sacral Therapy is practised by osteopaths, chiropractors, and naturopaths, as well as CST practitioners and quacks. It might be thought only patients with a particular interest would become involved, but the public are now being inveigled to offer endorsement through their laudable funding of charities such as the Royal Navy and Royal Marines Childrens' Fund. This recommends CST for the management of service personnel and their families suffering from post-traumatic stress syndrome, and actively raises funds for that purpose from the public. The charity should bear the opinion of Professor Edzard Ernst in mind: 'The notion that CST is associated with more than non-specific effects is not based on evidence.' [18]

Charities need to exercise critical analysis and be duly cautious of accepting implausible claims. They also need to be more circumspect in spending their charitable funds on implausible treatments. In 2011 The College of Medicine had its inaugural Conference at a venue arranged through a CST therapist who also delivered the opening address.

Shiatsu

By the turn of the first millennium, the underlying techniques of Japanese massage were mystical, often carried out by blind practitioners, *anma,* who incorporated elements of Chinese practice such as acupuncture. Tenpaku Tamai set down The modern principles of *Shiatsu Ryoho* in 1915 (Japanese: finger pressure way of healing). The Japanese Shiatsu College was founded by Tokujiro Namikoshi in 1940. In 1953, Namikoshi encouraged The Palmer College of Chiropractic to teach his methods. The Japanese authorities gave official recognition to Shiatsu in 1957. Today in Japan all practitioners must be licensed by the Japanese Ministry of Health.

There are currently two main schools of Shiatsu. The Zen style is based on traditional Chinese medicine including concepts of balancing life forces of *yin* and *yang.* Namikoshi's style also seeks to achieve a balance but additionally incorporates Western concepts of anatomy and physiology – rejecting *chi* and *meridians.* As with so many other CAMs, a plethora of variants on these two principal themes have developed and been promoted. Many involve 'bodywork' with meridians syncretised with Chinese *I-Ching,* the Book of Changes. Others lay emphasis on emotional work (*Shiatsu Yasuragi*), relate to Indian Tantric practice (*Tansu*) and other energy systems such as *Feng Shui.*

The practitioner is expected to diagnose diseases by touch and by feeling 'energy imbalances'. A skilled practitioner can identify sources of disharmony and then apply appropriate massage to achieve balance. The Shiatsu Society says the objective is to 'strengthen the body's natural ability to heal imbalance itself. It works on the whole person not just physical body, but also on a psychological, emotional, and spiritual being.'[19]

The Shiatsu Society UK reviewed outcome studies of Shiatsu in 2006 but found a lack of control and the blinding necessary for a formal scientific appraisal. There is no evidence that Shiatsu can treat any specific disease or provide more benefit than any other massage system.[20]

Qi Gong (Qigong or Ch'i kung)

Chinese: *Qi* or *ch'i* (pronounced 'chee'), 'breathing/ air' and 'the focus point for vital energy and spirit'+ *Gong,* 'force or power'. When combined: 'the manipulation of intrinsic energy within living organisms', and thus a system of medicine.[21] Qi Gong is practiced today in various forms, but all take their origin from the *Book or Canon of Internal Medicine* attributed to the Yellow Emperor Huang Di, the ancestor of the Huaxia Chinese, and founder of the Chinese civilisation. Styled 'Yellow' from his traditional, possibly mythical, birthplace near the Yellow river, tradition suggests he reigned from about 2697 to 2597 BC.[22]

Originally Chinese medical systems developed with shamanistic rituals, meditation and physical exercise. These evolved and became incorporated with religious beliefs such as Taoism. Four principle themes have emerged: Traditional Chinese Medicine applies the practice of Qi Gong in patient care; Chinese martial artists use

225

it to bring additional focus and 'energy' to their combative skills; both Taoists and Buddhists use Qi Gong to assist meditation; and Chinese moral philosophers apply Qi Gong as a fundamental principle in seeking harmony of *yin* and *yang*. At the time of the Cultural Revolution politicians sought to integrate these various themes as one system on a scientific basis. They were unsuccessful.

As a system of medicine, Qi Gong can comprise any of the four principal themes. Given the paucity of scientific evidence of effectiveness, other than anecdotal reports from patients that they have gained 'benefit', Qi Gong is regarded as being based on pseudoscience and remains an alternative medical system.

T'ai Chi Ch'uan

'Supreme Ultimate Fist' originated as a martial art, and finds expression in many ways, but is most usually seen today as a gentle exercise method based on based on posture, coordination and relaxation with elements of meditative calm. Exercise can raise arterial blood pressure, but the gentle exercise of T'ai Chi has been shown to lower it, improving health and psychological wellbeing. It is particularly suitable for the elderly.

Here 'chi' refers to the 'ultimate' and not the *ch'i* of the metaphysical 'vital force', which has never been identified physically. *Taiji* is the 'supreme ultimate', *wuji* – 'without ultimate, infinite'. In much Chinese and Taoist philosophy the symbol or diagram of 'ultimate power' is the circle divided into black and white halves by a curved line, and having a black or white dot on the contrasting halves. The *Taijitu*, represents the balance and harmony of *ying* and *yang*. 'The soft and pliable will defeat the hard and strong.'[23]

The underlying philosophy of T'ai Chi remains metaphysical and its theories are un-scientific, but the practice as it has developed during the twentieth century is of physiological benefit to stress management. T'ai Chi offers heightened expectances and enhanced placebo effects.[24]

Sceptics may think of these various Oriental techniques as *Fi Shi*.

Therapeutic Touch

'Touch' has been used to deal with disease for millennia. 'The Royal Touch' was credited with curing many cases of scrofula from the 11th to 16th centuries, but was then abandoned as the Enlightenment took force. During the 1970s Dr Dolores Krieger PhD, a registered nurse in New York, promoted 'health' as a harmonious relationship between an individual and the environment. She postulated that there exists a 'Human Energy Field' in which we all live and which can be manipulated by touch or even hands being placed near an individual. 'Healing' consists of using this method to re-channel the vital force and a healthy practitioner can transmit vital *pranic* energy to a patient. Martha Rogers, then Dean of Nursing at New York University, asserted that humans are themselves 'energy fields' and this accounts for the healers' ability to transmit forces. These ideas parallel the wisdom of ancient healers, Mesmer's animal magnetism ('everything in nature has a communication by a universal fluid, in which all bodies are plunged'), cranio-sacral therapy ('attunes subtle rhythms in the cerebro-spinal fluid') and Reiki ('spiritual energy can be transmitted').

Dora Kunz, President of the Theosophical Society, helped Krieger develop what has come to be styled as 'Therapeutic Touch'. TT purports to be 'scientific' – the alternate term 'laying on of hands' was deemed too mystical and redolent of faith healing. Many patients do 'feel better' after a consultation with such attentive caring practitioners and may feel warmth and other parathesiae during the 'therapy'. TT 'works' by type I placebo effects – and very comforting too. However, the human energy fields remain to be discovered and no TT practitioner has ever been able to identify such a field. No type II effects have ever been demonstrated. The James Randi foundation has offered $1.1 million to anyone who can demonstrate a human energy field. Only one person has taken up the challenge, and she failed. Although no such 'energy field' has been demonstrated, questions as to how such practices are to be distinguished from quackery and fraud remain unanswered.

An investigation published in the Journal of the American Medical Association concluded that 'Twenty-one experienced TT practitioners were unable to detect the investigator's 'energy field'. Their failure to substantiate TT's most fundamental claim is unrefuted evidence that the claims of TT are groundless and that further professional use is unjustified.'[25]

In a video offered on the internet by the College of Medicine, Dr Robin Youngson has revealed more of the value of therapeutic touch, claiming haemoglobin levels can be affected. No plausible objective evidence is offered.[26] Is that quackery? You must be the judge.

Alexander Technique
Frederick Matthias Alexander (1869-1955) was born in Tasmania and developed a career as an actor and orator in Australia. This was threatened during the 1890's when he began losing his voice and could find no cure from voice coaches or doctors. The Society of Teachers of Alexander Technique note that: 'It gradually became clear to him that stiffening his neck was part of a bigger pattern of tension involving the whole of his body. This tension pattern manifested itself at the mere thought of reciting.'[27] The possibility of a psychosomatic cause or variety of 'stage fright' appears not to have been further considered.

Alexander determined his posture and the tension in muscles and tendons required retraining. Not only did his voice improve but also symptoms of asthma. He opened a practice in London in 1904 to treat patients with similar problems and in 1931 founded a three-year training course for students of his technique. He published a number of books on his ideas and proposals – *The Use of Self* (1932) was particularly popular.

227

One of his first students was Irene Tasker who then set up a school to teach the technique to children in South Africa. In 1943 there was praise for Alexander's technique at the Transvaal Teachers Association meeting, with criticism of physical education methods then being used by Dr Ernst Jokl, the Government's Director of Physical Education. Jokal was not amused and went on to publish *'Quackery Versus Physical Education'* which described Alexander's methods as 'a dangerous and irresponsible form of quackery'. Alexander sued for libel.[28]

The legal defence team made much of of Alexander's claims that his method of gaining psycho-physical guidance under conscious control could render patients free of much disease. These claims were held to be preposterous. Nevertheless Alexander won the case with damages and costs. An appeal was lost, again with costs awarded to Alexander.

Alexander's principles were educational rather than medical, and only termed 'Technique' after his death. Specific exercises are not taught but rather clients learned to respond and react spontaneously to the various stresses of their lives and activity by 'constructive conscious control', and by 'end-gaining'- focusing on desired goals. Using the Technique does not cure or treat disease as such, but helps patients cope with difficulties of breathing, stress, and musculoskeletal problems such as back pain and arthritis. Nevertheless, some practitioners have now moved from educating the body to treating diseases. In 2008, the British Medical Journal reported a randomised trial which suggested significant improvement in low back pain with the use of AT. This trial was not placebo controlled – patients might have recovered in any event, with other forms of therapy or were simply reporting placebo effects.[29] There is no plausible evidence that specific diseases can be affected and that means AT has to be classified as a CAM.

Rolfing
Dr Ida Pauline Rolf (1896 -1979) was concerned that chronically disabled patients were not receiving treatment they needed and in the 1920's developed a system which she originally called *Postural Release* and later, *Structural Integration*. Her PhD in biochemistry entitled her to be styled 'Dr' although she never qualified in orthodox medicine.

After leaving the US in the 1920's Rolf studied homeopathy in Geneva and 'embraced a wide range of approaches including osteopathy, chiropractic medicine and disciplines of the mind including yoga and Korzybski's study of consciousness.'[30] Alfred Korzybski believed that the extent of knowledge is limited by both the nervous system and the structure of language, due to the 'consciousness of abstracting'. His ideas also influenced many science fiction writers including L. Ron Hubbard who founded *Dianetics* in the 1940's. Rolf founded the Guild for Structural Integration in the 1970's, devising a system of stretching and manipulation to help people achieve yoga positions. Her techniques to loosen the fascia which covers muscles became known as 'Rolfing'.

In the 1950's Rolf taught osteopaths in England, where she was a guest of John Bennett, a mystic and student of George Gurdjieff, a spiritual teacher of *The Fourth Way.* This offered a means of increasing self-awareness. By the 60's Rolf had returned to California and the Esalen Institute where Gestalt Therapy and Eastern thought were the order of the day. *Rolfing: The Integration of Human Structures* sets out her views as to how direct intervention by her methods can affect the evolution of the human species.[31] Normally ten sessions, each lasting an hour, will enable this integration. Some practitioners are gentler than others! There is no evidence-based published research to support use of the technique in any specific disease group.[32]

Bowen Technique

Thomas Bowen (1916-1982) was born in Victoria, Australia, to parents having emigrated from Wolverhampton. He went on to be actively involved in the Salvation Army. For many years, he was a general hand in a cement works, but over time developed a technique for dealing with the musculoskeletal problems of his colleagues.

Being profoundly deaf, Bowen did not talk much with patients and often saw up to fifteen patients an hour. They were told 'If I don't get you right in two sessions, go away and save your money'. His technique involved massage to tendons, ligaments and fascia by 'rolling moves'. This may only take a short while and the therapist then leaves the patient to have a break and rest, before another 'move'. Bowen held that the breaks allowed time for the body to heal itself, particularly by re-balancing muscle length. Although he appears to have used some osteopathic thrust methods, he strongly opposed other 'body work' techniques being used in conjunction with his own.

Bowen's work was reviewed by the Victorian Government Inquiry into Chiropractic, Osteopathy and Naturopathy in 1975. He told the Commission he was seeing 13,000 patients a year with an 80% success rate. This was due to having studied books on osteopathy and having 'a knack'. He applied to be a registered osteopath in 1982 but was unsuccessful.

As practised by Bowen, his technique involved 'seeing' what was wrong with the patient by using his fingers to 'sense the vibrations in musculo-skeletal tissue' and so determine what imbalance needed to be corrected in order that the body would heal itself. Bowen's method also applies finger touch analysis of a patient's entire skeleton in order to detect misalignments. These are then corrected by light, fast movements known as 'toggle-torque-recoil', which induce minute vibrations and allow the body to readjust itself. Patients hardly feel the force of the 'toggle'.

Many of Bowen's students were osteopaths and chiropractors who wanted to diversify their techniques. Bowen's 'knack' comprised 90% of his own method, based on A. T. Still's concept that 'structure governs function' and that disease requires structure to be corrected. Osteopath Oswald (Ossie) Rentsch controversially claimed that he had been commissioned by Bowen to document his technique. Certainly it has been Rentsch who has promoted the Bowen Technique worldwide. Together with his wife, Elaine, a Bach Flower Therapist, they introduced Bowen Technique to the US in 1990.

The Bowen Therapy Academy of Australia has trademarked the name 'Bowenwork' as a 'manipulative/body-based practice in the same category as osteopathy and massage.' It is postulated that gentle hand movements stimulate nerve pathways and cause a transitional state of realignment of microfibers within the nervous system to stimulate healing pathways. 'Conditions that are seen to respond well include: Crohn's disease, bed-wetting, scoliosis, haemorrhoids, infertility, uterine fibroids, asthma and anxiety.' There is no plausible scientific evidence offered in support of these prepostulations, and no indication of any better outcome than from regular physiotherapy. In the UK, physiotherapists are regulated by the Health & Care Professions Council, Bowen practitioners are not.

Reflexology and Zone Therapy

Dr William H. Fitzgerald, an ear nose and throat surgeon of Connecticut and London, initially discovered that pressure with a probe on the mucous membrane of the nose resulted in local anaesthesia. He identified many other areas in the ear, nose tongue and throat which gave similar results. In the 1910's and 20's he went on to identify areas or zones over many bony prominences where comparable results were achieved.

With Dr Edwin Bowers, Fitzgerald then postulated that the body can be represented by ten zones, each with concomitant representation on the foot. Why or how come there were ten he never explained. Fitzgerald developed his Zone Therapy on that basis, and the idea was taken up by a number of dentists and osteopaths.[33]

In the 1930's the term Reflexology was introduced by Eunice Ingham, a nurse and physiotherapist. She also postulated that the feet and hands represented reflex areas which linked to all parts and organs of the rest of the body. Appropriate attention by firm pressure with fingers and thumbs therefore affects the relevant part or organ, by 'improving blood circulation and balancing glands.'[34] There is no plausible evidence supporting this conjecture.

The International Institute of Reflexology emphasises on its website that: 'Reflexology does not purport to teach medical practice in any form. Reflexology is a unique modality in the health field. Its purpose is not to treat or diagnose any specific medical disorder, but to promote better health and well-being in the same way as an exercise and diet program...Reflexology can improve or eliminate many ailments during the course of four to six weekly treatments.' Amongst courses offered are those for 'improving fertility', back pain and 'emergency first aid'. That is of course a clear claim for diagnosis, treatment and cure and some might think the Institute's disclaimer is a 'quack Miranda warning' to avoid liability. If 'improving many ailments' is not 'treatment' – what is it?

The 'Original Ingham Method' is a registered trademark. Many other schools and teachers base their practice on the principles of Fitzgerald, Bowers and Ingham. There are a multiplicity of anatomical maps and diagrams of reflex areas, with little coherence and little agreement between the schools – though not all can be 'correct'. Light, heat, laser equipment and other paraphernalia may be purchased to assist the practitioner. Any camee considering such therapies will have to carefully consider the claims of the camists and enquire on what basis the particular reflex diagram they use has been established and how many patients they have treated whose disease or illness has not been affected. There is no plausible scientific evidence that reflexology is effective for any condition, beyond the placebo and comfort induced by massage. The many anecdotes mostly fail to distinguish between correlation and causation. The practice is 'alternative' – and will remain so until the stories of benefit are studied scientifically, reviewed by peers, and published in credible journals.

Techniques of massaging feet are relatively easy to learn and if aromatic oils are incorporated can be very comforting to patients. Many practitioners claim to help patients with serious chronic conditions and even cancer. No doubt they mean well, but they should explain that what they are doing is offering consolation, care and placebo. What they are not doing is affecting any disease process or 'improving any ailment'. If they claim to be offering 'Reflexology', by inference they are claiming to be doing just that. You must judge if this is quackery or fraud.

Nutritional Therapy
The word 'nutrition' has no generally agreed definition, and is certainly not protected in law. In the UK anyone can style themselves as a 'nutritionist', 'nutritional therapist' or 'consultant nutritionist'. And many people do. Some are misguided and deluded as to the value of their ministrations. Some are quacks intending to defraud the unwary by selling unnecessary supplements, vitamins, nutrients and 'natural' remedies. Some cause harm and are dangerous – as was exposed by the Consumer Association's *Which?* Report of February 2012 which found "High street nutritional therapists are a waste of money." Any one may purchase a T-shirt or coffee mug with the declaration they are a 'Nutritionist' – and a nice image of a plastic duck![35]

The web site www.nutritional-therapy.org.uk conflates 'Nutritional Medicine (biochemistry and nutrition)' with 'Natural Medicine (natural drug-free medicine)'. Nutritional therapy is described as being 'wholistic' (*sic*): 'Scientists as well as mystics agree that there is an energetic aspect to life. Disturbances in the energy fields lead to illness, and flower essences and homeopathy assist recovery.' Scientists' good names are being taken in vain. Whether naturopaths are happy for their beliefs to be syncretised with nutritional therapy is for them to decide.

Nutrition is clearly vital for health. That is a given – along with diet, exercise, stress reduction, removal of environmental toxins, weight optimisation and being nice to one another. Conventional practitioners attend to these issues, but without the un-scientific principles used by practitioners who style themselves as 'nutritionists'. A Thames Valley University course on 'nutrition' explains: 'Vitalism is the notion that

231

life in living organisms is sustained by a vital principle that cannot be explained in terms of physics and chemistry. This vital principle, often called "the life force", is something quite distinct from the physical body and is responsible for much that happens in health and disease.' An interesting faith for which there is no evidence. Which is why, for the protection of the public, 'nutritional therapy' is regarded as an alternative to science based healthcare.

UK patients who want dietary advice should see a dietician registered by the Health & Care Professions Council. Currently they are the only HPC registered, qualified health professionals that assess, diagnose, and treat diet and nutrition at an individual and wider public health level.[36] However, beware – 'nutritionists', and many other camists are trying to get their faiths recognised by the HPC.

On December 14th 2012 new EU rules on health claims came into force affecting claims for 'nutrition'. Here 'health' refers to a relationship between a food or ingredient and health, and 'nutrition' refers to the nutritional benefits of a food. Only claims that have been authorised by the European Food Safety Authority are now permitted. The Department of Health has emphasised that these regulations are designed to protect consumers from misleading or false claims and, as always, buyer beware.[37]

Dianetics
Lafayette Ronald Hubbard (1911-1986), a science fiction writer, published *Dianetics: The Evolution of Science* in the May 1950 issue of *Astounding Science Fiction*. It is said he had been influenced by Alfred Korzybski's *Science and Sanity: An Introduction to Non-Aristotelian Systems and General Semantics* (1933) which suggested it was possible 'to alter human behaviour in the direction of greater sanity.' Also in 1950 Hubbard published the handbook *Dianetics: The Modern Science of Mental Health* (Greek: *dia*, through + *nous*, mind). Hubbard advised readers he had discovered 'the dynamic principle of existence'. He did not reveal how this discovery was made, but attributed 'human aberration' to occult areas of the mind where cellular recordings termed 'engrams' were stored. These can be removed by the purchase of counselling courses and a process of 'auditing' until the purchaser is 'clear'. The American Psychological Association has pointed out 'these claims are not supported by empirical evidence of the sort required for the establishment of scientific generalisations.'[38]

The process of auditing is also helped by use of the 'electro-psychometer' or E-meter – a variety of the machine invented by Albert Abrams, instigator of Radionics. The United States Food and Drug Administration requires E-meters to indicate they are simply 'religious artefacts'. Science writer Martin Gardiner suggested any benefit of dianetics is as a result of faith healing.

Students commonly start by undertaking a free 'personality test' – and then purchase more courses as they progress up a hierarchy, reaching various levels of Operating Thetan (OT). Certain covert knowledge is not revealed until the student has been prepared by this gradual development, but book covers and advertising billboards available to the general public have depicted an erupting volcano. In Australia, a device on an advertising board regularly emitted smoke to add to the attraction. This is part of the knowledge imparted at level three of eight OT levels. Essentially: seventy-five million years ago a galactic overlord called Xenu transferred his planet's people to Earth in DC8 space planes. They were set down around volcanoes, which were subsequently detonated with hydrogen bombs. The insurgents' souls then entered humans as 'Thetans'. Perhaps utilising the Greek letter theta, used to mark death warrants. These souls now need to be cleared by the dianetic 'auditing' process. Hubbard did not explain how he knew this.[39]

The outcomes of dianetic auditing have not been reported in any form regarded as plausible by the scientific medical community and Dianetics remains a CAM – an alternative system for achieving mental health and wellbeing. A more complete account is given at www.xenu.net.

Applied Kinesiology

AK is a CAM which must be distinguished from 'kinesiology' which is the scientific study of movement (*kinesis,* movement). Kinesiology encompasses physics, mechanics, kinetics, physiology and psychology and forms the basis for further scientific study of human movement in sport, exercise, work, and health. Physiotherapists (physical therapists in the US) base their profession on science. Conversely, 'Applied Kinesiology' is a diagnostic method employed by some chiropractors and other camists. As such, AK is 'alternative', for there is no reproducible credible scientific evidence of its benefit. The title 'kinesiologist' is not legally protected, but camists who claim they practice 'kinesiology' are being intentionally deceptive unless they have specifically studied human kinetics to a professional level.

George J. Goodheart devised AK in 1964 as a method of muscle testing 'based on chiropractic principles'. The use of the term 'kinesiology' was then appropriated for AK. Goodheart contended that organ dysfunction could be identified by weakness in certain muscle groups due to 'the viscerosomatic relationship'. The AK practitioner tests muscles for their strength and tension against resistance – said to indicate mental stresses, sub-optimal balance and nutritional deficiencies such as those of manganese and magnesium. Practitioners believe there is an innate intelligence or 'force' which appropriate chiropractic can then adjust and that together with manipulation, meridian therapy and nutritional counselling 'balance' can be regained. The purchase of nutrients from the practitioner is frequently recommended. No reputable scientific journal has ever published a paper supporting the validity of these approaches.

More recently, there has been a fashion to wear silicone bracelets, some containing magnets or holograms, which are claimed to improve stamina, power, balance and wellbeing. Tests to 'prove' their effects are similar to those used in AK, and frequently invoke the ideomotor response. The bands have been popular with a wide range of people from sportsmen and women to politicians, as well as patients suffering from genuine symptoms. The manner by which they work, by suggestion and placebo effects, has been well demonstrated on a number of web sites and by magicians such as The Amazing Randi and Banachek (born Steven Shaw 1960 in the UK, and now based in the US).[40]

Inevitably, variants have emerged such as Contact Reflex Analysis which has been accepted as being 'within the legitimate scope of chiropractic' by some US licensing boards. Its originator, chiropractor Dick Versendaal (1937-2014) taught how to assess reflexes 'similar to acupuncture points and meridians' generated when AK moves were carried out. 'Allergy reflexes' are a particular feature as '80% of diseases are due to allergy'. A 'management plan' can then be devised, usually involving the purchase of 'supplements'.[41]

Ideomotor Response

Priests of ancient wisdom employed automatic or mediumistic spirit writing as a means of contacting the dead. An oracle or seer's use of a pendulum to answer questions was recorded in the third century A.D (*Ideo*, idea + Latin: *movere*, to move). Similar methods are used today in the course of magical entertainments, for dowsing, and in use of the Ouija board. Well-known to students of the occult since its commercial development in the 1890's, the concept of ouija suggests a test subject can unconsciously give a degree of muscular action and movement simply by mental imagery and thinking of the idea. Now a registered trademark, its originators claimed the word 'ouija' was derived from ancient Egyptian, but probably it was the combination of the French and German for 'yes' which caught the ear.

Dr William Carpenter (1813-1985) studied at University College Hospital in London and was elected a fellow of the Royal Society in 1844. His early academic studies were on comparative neurology, and in the 1850's he set in train what has become the theory of adaptive unconsciousness. Unconscious prejudices and perceptions may be in progress without an individual being aware of them and can have a significant effect on movement.

At that time, Cartesian dualism was popular – it has only been in the last fifty years that the cognitive sciences have taken Carpenter's unitist approach to mind and body on board.

Carpenter's friendship with Dr James Braid, the surgeon who developed the scientific principles of hypnotism, allowed cross fertilisation of ideas. Braid himself sought to induce hypnosis by inviting the subject to concentrate mentally – the same principles of suggestion found expression in the ideomotor response which induces and arrests movement.

The term 'ideomotor response' was first used scientifically by Carpenter in 1852 following tests on the effects of the unconscious mind on emotions, muscles and movement. The ideomotor response is not a CAM in its own right, but a technique which has been used in various ways by many CAMs such as in the muscle testing of Applied Kinesiology, chiropractic techniques, pendulum dowsing, the 'pulse diagnosis' of Traditional Chinese Medicine, the rubbing plates of Radionics and other systems of 'energy medicine'. All may produce a demonstrable response which enhances placebo effects.

One such effect is 'table turning' during séances. Demonstrated by a group of people seated around a table with their palms flat on the top, the table may suddenly and unaccountably move. This was initially held to be due to the combined influence of electricity and magnetism. In the 1840's, Karl von Reichenbach claimed this *odic force* represented the vital force of life. Taking the name from Odin, the Norse god of wisdom and war, von Reichenbach carried out scientific experiments on the forces of electricity and magnetism but was unable to establish the connection. That was left to the later work of Michael Faraday and the equations of James Clerk Maxwell.

Von Reichenbach suggested that the odic force was related to the mesmeric force responsible for hypnotism. He explored similarity with *qi* and *prana*, but no credible scientific explanation was ever offered and interest faded. After Faraday's discovery, it was electro-magnetism which many held to be the origin of any odic force, as well as coloured aura around people, animals, magnets and crystals and spirits summoned up by psychic mediums.

Sir Michael Faraday carried out an ingenious controlled study on table-turners in 1853. He covered a small table with a stack of cardboard sheets, a vertical line being marked on one side. The table sitters placed their palms on top and concentrated. When eventually the table moved, examination of the angle of the marked line showed that the cardboard pile, and hands, had moved before the table – rather than the table having moved before the hands. He concluded that the sitters were unconsciously pushing the table in the expected direction – even though each individual was quite convinced they were applying no such force. Fake mediums of course had secret confederates to assist in this fraud.[42]

Similar effects, and the influence of suggestion, are demonstrated today by magicians and by hypnotists. Their methods would probably fool even Faraday. Certainly Faraday's report convinced most of his colleagues that table turning did not stem from a new physical force or psychic power. There is no substitute for science, but may the Force be with you!

Tar -Water

The pine cone appears in the most ancient of art works. Assyrian and Babylonian kings carried staffs capped with pine cones symbolising the regeneration demonstrated by cones' repeated opening and closing. Some scholars suggest that the later Jewish esoteric Kabbalah Tree of Life was based on the Assyrian pine. Since the times of ancient Greece, pine tar obtained from the wood of pine trees, has been recognised for its value as a mild bactericidal and as water proofing for ships and roofs. One of the popular remedies of the Middle Ages was pine tar dissolved in water. A Finnish proverb has it that 'if sauna, vodka and tar won't help – the disease is fatal.'

Dr George Berkeley (1685-1753), the Bishop of Cloyne in Ireland, published *Siris: A Chain of Philosophical Reflections and Enquiries concerning the Virtues of Tar Water and Diverse other Subjects* (1744). Pine water was thought to contain the 'ethereal essence' of sunshine, could treat most diseases and assist 'lift the mind to God.' The Greek mythological character Siris was associated with pine trees.[43]

Berkeley's work is an example of philosophical 'bait and switch' still prevalent today. It begins with an extensive, though un-scientific, treatise on health and the benefits of tar water – but ends with a discourse on the soul, the Holy Spirit and the Trinity: 'It was a doctrine of ancient sages, that the soul was the place of forms, as may be seen in the twelfth book of the arcane part of divine wisdom, according to the Egyptians' (Latin: *arcana*, secrets).

Berkley suggested a pint of tar-water a day would act as a universal panacea (*Panacea*, the goddess of healing all things). His list of diseases which could be cured was extensive and included impurities of the blood, small pox, pleurisy, erysipelas, hysterics, gout and fevers. He also considered that mercury, then a component of many medicines, could cause 'great mischief 'and opined: 'No medicine can withstand the execrable plague of whisky spirits, distilled from malt, which operate as a slow poison, wasting the health and strength of the body and soul....'

As Berkeley was well regarded as a serious and pre-eminent metaphysical philosopher, pondering the meaning of life and the universe, it was inevitable that attention was paid to his opinions, even on disease and medicine. Dr Thomas Reeve, physician at St. Thomas' Hospital, London, demurred from his opinion on tar water and published *A Cure for the Epidemical Madness of Drinking Tar Water*. He addressed Berkeley directly: 'Thus in your younger days, my Lord, you made the surprising discovery of the *unreality* of matter, and now in your right old age you have undertaken to prove the *reality* of a universal remedy. An attempt to talk men out of their reason did of right belong to that author who had first tried to persuade them out of their senses.'

Dr Oliver Wendell Holmes said 'Berkeley held two very odd opinions; that tar water was everything, and that the whole material universe was nothing.' Dr Worthington Hooker pointed out that Bishop Berkeley had evidently forgotten that human illness had an overall tendency to recover. The fact a patient had drunk tar-water did not necessarily mean the tar-water had caused the recovery. Berkeley had just not appreciated the necessary analysis when considering cause and effect. As Hooker opined: 'The history of medical delusions most copiously illustrates the truth – that folly is very far from being confined to fools.'

Charles Dickens had Young Pip receiving doses of tar-water in *Great Expectations*. Today tar water is largely unheard of, but this brief review serves to indicate how healing traditions can be established by an 'authority' – if only for a while. Today we would regard such promotion as quackery but the social and theological standing of the good bishop assuaged many concerns. In medical matters he was a fool to himself more than anything else. As a quackademic autoquack he is not alone.

Aromatherapy

Medieval alchemists' principal interest was in turning base metal into gold, but their techniques were also applied to plant and animal matter. Many ancient peoples knew of the existence of oils in plants – liquids at room temperature and immiscible with water. In the 11th century, Avicenna used steam distillation and dissolved oils in solvents such as alcohol and ether. By the turn of the 13th century Ibn al-Baitar, an Andalusian doctor and alchemist, described numerous such distillations in an extensive therapeutic *materia medica*. These volatile or ethereal oils, *aetherolea*, were used as medicines either by direct application or in compound preparations. Many were also valued as soaps, perfumes and flavourings. The process of distillation extracted the essence of the plant and some oils were referred to as 'essential'. Use of this word does not imply these oils are vital and indispensable but simply that they are a principal element. Nevertheless, the implications of the word are not lost to the marketing department of modern manufacturers. Other oils are described as absolutes, fragrant, carriers and herbal.

René-Maurice Gattefossé published *Aromathérapie: Les Huiles Essentielles, Hormones Végétales* in 1937, and the term 'aromatherapy' became applied to a range of treatments utilising these various oils. Many oils are held to have mind altering properties and to effect emotions and spiritual awareness. Reduction of anxiety, enhancement of energy, relaxation and pain relief may all be affected by chemical influence on the brain's limbic system, but at present the pharmacology has not been established and there is no scientific evidence of worthwhile direct effects of these oils on specific diseases. Conversely, harmful side effects have been identified. Some therapists claim the oils represent distilled 'life force' and that their use can 'balance the body's energies'. Ask for substantiation of any such claims – they may be fraudulent. Evidence is awaited and for the present, aromatherapy remains an alternative system for treating disease and illness – condimentary but not therapeutic. Pleasant aromas may well affect mood and be comforting for patients – enhancing the benefits of having the attention of a caring empathic therapist. These are placebo effects and expectation responses. Providing patients understand there is no evidence that diseases will be affected, there can be little objection to the use of oils – but patients' full understanding on that point and informed consent is a paramount consideration.

Anthroposophical Medicine

During the latter half of the 19th century, various esoteric and occult orders became popular. The Theosophical Society was founded in New York by Helena Blavatsky in 1875 to promote interest in the 'complementary aspects of spirit and matter' and search for 'Truth'. The Society's seal incorporated the Star of David, Ankh, Aum and

Swastika. In 1911 the Theosophical Society in England laid the foundation stone for its new headquarters in Tavistock Square, London. Its president, Mrs Annie Besant became active in the National Secular Society and was a friend of its architect, Sir Edwin Lutyens. The war intervened, the Society could not complete the building and it was sold to the British Medical Association for its own headquarters – now BMA House. Some suggest the spirit of Theosophy lingers on and that the ghost of Besant even now haunts the fifth floor, still searching for Truth.

Rudolf Steiner (1861-1925), became the German Theosophical Society's General Secretary in 1902. He was an Austrian architect, philosopher and social reformer who had 'spiritual experiences' when a child. Following a schism in 1913, Steiner formed the Anthroposophical Society and founded schools based on his own philosophies of astrology, clairvoyance, esoteric practice, 'spiritual science' and his belief in reincarnation, gnomes, spirits and karma. The basic educational theory being that children have an innate spirit that has been through previous lives and which evolves karmically into a 'Germanic-Nordic body' before returning to the spirit world. The teacher has 'a sacred task in helping the child's spirit grow.'[44]

The first Steiner school was opened in 1919 to serve the children of employees of the Waldorf-Astoria cigarette factory in Stuttgart. In the US and continental Europe today they are known as Waldorf Schools – in the UK, Steiner Schools. The websites and promotional material generally do not make clear their association with Steiner's Anthroposophic philosophy and practice, nor that children are taught in a milieu of spirits and physical reincarnation. Steiner's work has been reviewed by Frederick Amrine in *Being Human:*

> The results of Steiner's researches yielded many profound insights into human nature and the history of the world. First and foremost, Steiner recovered and explicated the ancient mystery – knowledge that human nature is triune, comprising not only body, but also soul and spirit. Only at the end of his life was Steiner able to devote full attention to the second great task of his professed mission: communicating the reality of reincarnation and karma in a form appropriate for the West. Steiner worked with medical doctors to create new kinds of "Anthroposophical extended" or "complementary" medicine: Hauschka is now also considered by many to be the ultimate in cosmetics. Dozens of communities here and abroad, notably the Camphill movement, are working out of Anthroposophical insights to meet the special needs of children and adults.[45, 46, 47]

Steiner believed that humans existed in a spiritual hierarchy which was based on skin colour: black people were spiritually lazy – blond haired blue eyed Germanics were the most spiritually advanced and it was their destiny to lead humanity through to spiritual maturity. He believed in quack medicine, spiritual dance rituals and a false history based on Atlantis. His beliefs in anatomy, biology, mathematics and history were all of an occult, pseudo-scientific and superstitious nature.

Steiner also actively promoted organic farming and ecology and in 1924 devised the term 'Bio-dynamics' to describe how farming can be based on astrological, magical, mystical and cosmic forces and how Anthroposophy can enable science to maintain contact with the spirit world. 'Everything that lives in the siliceous nature contains forces which comes not from the Earth but from Mars, Jupiter and Saturn.'[48]

The website of the Biodynamic Land Trust tells us:

> Biodynamic farmers and growers recognize that the life of a farm is open to wider influences. The more subtle rhythms associated with the sun, the moon and the planets form the basis of an annually produced planting calendar. This guides growers towards appropriate times for cultivation and sowing for optimal quantity and quality. Profound social change is now being triggered by new approaches to biodynamic, organic, and sustainable and community-supported forms of farming practice. Biodynamics calls for new thinking in every aspect of the food system, from how land is owned to how farms are capitalized to how food is produced, distributed and prepared. Biodynamics, then, is a type of organic farming that incorporates an understanding of 'dynamic' forces in nature not yet fully understood by science.[49]

The Biodynamic Sowing and Planting Calendar sets out astrological tables, showing the positions of the Moon, stars and planets and advising when it is allowable to plant and harvest various crops. In August 2012, the UK found Mars and Saturn in the 'cold constellation of Virgo', Mercury was supported by the watery influence of Uranus in Pisces, and 'Pluto in Sagittarius may bring some warmth.' The creation of various 'dynamized' manures is a central tenet of bio-dynamics. These are recipes, often using dung and other ingredients packed in animal skulls and cow horns, buried by ritual using dowsing to avoid ley lines and creating magical preparations that capture the life forces needed for plants.[50]

The Soil Association was founded by proponents of bio-dynamics. Bio-dynamics parallels modern organic farming, but is more esoteric, relies on *chi* or 'life energy' and seeks to have the best of both worlds by achieving balance between the physical and non-physical realms. The Soil Association web site proclaims it was 'founded in 1946 by a group of far-sighted individuals who were concerned about the health implications of increasingly intensive agricultural systems following the Second World War' Amongst those individuals, Lady Eve Balfour is cited as being a principal founder. When she addressed the International Federation of Organic Agriculture Movements in 1977 she commented: 'I do not know where or when the ideas that have brought us together were first called a movement, but I have little doubt that the main inspiration derived from the work of the early research pioneers in the first quarter of this century, though this is not to discount the influence of one of the most important, who was even earlier, namely Rudolf Steiner.' She went on to say 'A substance may be the same chemically but very different as a conductor of living energy. The hypothesis is that energy manifesting in birth, growth, reproduction, decay, and rebirth, can only flow through channels composed of living cells, and that when the flow is interrupted by inert matter it can be short-circuited with consequent damage to some part of the food chain, not necessarily where the block occurred.

The Anthroposophical Society's research establishment at Dornach has provided some evidence in support of such a view.'[51]

For many years the editor of the Soil Association's journal was Jorian Jenks, a former member of the British Union of Fascists and campaigner on behalf of farmers and farm workers.[52] Between 1995 and 2010 the Director of the Soil Association was Patrick Holden, a biodynamic farmer. The Soil Association holds conferences on Bio-dynamics such as *'The Future of Agriculture: A Biodynamic approach'* and assists the marketing of 'organic foods'. 'For foods to be labelled as organic, at least 95% of the ingredients must come from organically produced plants and animals, that is, food which is produced using environmentally and animal friendly farming methods on organic farms. These methods are legally defined and any food sold as 'organic' must be strictly regulated'.[53] The Soil Association (Patron, HRH the Prince of Wales) does not repudiate Steiner's magical and esoteric philosophy nor deny its influence on the Association, regularly holding meetings with the Biodynamic Land Trust.[54] In November 2014, four of the Soil Association's trustees resigned as they 'question the presence on the management committee (with an attendant reputational risk) of a non-organic farmer and a doctor who publicly attacks an important tool of organic animal husbandry (homoeopathy).'

The Camphill Trust and communities, 'inspired by Rudolf Steiner's philosophy of anthroposophy' were founded outside Aberdeen in 1940 and now provide homes for people with learning disabilities and other special needs enabling them to live 'in an atmosphere of mutual care and respect.'[55]

The word 'theosophy' (divine wisdom), was once synonymous with 'theology' and then became associated with those who possessed Gnostic or esoteric knowledge of enlightenment leading to salvation. The basic precepts were set down in *Arbatel,* a book on white magic which was popular in the late sixteenth century. Paracelsus contributed to the developing movement, which reached its apogee with the works of Jakob Böehme. Perhaps this is why Paracelsus has been regarded by many as a quack. After a vision in 1600 Böehme wrote *Aurora* (1612) and *The Three Principles of Divine Being* (1619) He included esotericsm as a principle component of his system which he claimed gave a more profound understanding of nature than that of Aristotle.

Steiner initially saw Anthroposophy as a 'spiritual science' (an oxymoron) and he went on to apply its principles in architectural design and the performance arts. Steiner claimed to be a clairvoyant in the fields of culture, philosophy, politics and economics and developed the *Threefold Order* to utilise these insights as the *Threefold Commonwealth* of the State, Economics and Culture.[56] Currently this term is reflected in the Triodos Bank which lends to many alternative medicine businesses on the basis of its own Anthroposophical underpinning. Both the Triodos Bank and Soil Association use variants of the trefoil as their logos. Steiner also coined the term *eurthymy* to describe the harmonious rhythm and movement practices that he propounded.

In conjunction with Dutch gynaecologist Ita Wegman, Steiner founded a school of Anthroposophical Medicine in the 1920's, giving four seminal lectures to doctors in 1922. Anthroposophical medicine is based on herbs, massage, exercise and metaphysics and is integrated with homeopathy and art therapy. Disease results from behaviour during past lives and so conventional medicine may not be necessary – a potentially dangerous suggestion. He also taught that the heart is not a pump, but rather that blood circulates because of its 'spirit'.

Anthroposophic doctors hold that cancerous cells develop 'parasitically,' much as does mistletoe when growing on its host tree. The use of mistletoe in the treatment of cancer is therefore encouraged. Ita Wegman developed *Iscar* and *Iscador* a fermented extract of mistletoe in 1917, and opened a clinic in Switzerland to apply her methods (*Ixos,* mistletoe). The doses of extracts used vary, some being homeopathic. The latter contain no therapeutically active principle, but other doses contain viscotoxins, mistletoe lectins and their isoforms. The US Federal Drugs Administration and UK Medicines Agency have not cleared them for use in cancer therapy – to date, available preparations simply have not met the required standards. Ita Wegman later co-founded the naturopathic medicine, homeopathic remedy and health products company Weleda.

Anthroposophic doctors are conventionally qualified, but they generally reject the benefits of vaccination – a policy that places whole communities at risk. With emphasis on the karmic destiny of patients, spirits, reincarnation and a lack of plausible results for the methods employed, AM remains a CAM. It is supported by some state authorities which, being democratic, do what they can to give patients what they want. State support does not imply scientific credibility or endorsement of the practices.

Perhaps understandably, many anthroposophic doctors do not want patients to fully appreciate the implications of their faith, and try to present their system as being 'a patient- centred and whole-systems approach' and part of 'integrated medicine'. Whether such flights of metaphysical fancy can be integrated with the demands of evidence-based medicine, without undermining the benefits of modern methods has to be considered by any camee considering such an approach. Patients must ensure they are fully informed about anthroposophy. It may not mean what it says on the tin. Likewise, parents considering Steiner schools for the education of their children must ensure they are fully informed – websites for Steiner schools are often coy about their anthroposophical underpinnings.[57]

Environmental Medicine
Dr John Snow (1813-1858) had the perspicacity to identify London's Broad Street water pump as the source of a cholera outbreak in 1854, and developments under his stimulus led to a more scientific approach in public health medicine. The medical aspects of public health practice are described as 'the art and science of improving the community's health through the organised efforts of society'.

'Environmental Medicine' is a developing field in CAM involving the interactions between environment and human health, and the role of the environment in causing or mediating disease for individuals. Practitioners are concerned about 'environmental stressors' such as allergens, toxins and electromagnetic fields, whether from power lines or Wi-Fi. EM is 'alternative' because in very many cases there is absolutely no evidence whatsoever for disease or distress to have been caused by these mechanisms. Practitioners who claim they can alter such stressors provide no plausible evidence of such abilities, are taking advantage of the vulnerable and may be quacks or even frauds. For example, 'Electro-sensitivity' is very real to those who believe they suffer from it, but careful tests have yet to identify any problem in reality. The issue remains one of belief, and treatments other than psychological are alternative to science based conventional medicine. As Witthöft and Rubin suggest: 'Media reports about the adverse effects of supposedly hazardous substances can increase the likelihood of experiencing symptoms following sham exposure and developing an apparent sensitivity to it. Greater engagement between journalists and scientists is required to counter these negative effects.'[58]

You must be the judge about 'electrosensitivity' but beware, and consider the Quackometer's view.[59]

Qualia Medicine
The earlier section on Descartes noted the use made by some philosophers of 'qualia' – the sense of what it is to have an experience. Perhaps inevitably some physicians have attempted to fashion an approach to medicine based on 'Qualia' and incorporate quarks and quanta as a three-in-one which provides the best appreciation of reality. Deepak Chopra advises: 'Matter and energy aren't enough to explain the universe. We propose that a third element, qualia, must be added before anything approaching a unified description of reality will ever be possible...As hard as it may be for physicalists to accept, there is no sunset, cloud or mountain, electron or galaxy independent of a unified state that must include an observer and the process of observation... Qualia medicine could one day explain spontaneous remission of cancer, for example...present mind-body phenomena like the placebo effect will expand. Instead of being peripheral to 'real' medicine (i.e. drugs and surgery), the mind-body connection will be central to prevention and wellness.'[60]

Let us hope so, but when considering healthcare and well-being, suggestions that the trinity of quarks-quanta-qualia provides any substantial benefit smacks more of sharp branding and marketing based on the coincidence of 'qu-' initiating those buzz words.

Crystal Healing
A crystal is a solid with molecules, atoms or ions arranged in a regular form and with symmetrically arranged faces (periodic in three dimensions). That is all there is to it, but many camees and camists find these features strangely attractive and claim they can 'resonate with natural vibrations' and engage 'healing properties' by placing crystals on affected parts, relevant chakras or simply by handling them. There is no

evidence to support claims that: 'Rose quartz works with the emotional body; citrine rejects negative energy; black tourmaline is very grounding, while celestite connects you to the "angelic realms."'

This type of sympathetic magic has been seen in many cultures including the Chinese, who have ascribed these powers to crystalline jade, and Hopi Americans and Hawaiians, for whom quartz holds significance. There is no rational explanation of the nature of the 'energies' claimed by practitioners nor plausible evidence of any benefit for patients beyond those achieved by placebo effects.

Christopher French, professor in the Anomalistic Psychology Research Unit at Goldsmith's University of London, views any benefit experienced as the result of suggestion. Paediatrician Paul Offit agrees, pointing out: 'The placebo effect is often dismissed as "just in my head" and that's seen as dismissive. But the mind can be a powerful healing tool.'

Use of crystals would not matter if it were not for the fact that some patients defer seeking conventional medical care and spend time and money needlessly. And given some practitioners have set up charities to seek financial support from businesses and the public generally, we must all question these claims more critically.

'Biofield Therapies' and 'Energy Medcine'

Many CAMs purport to engage with 'energies', though not those recognised by conventional science. Some are considered in chapter 14, but here, an insight into the mindset of those involved in research into such concepts is offered by a Roundtable Discussion reported in The Journal of Alternative and Complementary Medicine:

> We should begin with a few definitions: Biofield therapies, which most commonly include external Qigong, Healing Touch, Johrei, Reconnective Healing, Reiki, and Therapeutic Touch, are a family of health care practices that involve either, or both, hands-on and hands-off treatment...We infer that such healing can occur since living systems coexist within and co-contribute to a biofield, which we define in terms of electric, magnetic and electromagnetic fields as well as subtle energies (energies that appear to exist but have not yet been measured).[61]

If they have not been measured, no such inference can be drawn – measuring observations is how real science works. Biofield Research is further described on a website of that name: It combines 'Computer technology with reflex-zone and meridian studies in three visual formats: Aura representation of your personal electromagnetic field, Energy Flow Activity and bio-energetic readings of 45 Body Zones.'[62] There is no plausible evidence humans have a 'personal electromagnetic field' nor that any of these techniques can diagnose or affect disease pathology. Use of undefined sciency sounding words is the hallmark of a quack.

Other 'Energy Medicine' and 'Energy Psychology' methods include Emotional Freedom Techniques (EFT), Thought Field Therapy, Theta Therapy and the Tapas

Acupressure Technique (after acupuncturist Tapas Fleming). Essentially these techniques use hypnosis, but practitioners are in denial of this. Keen to have their views more respected and asserted, enthusiasts represented by the Association for Comprehensive Energy Psychology (ACEP) have asked Wikipedia to 'create and enforce new policies that allow for true scientific discourse about holistic approaches to healing.' Wikipedia co-founder Jimmy Wales refused, pointing out:

> 'Wikipedia's policies around this kind of thing are exactly spot-on and correct. If you can get your work published in respectable scientific journals – that is to say, if you can produce evidence through replicable scientific experiments, then Wikipedia will cover it appropriately. What we won't do is pretend that the work of lunatic charlatans is the equivalent of "true scientific discourse." It isn't.'[63]

Gwyneth Paltrow's 2014 'conscious uncoupling' from husband Chris Martin was said to have been managed by EFT. This is a method of counselling in which the patient taps or rubs 'end points of the body's energy meridians to remove energy blockages.' On hearing this, many people's occipito-frontalis muscles reflexly contracted.

Holistic Medicine

Camists use a variety of words to describe their practices and have them distinguished in the crowded healthcare market place. Most who are not registered medical practitioners avoid blatant suggestions that they are, though many are prone to imply they have comparable status and some like to style themselves as 'doctor'. They nevertheless have beliefs and faith in one or more systems which are regarded by the general scientific and medical community as 'alternative'. That title may be thought pejorative, and 'complementary' and 'integrated' (or 'integrative') are now more regularly used. 'Condimentary' may yet catch on to imply the pleasure gained from camistry. One adjective which is becoming more regularly used is *holistic*, taken by some as a synonym for 'integrated' and some even claim they practice 'Holistic Integrated Medicine'.

In healthcare the term *holistic* is used with various definitions and implications in support of marketing different camist services but its meaning is reasonably expressed by The American Holistic Medical Association: 'The primary goal of holistic medical practice is the conscious pursuit of the highest level of functioning and balance of the physical, environmental, mental, emotional, social and spiritual aspects of human experience, resulting in a dynamic state of being fully alive. This creates a condition of well-being regardless of the presence or absence of disease.'

This is of course a goal of all healthcare practitioners, though most conventional practitioners specialise in one domain, disease or illness. The field of 'health' is simply too vast to do otherwise effectively. This is why a scientific approach is so essential. Holistic and 'integrative' practitioners are content to endorse, incorporate or even use alternative medical systems for which there is no credible evidence for the effects claimed. Which is why they are 'alternative' and cannot rationally be 'integrated' with conventional medicine.

The AHMA contends: All people have innate powers of healing in their bodies, minds and spirits. Holistic health care practitioners evoke and help patients utilize these powers to affect the healing process.' Sadly, no scientifically derived plausible evidence in support of that contention is available. Holistic practitioners use a wide variety of different alternative medical systems, but rarely offer any explanation of their differences or the basis for choosing one over the other. Marketing can be persuasive, which is why these titles are conjured, but in the absence of plausible evidence for the claims made, it is hard to distinguish a sincere practitioner (who is deluded) from a quack (who is deceptive) and from a fraud (who is dishonest). You must be the judge.

Cancer surgeon Professor Michael Baum advises: 'Alternative versions of holism are arid and closed belief systems, locked in a time warp, incapable of making progress yet quick to deny progress in the fields of scientific medicine'.[64]

Railroad Therapy
Websites describe numerous stories of strange, bizarre and irrational therapies. Camees and placebists are encouraged to make their own enquiries and draw their own conclusions but an example follows of the lengths desperate people will go to if they are unable to gain benefit from orthodox care – either because they cannot afford it, or because orthodox mechanisms of action are not adequate.

Associated Press has reported that sick Indonesians who are unable to afford doctors and prescription medicines feel they have only one option: Electric Railroad Therapy.[65] For thirteen years Sri Mulyati has had diabetes with associated high blood pressure, sleeplessness and high cholesterol. She simply cannot afford orthodox healthcare, but she had heard of a man paralysed by a stroke who was intending suicide, but who found relief as he lay on the railroad track. Sri has told how she too lays down across railroad tracks at Rawa Buaya to experience the electric current – which increases as the trains approach. She certainly experiences mild shocks and spasms, but is able to scramble clear before being struck. For her, 'it works.'

Sri, and many like her, regularly undergoes this therapy in spite of government opposition. Desperate she may be, but simply by the exercise of going to the tracks and escaping the train she will be getting good aerobic activity which is part and parcel of a holistic approach to diabetic care. Psychologically at least she will feel more positively engaged in her own health care. Do not try this at home.

Condimentary Medicine
Condiments add flavour and pleasure to a recipe (Latin: *condire*, to season). By definition, 'Complements' as in 'complementary medicine', complete and make recipes whole. Complements are not needed for modern medical recipes – which are designed to be complete as they are. Use of the term 'condimentary' represents a more honest representation of what CAM is doing – providing pleasure but

245

without significant effect on pathology. What practitioners generally do not tell you is how CAM works. Patients do benefit from supplementary, complementary and alternative medicine products and practices. But unless and until plausible evidence is adduced, their role in health and well being would be clearer if they were referred to as 'condimentary.' The practitioner must be distinguished from the practice, the therapist from the therapy. Patients would then be better enabled to decide whether or not to spend time, trouble, and money on them – or whether to use available funds to obtain better conventional treatments and support from orthodox practitioners and placebists.

Endnotes to Chapter 14

1. J.U. & C.G. Lloyd Bulletin No. 11 of the Lloyd Library Reproduction Series No.7 1909. www.swsbm.com.

2. J. C. Hubbard. Eclectic Medical Association: Presidential Address 1934. www. henriettesherbal.com/eclectic/journals.

3. History of Stanford Medical School and predecessors. http://elane.stanford.edu/wilson/ Chapter 26.6.

4. Albert Abrams: *Two Electronic Diagnoses: The Reactions of a Guinea Pig and a Sheep,* in the *Reaction of Abrams. JAMA* 79, no. 27, 1922.

5. Austin Lescarboura 'Abrams Investigation'. *Scientific American* 131, no. 3 (March 1924): 159.

6. www.radionic.co.uk.

7. hhhp://www.chiroweb.com/archives/09/14/15.html.

8. www.dynamicchiropractic.com/mpacms/dc/article.php?id=44416.

9. Paulette Cooper .*The Scandal of Scientology*. New York: Tower Publications 2007.

10. Sebastian Kneipp. *My Water Cure* and *Thus Thou Shalt Live*. www.archive.org/stream/ mywatercureastes00kniiuoft#page/n7/mode/2up.

11. Benedict Lust. Editorial, *The Naturopathic and Herald of Health*. Issue 1 January 1902.

12. http://www.gncouncil.co.uk/.

13. www.chicagohealers.com/naprapathy.

14. *Tarbell's Course in Magic,* Tarbell System Inc. 1927, in seven volumes. Louis Tannen, New York

15. www.mctimoney-college.ac.uk/biography-of-john-mctimoney.

16. Theodore Jordan, *Swedenborg's influence on Sutherland's primary respiratory mechanism model cranial osteopathy.* The International Journal of Osteopathic Medicine. Vol 12. September 2009.

17. Kazanjian Λ. and others. *A systematic review and appraisal of the scientific evidence on craniosacral therapy.* BCOHTA, May 1999.
Prof. Edzard Ernst. *Craniosacral therapy: a systematic review of the clinical evidence*: Focus on Alternative and Complementary Therapies, Volume 17, Issue 4, December 2012.
Paul Posadzki, Myeong Soo Lee, and Edzard Ernst. *Osteopathic Manipulative Treatment for Pediatric Conditions: A Systematic Review.* Pediatrics Vol. 132 No. 1 July 1, 2013.

18. www.chirokinetictherapy.com and www.imperfectlynatural.com/articles-1/measles-vaccination-david-stevens.

19. www.shiatsusociety.org/public/downloads_public/Shiatsu%20Systematic%20 Evidencee%20Review%20Complete.

20. Robinson,N., Donaldson J. and Lorenc A. *Shiatsu: A Review of Evidence.* London: Thames Valley University. 2006.

21. Cohen K.S. *The Ty of Qigong: The Art and Science of Chinese Energy Healing.* Random House Canada. 1999.

22. Veith Ilza; translator. *The Yellow Emperor's Classic of Internal Medicine*, revised paperback edition. Berkeley: University of California Press. 1972.

23. Lao Tzu. *Tao Te Ching.* 6th century BC.

24. Lu X, Hui-Chan C, Tsang W, *Tai Chi, Arterial compliance and muscle strength in older adults.* European Journal of Preventative Cardiology 4th April 2012.

25. Linda Rosa; Emily Rosa (age 9); Larry Sarner; Stephen Barrett: *A Close Look at Therapeutic Touch.* JAMA 1998; 279(13).

26. www.collegeofmedicine.org.uk/why-compassionate-care-saves-time-money. 2012.

27. Michael Bloch *FM: The life of Frederick Mattias Alexander.* Little, Brown. London 2004.

28. *The Star, Rand Daily Mail.* Johannesburg. 16th February-4th March 1948.

29. Little, P. et al, *Randomised controlled trial of Alexander Technique (AT) lessons, exercise, and massage in chronic and recurrent back pain.* British Medical Journal, August 19, 2008.

30. www.rolfing.org.

31. *Rolfing: The Integration of Human Structures.* Harper and Row, 1977.

32. Jones, T.A. *Rolfing.* Physical Medicine and Rehabilitation Clinics of North America 15

(4): 799-809 2004.

33. William Fitzgerald, Edwin Bowers, *Zone Therapy or Relieving Pain at Home*, I. W. Long, Columbus, Ohio, 1917.
The founder of Naturopathy was impressed. Benedict Lust later wrote *Zone Therapy or Relieving Pain and Sickness by Nerve Pressure* . Benedict Lust Publications, New York City, 1928.   See also: Laura Norman with Thomas Cowan, *The Reflexology Handbook, a Complete Guide*. Piatkus.1989.

34. Patricia Benjamin, *Eunice D. Ingham and the development of foot reflexology in the US.* American Massage Therapy Journal, 1989 and www.reflexology-uk.co.uk.

35. Duck tee shirts can be obtained from www.badscience.net.

36. www.bda.uk.com.

37. 2012 regulations based on Regulation (EC) no 1924/2006 of European Parliament.

38. Lucy Freeman, *Psychologists Act against Dianetics*, New York Times September 9th, 1950.

39. www.xenu.net/archive/oca/gardner.html.

40. www.youtube.com/watch?v=Piu75P8sxTo.

41. http://paulharrisonline.blogspot.com/2011/05/power-band-bull.html.

42. Illustrated London News, 1853.

43. George Berkley. *Siris.* paragraph 269. Siris was a very naughty boy. Greek mythology has it that he was an outlaw who tied travellers to bent pine trees which he then loosened, tearing them apart. *Siris* was also Ethiopian for the Nile, where sunshine and water achieved fertile conjunction.

44. Anna Giesenberg, *Spiritual development and young children*; European Early Childhood Education Research Journal (2000) 8(2) 23-27. Also www.dcscience.net/?p=3528.

45. Frederick Amrine. *Discovering a Genius*. Being Human. February 2011.

46.www.anthroposophy.org/fileadmin/nfm/bh-1/being-human-2011-01-Amrine-Discovering.pdf.

47. www.quackometer.net/blog/2013/01/steiner-academy-bristol-a-challenge.

48. www.rsarchive.org/Search.php.

49.www.biodynamiclandtrust.org.uk/about/what-biodynamic-agriculture-and-horticulture.

50. www.quackometer.net/blog/2012/07/is-biodynamic-farming-vegan.html.

51. Eve Balfour. *Towards a Sustainable Agriculture.* 1977. http://journeytoforever.org/farm_library/balfour_sustag.html. In which Balfour cites Steiner's eight lectures on Agriculture in 1924. English translation: Bio-Dynamic Agricultural Association, 1974.

52. www.facebook.com/pages/Soil-Association/105542389479699?v=desc.

53. www.soilassociation.org/farmersgrowers/newsandevents/articleid/2580/the-future-of-agriculture-a-biodynamic-approach.

54. Personal communication, The Soil Association, 2013.

55. Readers who wish for a more complete account of these beliefs might refer to Peter Staudenmaier, *Anthroposophy and Ecofascism.* www.openwaldorf.com/anthroposophyandecofascism.pdf.

56. Rudolf Steiner. *The Mission of the Individual Folk Souls in Relation to Teutonic Mythology.* London 1970.

57. Nick Nakorn: http://nicknakorn.wordpress.com/2010/07/13/can-we-trust-the-soil-association/.

58. Witthöft M, Rubin GJ. *Are media warnings about the adverse health effects of modern life self-fulfilling? An experimental study on idiopathic environmental intolerance attributed to electromagnetic fields (IEI-EMF).* J. Psychosom. Res. 2013 Mar;74(3):206-12. doi: 10.1016/j.jpsychores.2012.12.002. Epub 2012 Dec 23.

59. www.quackometer.net/blog/2013/03/the-bbc-will-make-you-sick.html

60. www.sfgate.com/opinion/chopra/article/From-Quanta-to-Qualia-The-Mystery-of-Reality-4025712.php#ixzz2H12Tx0gq.

61. Richard Hammerschlag, Shamini Jain, Ann L. Baldwin, Gloria Gronowicz, Susan K. Lutgendorf, James L. Oschman, and Garret L. Yount. The Journal of Alternative and Complementary Medicine. December 2012, 18(12): 1081-1086.

62. www.biofieldresearch.com. More techniques which might best be described as *Fi Shi.*

63. http://arstechnica.com/science/2014/03/wikipedia-founder-calls-alt-medicine-practitioners-lunatic-charlatans/

64. Professor Michael Baum in *Healing, Hype or Harm*, edited by Edzard Ernst. Imprint Academic, Exeter. 2008.

65. http://news.yahoo.com/desperate-sick-indonesians-railroad-therapy-093553280.html.

Chapter 16

Faith, medicine and magic

Faith is the substance of things hoped for, the evidence of things not seen...
Epistle to the Hebrews[1]

Imagination is next akin to a miracle – working faith.
Francis Bacon

Nothing is so firmly believed as that which is least known.
Michel de Montaigne[2]

The fact that a believer is happier than a sceptic is no more to the point than the fact that a drunken man is happier than a sober one.
George Bernard Shaw

Insofar as religion consists in a way of feeling, rather than in a set of beliefs, science cannot touch it.
Bertrand Russell

Faith is a positive, hopeful attitude that is willing to dissent from convention, common sense, reasonability. It is a form of hope that sticks its neck out. But is this such a good thing? Not necessarily: there are great dangers here ... Hitler's evil creed was a form of faith, and so was Karl Marx's 'science'.
Theo Hobson[3]

There has always been a close association between religious beliefs and the practice of health care. All religions express pastoral concern for humankind in general and for the welfare of their adherents in particular. In order to assist the reader to place their own beliefs and understanding of science and religion in context, a few of the better known religions which are especially associated with health care are reviewed.

By definition, there can be no rational proof of a faith-based belief. Doctors and other health care professionals are obliged by their professional ethics not to proselytise in support of their own beliefs, nor 'to express to patients, personal beliefs including political, religious or moral beliefs, in ways that exploit their vulnerability or that are likely to cause them distress.' [4]

From time immemorial, diseases, distress and disabilities have been healed by appeal to deep emotional, transcendent and psychological responses referred to as 'spiritual'. Charismatic members of early human civilisation developed prayers, dances, and rituals to induce the healing processes. Some aspects of this style of healing are discussed in the section on Traditional Shamanic Medicine.[5] Later, as religions became organised and were ascribed by prophets and priests to explicit deities, so specific prayers and practices developed to secure their divine intervention. The Greeks established temples dedicated to their gods where personal intercession was sought. For health and healing, Asklepios was the leading figure, along with his daughters. In 293 BC the Romans dedicated a temple to Aesculapius (the Latinised spelling) on Tiber Island in Rome where there is a hospital to this day.[6]

Spirits have been part of human experience from the ancient of days (Latin: *spiritus, breath*). Early humans were only too well aware of their physical bodies but also believed in a non-corporeal breath, vital spark, or animating energy which gave rise to the emotions, thoughts and the intellect. Some felt these spirits or souls continue to exist after death. Each religion has considered these philosophies and each has devised its own account. Ghosts, demons, or deities have all been invoked at various times. Religions suggest meaningful contact may be made through the vicarious intercession of priests. Some people, such as Abram, Moses, Mohammed, Sun Myung Moon and Joseph Smith have claimed they have had direct personal contact with the divine. Some claim to have been granted the 'gift' of healing. Luke records Jesus' healing powers. After his resurrection, Jesus gave a Great Commission to his disciples 'to go out to all nations and in my name, they will drive out demons and when they drink deadly poison it will not hurt them; they will place their hands on sick people and they will get well.'[7]

In all religions, prayers are regularly offered in order that God or gods will assist the recovery of those who are suffering illness. Moses set down Yahweh's law in Leviticus 20:6, 'I will set my face against the person who turns to mediums and spiritualists ...' Other faiths, including the Sufi tradition within Islam and Hinduism, have a basis in animism with regular contact with spirits. In *Religion for Atheists,* Alain de Botton advises 'that religions merit our attention for their sheer conceptual ambition; changing the world in a way that few secular institutions ever have.'[8]

In addition to the spiritual, some organised religions have paid particular attention to health and physical wellbeing. Their systems are worthy of note and give some insight into the mindset of people of faith. There can be no doubt that belief systems can give rise to powerful psychological and emotional experiences which can be of the most intense kind. Teresa Sánchez de Cepeda y Ahumada (1515-1582) was a Spanish mystic who had spiritual experiences, visions, transports and raptures, which she referred to as 'ecstasies' (*eksatsis*, entrancement). In some she envisioned an angel: 'I saw in his hand a long golden spear with tip of fire....he appeared to me to be thrusting it at times into my heart, and to pierce to my entrails...the pain was so sharp, that it made me utter several moans.'[9] Giovanni Bernini's statue *Ecstasy of Teresa* (1646) can be seen in the basilica of Santa Maria della Vittoria, Rome and has given rise to other interpretations of Teresa's experiences. As a lady customer said when Harry met Sally in a diner: 'I'll have what she's having.'

Animism
Spirits have governed the world of humans, plants, other natural life and even apparently inanimate features such as rocks, mountains and rivers ever since *homo* became *sapiens*. The term 'animism' was introduced by Georg Ernst Stahl, circa 1720, to refer to the 'doctrine that animal life is produced by an immaterial soul' (Latin: *animus*, soul, life). In *Primitive Culture* (1871) anthropologist Sir Edward Tylor identified many indigenous peoples for whom non-human entities – animals, plants, inanimate objects, and natural phenomena also possess a spiritual essence. Shamans and witch doctors claim particular skills at entering the spirit world to obtain healing for their clients.

Christian Science
Like Teresa, Mary Baker (1821-1910) had been unwell for most of her life and often bedridden. No orthodox doctor seemed able to help. In the early 1860s a combination of homeopathy from Alvin Cushing, magnetic healing from Phineas Quimby and divine revelation after intense Bible study, set in train 'self-healing.' Convinced that 'there is but one creation and it is only spiritual' she followed her own logic to believe all sickness was in the mind and the result of fear, ignorance or sin. In *Science and Health with Key to the Scriptures* (1875) she urged that the illusion of sickness and pain could be dealt with by 'mind healing'. Baker is now generally known by the name of her third husband as Mary Baker Eddy.

Phineas Quimby (1802-1866) initially trained as a watchmaker and was then taught to be a magnetic healer and mesmerist by Charles Poyen in the 1830s. His papers were collected in *Health and the Inner Life: An Analytical and Historical Study of Spiritual Healing and Theories.* Quimby researched the mental and placebo effects of the mind, noting that some medicines appeared to cure patients of disease, yet had no intrinsic value. His system, sometimes referred to as *Quimbyism,* was a healing method with incidental religious teaching. Although Baker Eddy studied with and was treated by Quimby, the system she developed was a religious teaching with an incidental healing method. In *Science and Health,* a chapter titled *Animal Magnetism*

Unmasked warned that animal magnetism could lead to 'moral and physical death' of both practitioner and subject. It was Quimby who first coined the term 'Christian Science'.

Mary Baker Eddy founded the First Church of Christ, Scientist, in Boston (1879) and the Massachusetts Metaphysical College (1882) – teaching the principle which she regarded as scientific: *'Patient, heal thyself.'* Many of her students were women who generally found entry to the orthodox medical profession very difficult at that time. Mark Twain regarded her as 'the queen of frauds and hypocrites.' Today, Christian Scientists utilise modern medical practices, but continue to place great reliance on prayer.

Seventh Day Adventists
William Miller was a Baptist layman who declared in 1822 'that the second coming of Jesus Christ is near ... on or before 1843.' In 1840 his views were preached throughout the United States, and rapidly, the world. There was a Great Disappointment as 1843 passed uneventfully but the Second Advent was expected in due course, if not capable of accurate prediction. Adventists declare 'a gospel of health' with hydrotherapy a principal recommendation – a development of Vincent Priessnitz's cold water cures of mid nineteenth century Europe.

In 1866 the Adventists founded the Western Health Reform Institute at Battle Creek, Michigan. In 1875 Dr John Harvey Kellogg graduated from New York University Medical College and became the Institute's Superintendent. John's brother William, its book keeper, developed the cereals business bearing their name. After it was burnt down in 1902 the Institute was renamed Battle Creek Sanitarium with health resort facilities and special emphasis on rehabilitation (Latin: *sanitas,* health).

Kellogg used a variety of treatments, particularly nutritional diets, enemas, colonic massage, physical exercise and careful hygiene. He referred to his method as 'a composite physiologic method comprising hydrotherapy, phototherapy, aromatherapy, electrotherapy, mechanicotherapy, dietetics, physical culture and health training.' Although popular with affluent patients, the Wall Street crash of 1929 took effect and the 'San' entered receivership in 1933. It is now run by the US Army.

Scientology
Originating with the works of science fiction author and fantasist Lafayette Ron Hubbard (1911-1986), *Dianetics* was proposed as a system to restore mental health and is reviewed in the previous chapter. Hubbard was challenged by authorities who were concerned that he was practising medicine without a licence. To obviate this problem, in 1953 he incorporated the Church of Scientology, the Church of American Science and Church of Spiritual Engineering. Dianetic auditors were now legitimately ministering to their flock. Not all governments have granted the status of being a recognised church (France, and Germany have not, the UK did so in December 2013 but appeals against this are in hand). Some countries

allow the organisation to be tax-exempt. Scientology was banned in Western and South Australia in the 1960s as being a sham religion but changed its name to *The Church of the New Faith* in 1969. As such, an appeal to the High Court of Australia was successful and tax exempt status was established in 1983 – judges opining: 'Charlatanism is a necessary price of religious freedom and if a self-proclaimed teacher persuades others to believe in a religion which he propounds, lack of sincerity or integrity on his part is not incompatible with the religious character of the beliefs, practices and observances accepted by his followers.'

The word *Scientology* seems to have first been coined by poet Allen Upward in his book *The New World* (1901) as meaning 'science elevated to unquestioning doctrine'. In 1934 the philosopher Anastasius Nordenholtz used the term to mean 'science of science'. Hubbard may not have been aware of either of these earlier uses. Today the Church has diversified and is active in literacy, business administration and drug rehabilitation as well as personality assessment and mental health. It is often seen as being antithetical and in opposition to orthodox psychiatry.

The Church of Jesus Christ of Latter Day Saints
A Christian revival movement in the first half of the nineteenth century led to many other new American denominations, such as that of the LDS, often known as Mormonism. Mormons believe that in 1823 religious revivalist Joseph Smith (1805-1844) was visited by an angel called Moroni, the son of the prophet Mormon, who had been sent from a god whose throne is near a planet or star called Kolob.[10]

The angel directed Smith to buried gold plates on which was set out the history of the Nephites and Lamanites, lost tribes of Israel. In 600 BC these tribes had emigrated to America and were the ancestors of today's native North and South Americans. Shortly after his resurrection, Jesus of Nazareth himself had visited America to spread his gospel.[11]

Fortunately, divine inspiration enabled Smith to translate the plates and set down their texts as *The Book of Mormon*. This led to the founding of the Church of Latter Day Saints in 1830.

As well as practicing polygamy, Smith's disciples should avoid tobacco, alcohol, hot drinks, wear certain undergarments and eat meat only sparingly. For some reason, God's Word of Wisdom in respect of polygamy has more recently been set aside by the Church's elders. The Prophet Joseph Smith's writings confirmed the efficacy of faith healing and he is said to have cured malaria by prayer. Church Elder Brigham Young advocated healing by women members – though later only male priests were deemed to have the appropriate authority. The Church offers Priesthood Blessings to cure some diseases, though these seem to be of the self-limiting variety.[12]

Many of America's new immigrants found traditional European churches fossilised, unexciting and not able to represent the frontier spirit which had drawn them to the West. New churches were founded by those who thought they could communicate with spirits, gods and angels. Emanuel Swedenborg (1688-1720) thought so and he influenced many philosophers and medical practitioners, including those who were beginning to use the methods of Mesmer, de Puységur and Braid to induce the trances which allowed contact with supernatural entities and spirits.

The Supernatural

The placebist will respect patients with any belief, or none, and will recognise that many religions distinguish between the 'spirit' which is the vital energy present in all living things, and the 'soul' which is eternal and mediated by a deity. Detailed metaphysics need not concern the practical placebist, but consideration of some stories about spirits, ghosts and the supernatural gives insight to the mindset of a number of patients who are attracted to supernatural or occult systems of medicine.

After his wife Elizabeth died in childbirth in 1757, William Kent had an affair with his sister-in-law Fanny – a crime under Canon Law of the time. William and Fanny moved to London and took lodging in Cock Lane, but fell out with the landlord when he learned they were not married. Strange rapping and scratching noises were then heard, and it was claimed the ghost of Elizabeth had been seen. After Fanny died of small pox, the landlord and his eleven year old daughter claimed to have seen her ghost also, who declared she had been poisoned by Kent. Crowds, including royalty, paid the landlord an admission fee to visit the scene of the famous Cock Lane Ghost.

A commission, including Dr Samuel Johnson, was set up to investigate these claims. Eventually a hoax was declared, the noises having been made by a small piece of wood secreted by the child. The perpetrators were tried by the Lord Chief Justice himself, were convicted and Kent was awarded damages for having been libelled by the claimed 'ghost'.

But not only had the gullible public been taken in. The local priest, having leanings towards Methodism, believed in ghosts and it had been his belief which led to public castigation of Kent as a murderer. John Wesley, although an Anglican Vicar, laid greater emphasis than most on the supernatural, witchcraft and magic. He felt he had been haunted as a youth and belief in the supernatural became a tenet of the church he founded. His supporters gave greater credence to the Cock Lane events than did more conventional Anglicans. Horace Walpole attended an assembly and thereafter accused Methodists of actively seeking to establish the presence of ghosts – much as today's camists actively seek to establish the presence of 'energies', 'spirits', 'intelligences' and 'forces' in the domain of camistry.

With caution at first, newspapers eventually poured scorn on the credulity of those who had been taken in, including Johnson. Satirical prints became popular – Oliver Goldsmith published *English Credulity* and William Hogarth, *Credulity, Superstition and Fanaticism*. By the nineteenth century Charles Dickens was making references to the Cock Lane Ghost in a number of books. We still benefit from the insightful investigations of rational journalists.

255

Catherine and Margaret Fox

Brought up in New York, in 1848 the sisters reported knocking or tapping in their house, as if furniture was being moved. Their mother could not believe the girls were up to mischief, and ascribed these weird sounds to the spirit of a pedlar, murdered in the house some years before. The sisters' first report is often regarded as the date of the initiation of *Spiritualism* as a defined movement. Many of their supporters were Quakers, who took up a number of contemporary causes including the abolition of slavery and advancing women's rights. The Fox sisters demonstrated their gifts at assemblies, styled 'séances' (French, from the Latin: *sedere,* to sit). As at Cock Lane, the donations they received provided a substantial living but in 1888 Margaret Fox confessed their whole performance had been a fraud and hoax. The original knocking had been produced by bumping an apple on the floor. Later they had learned to click their fingers and covertly tap their feet to produce the mysterious sounds. However, by now the idea was so implanted amongst the general public that their confession was largely ignored. A similar response is often seen when hoaxers confess – exemplifying classic confirmation bias in which information is interpreted in a biased way so as to confirm beliefs already held. Crop circle makers who confess their hoaxes are often told 'Ah, but the aliens made you do it.' Perhaps they did – it cannot be proved they did not.

Charles Grafton Page (1812-1868)

Page practiced as a qualified doctor in Virginia but was also an advocate for patent applications. He was well used to detecting fraud in science and was a dedicated scientist in America's first rank. Particularly interested in electromagnetism, he invented a number of electrical devices and developed an early form of electrotherapy which gave patients a mild shock.

Page attended performances by the Fox sisters and applied his knowledge of medicine, electricity and fraud investigation. The fact that he was a talented ventriloquist also helped. Ventriloquism is regarded as a branch of the modern magic arts, for it involves methods such as misdirection and illusion which is fundamental to magical technique. Magicians should not expose their secrets but it can be revealed that Nooky Bear, Archie Andrews, Lefty and Lord Charles did not actually speak – they were dummies. Promise not to tell.

Page soon analysed how the Fox's illusions were created:

> 'The prime movers in all these marvels are *impostors* and their disciples, *dupes.* While the former are filling their coffers at the expense of the latter, they must often indulge in secret merriment at the credulity of their adherents, and particularly at the grave discussions of the learned clergy and others upon electricity, magnetism, the new fluid ... or the devil's immediate agency. The instant the idea of the superhuman gets possession of the mind, all fitness for investigation and power of analysis begins to vanish and credulity swells to its utmost capacity. The most glaring inconsistencies and absurdities are not discerned and are swallowed whole.'
> [13]

In America, the Seybert Commission (1887) investigated a number of spiritualist mediums and a wide range of spiritualist phenomena, including rapping on tables; spirit writing on school slates; spirit photography; the manifestation of 'ectoplasm'; psychic surgery and communication by mediumship with spirits of the departed themselves. Although many members of the commission were supporters of spiritualism, they found no genuine mediums.

These considerations should be borne in mind not only by those interested in spiritualism, but also CAM in general because the psychological drivers of those interests are comparable and may be identical.

Spiritualism itself has evolved and developed, and currently may be found in three principal movements: *Syncretism* – refers to the style of philosophy which seeks a combination of various schools of thought and an inclusive approach to all faiths. Some have likened it to the New Age movement. *The Spiritualist Church* is more formally organised along the lines of Christian denominations. It offers training for mediums and most churches are affiliated with the National Spiritualist Association in America or the Spiritualists National Union in the UK. *Survivalism* is a term preferred by a number of spiritualists who have a belief in the survival of the conscious-self after death, in out-of-body experiences and in mediumship as a means by which the other world may be experienced. They hope to secure the benefits of 'both worlds'.

Some mediums may have genuinely believed they could contact 'the other side'. Some still do. Others found they had gifts of showmanship and fraud was never far from the surface:

Ira and William Davenport
These American magicians performed as the Davenport Brothers in the latter half of the nineteenth century. Noting the success of the Fox sisters they developed an act promoted by Dr J.D. Ferguson, a Spiritualist who supported the brothers' claims that their effects were due to spirit powers – an assertion he robustly proclaimed as only a revivalist could. The American Civil War of 1861 to 1865 left many bereaved families who were desperate to contact their loved ones who had passed 'to the other side' – and business flourished.

The Davenport's Spirit Cabinet was a large wooden box set on trestles in which both brothers were seated. Their hands and feet were bound and tied to the box with rope. To ensure nothing untoward could take place, a committee of audience members surrounded the cabinet. Various musical instruments and bells were placed inside and the lights were dimmed as 'the spirits refuse to work in light.' The brothers entered a trance and as soon as the doors were closed, the spirits played the instruments, rang the bells and even tossed them out of the open top. The committee threw open the doors. The brothers remained entranced and firmly tied and bound to the seats. The gullible audience could only assume 'spirits' had been at work. The act was very successful and was introduced to England where spiritualism had captured interest.

'The Ghost Club' was established in London in 1862. Its objectives were, and still are, to carry out investigation and research into ghosts, psychic and paranormal activity. The club investigated the Davenport's claim that they could contact the dead but the results were never published. Perhaps this was because some members believed in spiritualism and the results were not supportive. This is publication bias. In 1882 the Society for Psychical Research was founded with emphasis on investigations carried out 'in a scientific and unbiased way.' Initially there were a number of spiritualist members, many of whom resigned when fraudulent mediums were exposed. It was one of the SPR founders, Frederic Myers, who coined the term 'telepathy'. Later SPR members included the Reverend Charles Dodgson, better known as Lewis Carroll and Sir Arthur Conan Doyle who wrote *The History of Spiritualism* (1926). 'Psychical' refers to supernatural and paranormal activity and should be distinguished from 'psychic' which now refers to the activity of the mind (*Psyche* was the goddess of the soul and *psyche* also means butterfly, which changes from a caterpillar to a beautiful insect).

Exposing fraud

John Nevil Maskelyne (1839-1917)
As a young watchmaker in Cheltenham, England, Maskelyne attended a Davenport séance in 1865. He felt chagrin when asked to repair a mechanical device and realised it was being used to make the rapping noises at the séances. As an invited member of the stage committee surrounding the Spirit Cabinet he saw how the illusion was created. Three months later he and his friend, cabinetmaker George Cooke, gave a demonstration of a 'séance in open daylight, showing the possibility of accomplishing, without the aid of spiritualism, not only all the Davenports' tricks but many others.' The brothers left England four weeks later.[14]

Maskelyne and Cooke became professional magicians and entertainers. One of Maskelyne's most notable inventions was the *Box Trick* in which he made an instantaneous escape from a roped and locked trunk. Later they presented a rapid substitution of the magician sitting on the trunk with a young lady from the inside. Now known as *Metamorphosis*, the illusion has been a favourite of numerous magicians since, including Houdini. Maskelyne used his watch making skills in many of the illusions he invented – his most useful device was the Patented Coin-Operated Mechanism. Anyone with the need could drop a penny in the slot and the door to the public convenience would open – as if by magic. Being able to 'spend a penny' was a valuable contribution to public health.

For a time, a principal component of Maskelyne and Cooke's act was to expose fraudulent spiritualists, mediums and psychics. In 1870 they presented a private show for the Prince of Wales, explaining they were performing illusions and were not in harmony with vital spirits. They afterwards advertised themselves as 'Royal Illusionists' and as 'Anti-Spiritualists'. Their shows at the Egyptian Hall in Piccadilly did much to help vulnerable members of their audiences avoid being gulled and cheated by fraudsters, though they always invited the audience to make up their own minds. With only two hundred seats the Hall was no bigger than The Magic Circle's present theatre at the Centre for Magical Arts in London but became famous as 'England's Home of Mystery.'

With an eye out for new attractions, other magicians offered similar demonstrations. Most magicians are very honest. They tell you they are going to fool you – and then they do so. A magician who claims his skills are as a result of supernatural assistance is simply a fraud – and in the field of health care, whether mental, emotional, psychological or physical – a quack. Though exposure of a magician's secrets is anathema to magicians, a number of have offered séances coupled with exposure of the fraudulent methods of spiritualists. Members of societies such as The Magic Circle undertake not to expose methods to anyone who is not a magician. Nevertheless, with so many vulnerable people being gulled into parting with money in order to establish contact with their dear departed, some of the most eminent magicians developed good careers exposing this quackery.

Erich Weiss (1874-1926)
Weiss became best known as the magician and escapologist Harry Houdini, but also as the debunker of psychics and mediums. Sir Arthur Conan Doyle, who had trained as a doctor, was a committed spiritualist and believer in fairies. He thought his friend Harry was himself a medium and Doyle was critical at his lack of integrity in admitting it. Houdini arranged with his wife Bess, that after his death, if it were possible, his spirit would return and give her a code word during a séance. It never has, but Houdini Séances are still held by magic societies around the world on the anniversary of his death every October 31st and magicians live in hope.

One technique commonly used by fraudulent mediums and psychics goes under the heading of 'cold reading'. It is surprisingly easy to question a subject and get information which can then be fed back in a way which leads them to believe the medium has the assistance of the supernatural. 'Hot reading' involves covert access to information such as sources based on the Internet, or simply having assistants overhear conversations in the theatre lobby, pre-show.

A number of fraudsters have been debunked, but desperate folk prefer not to notice. Séance demonstrations by magicians are illusions but unless they are declared as such, they are not part of modern magic because fraudulent deceit of vulnerable and gullible people is involved and is anathema to ethical magicians. Genuine psychics communicate with the dead by supernatural means and cannot be challenged as being frauds without running the risk of being sued for libel. Under UK libel law the burden of proof lies with the accuser having to prove the claim. If a psychic simply states 'I can communicate with the dead', science will have a hard time proving they cannot achieve this feat. Of course, if an investigator can prove there has been covert radio communication or phone hacking that might be different. As ever, you must be the judge.

J.N. Maskelyne founded The Magic Circle's Occult Committee in 1914. Today's Paranormal Investigation Committee continues under the chairmanship of David Berglas to 'To investigate claims to supernatural power and to expose fraud.' The Society of American Magicians has had an Occult Investigation Committee since the time of Harry Houdini. Magicians who are legitimate in offering their mysteries as entertainment will have their secrets preserved but fraudulent claims to be using supernatural forces will be exposed. 'International Man of Mystery' David Berglas gave a séance at the Magic Circle's Centenary Conference in which he demonstrated table tipping and levitation. Derren Brown has reproduced the Davenport Brother's Spirit Cabinet illusion on television. Tommy Cooper only lasted a second in the box before lurching out declaring 'Ooh – it's dark in there!'

Randall James Zwinge (b.1928)
Magician 'The Amazing James Randi', has set up an Educational Foundation in order to expose fraud in the area of paranormal, psychic and supernatural claims, to promote critical thinking and to enable people to defend themselves against pseudoscientific claims (*para*, beyond. Latin: *super*, above). The JREF has a million dollar challenge to anyone who can produce evidence of paranormal activities including mediumship, homeopathy, Reiki and 'effects which lie outside the range of normal experience or scientific explanation.' A million euros is also on offer on a similar basis through the Association for Skeptical Enquiry. The awards remain unclaimed. Magicians are quite prepared to mislead and misdirect patients with sleight of hand and sleight of mind, but only as honest entertainment. Not as part of a fraudulent act.[15]

Derren Brown (b.1971)
The psychological illusionist and 2012 winner of The Magic Circle's Maskelyne Award for contributions to British Magic Arts has explored *Fear and Faith* in TV programmes. Brown was able to demonstrate how an atheist scientist discovers god, the psychological basis of religious belief, and how a new drug completely removes fear. Were these outcomes the result of hypnosis? The use of advanced placebo effects? Impudent thaumaturgy? You must be the judge – but have faith.

Respecting faith, beliefs and CAM

Freedom of thought, conscience and religion is now guaranteed by article 9 of the European Convention on Human Rights. 'Twas not always thus. The last executions for witchcraft in England were in Exeter in 1682, and the last man to be hanged in Britain for blasphemy was eighteen year old Thomas Aikenhead in Edinburgh as recently as 1697. Although the freedom to hold religious views is absolute, article 9 makes it clear that the freedom to manifest one's religion is subject to certain limitations, including those designed to protect the rights and freedoms of others. Article 19 of the Universal declaration of Human Rights includes the right 'to seek and impart information and ideas through any media', but there is no right not to be offended or hear contrary opinions.

Respect for people's freedom of belief does not imply respect for those beliefs, or that people are free to act on those beliefs without constraint. Likewise, the expression of opposition to any beliefs, whether religious or concerning medical care, is vital to critical discourse. This can create a problem for those who wish to see CAM 'integrated' with conventional medicine, because too close an involvement with irrational and implausible faiths and teachings encourages a flight from science and corrupts the attempts of conventional healthcare professionals to advance evidence-based medicine.

If we take it that a religion defines an organised cultural approach to a deity, CAMs are not religions – but they do require a belief in unconventional, non, pseudo, or even anti-scientific precepts. To that extent they are irrational, based on faith and comparable considerations in respect of 'respect' can be applied. Many who demand 'respect' seek to prevent criticism or satire. Respect is not synonymous with tolerance or deference. Camists who demand respect for their beliefs are actually seeking deference, reverence, regard, esteem and approbation for themselves. That may not be appropriate. Not all beliefs should be respected – racism and sexism are certainly not. A person's right to believe unwise or irrational things must be respected and so should the person. But that does not mean the belief is endorsed and should not be challenged by critical and rational analysis.

When Elizabeth was crowned on June 2nd 1953, the Queen made her Coronation Oath in which she was asked: 'Will you to the utmost of your power maintain the Laws of God and the true Profession of the Gospel? Will you to the utmost of your power maintain in the United Kingdom the Protestant Reformed Religion established by law? Will you maintain and preserve inviolably the settlement of the Church of England, and the doctrine, worship, discipline and government thereof, as by law established in England?' She replied: 'All this I promise to do.' Whether Prince Charles will in all good conscience feel able to take this oath, given his professed hope that he would rather see his role as 'Defender of Faith, not *the* Faith', remains to be seen. It is hard to see how encouragement or support of any other faith is compatible with the obligation to do all in his power to maintain and preserve the protestant reformed religion and settlement. No doubt in due time he will explain, or seek to have the settlement altered.[16] Prince Charles' faith in the value of unconventional treatments was explained when he addressed the BMA in 1982:

> I suppose, too, that human nature is such that we are frequently prevented from seeing that what is taken for today's unorthodoxy is probably going to be tomorrow's convention. Perhaps we just have to accept it is God's will that the unorthodox individual is doomed to years of frustration, ridicule and failure in order to act out his role in the scheme of things, until his day arrives and mankind is ready to receive his message; a message which he probably finds hard to explain himself, but which he knows comes from a far deeper source than conscious thought.

Bear in mind that science-based medicine was unorthodox until the twentieth century, but is conventional today. William Harvey, Charles Darwin, Ignaz Semmelweis and many others were ridiculed at first, but it is now science which provides rational messages.

Humanism and Secularism

In order to provide context and balance, this chapter closes by offering quotes from authors who have considered different belief systems but which are not religious:

'Humanism in the modern sense of the term is the view that whatever your ethical system, it derives from your best understanding of human nature and the human condition in the real world. This means it does not premise putative data from astrology, fairy tales, super-naturalistic beliefs, animism, polytheism, or any other inheritance's from the ages of humankind's remote and more ignorant past.' A. C. Grayling.[17]

'The humanist view of life is progressive and optimistic, in awe of human potential, living without fear of judgement and death, finding enough purpose and meaning in life, love and leaving a good legacy.' Polly Toynbee, President, British Humanist Association, 2012.[18]

'Humanism is a philosophy of service for the greater good of all humanity, of application of new ideas of scientific progress for the benefit of all.' Linus Pauling, Nobel Prize winner.

George Holyoake had been the last person convicted in the UK for blasphemy in a public lecture in 1842. In 1851 he coined 'secularism' to describe a philosophy which requires the separation of government or institutional organisation from religion or religious beliefs (Latin: *in saeculo*, in the world). Secularism is termed 'laicism' in France and some other European countries (*laikos*, of the people). The formal status of France, Spain and Israel are as secular states. Many secularists are atheists or humanists, but some may be devoutly religious. All believe in freedom of religion but that religion should remain a personal matter and not impinge on the state or society in general.

Philosopher Stephen Law advises: 'Humanism involves a commitment to secularism…but a secular society is not necessarily a society in which there is little or no public manifestation of religious belief… simply one in which the state itself takes a neutral view with respect to religion.'[19]

Delivering the British Humanists Association's Voltaire Lecture in 2015, Bonya Roy, whose husband Avijit was hacked to death in Bangladesh for writing a blog reflecting humanist values, said: 'It is not just ourselves, but each other, every trafficked slave, every murdered writer, every lost and lonely mind, that are important and have value.' Human beings have yet some way to evolve.

Endnotes to Chapter 16

1. New Testament, King James Version, often attributed to Paul, Letter to the Hebrews 11:1, c. 63AD.

2. Michel de Montaigne, essayist (1533-1592).

3. Theo Hobson, *Faith*, Acumen Publishing, Durham, 2009.

4. General Medical Council, *Good Medical Practice,* 2006.

5. *Iatros*, healer, hence *iatrogenic* for harm resulting from the ministrations of healers themselves.

6. Asklepios bore a staff with single serpent entwined which has become the worldwide symbol of medicine. The staff with two serpents and wings, the caduceus, was the Greeks' symbol of Hermes (the Romans' Mercury), messenger to the gods and a player of tricks and scams. The caduceus had nothing directly to do with medicine until American Army orderlies who carried messages and communications to medical personnel adopted it as the symbol for their units and uniforms. Its use in medicine is misleading, unless the intention is to convey trickery.

7. Mark 16:15-18 and *The Great Commission.* Matthew 28:16-20. New International Version, 1966.

8. Alain de Botton. *Religion for Atheists*. Penguin Books, London 2012.

9. E. Allison Peters, translator. *The Autobiography of Teresa of Ávila.* www.jesus.org.uk/ vault/library/Teresa_life.pdf. 1995. Chapter XX.

10. The astronomical identity and position of Kolob is unknown. Joseph Smith: *Book of Abraham*. Times & Seasons, Nauvoo, Illinois, 1842. The name designates Utah's Kolob Canyons. Please do not spell it backwards, beliefs must be respected.

11. *Book of Mormon.* 3 Nephi 11 to 3 Nephi 26.

12. *Book of Mormon.* 9:19; LDS Doctrine & Covenants (originally 1835), Salt Lake, Utah, 1921. 35:9 and 46:19..

13. Charles Page: *Psychomancy: Spirit-rappings and table-tippings exposed.* D. Appleton & Co. New York. 1853.

14. Michael Bailey: *The Magic Circle: Performing Magic through the ages.* Tempus Publishing, Stroud, 2007. The American Davenport Brothers should not be confused with the British family of the same name which runs a prominent firm for the supply of magic books and paraphernalia from its shop at Charing Cross, London.

15. www.randi.org.

16. www.princeofwales.gov.uk.

17. A.C. Grayling. *Against All Gods.* Oberon Books, London, 2007.

18. www.thinkhumanism.com/humanist-quotes.html.

19. Stephen Law, *Humanism*, Oxford University Press, 2011.

Part Three:
The Real Secrets Revealed

Chapter 17

How Alternative Medicine works

Know thyself.
Ancient Greek maxim

To thine own self be true
Polonius[1]

The brain is very good at deluding itself.
Daniel Levitin, Neuroscientist

Reality is plastic. We do not see our immediate world as it is, but as it was a split second ago. Nerve signals when we sense the external world, think, dream and imagine are travelling at about 270 miles an hour. The speed of thought is orders slower than the speed of light, and continues even when we are asleep. Alive, we dream.

Little packets of energy, connected to each other by nerve cells of the brain, give us the experience of our mind. There are a thousand trillion nerve connections in our brains This is the number of seconds in 30 million years. The reader will have to await further research for deeper explanations of how a mind is created, but no 'vital force' has been identified. Julian Huxley noted: 'We do not explain how a railway steam engine works by saying it is due to a 'locomotive force'. Why then do we explain how the brain works by suggesting a 'vital force?'[2]

The packets of energy result in an electric current being propagated to the next cell by organic molecules. There are more than fifty neurochemicals including catecholamines; glutamate; oxytocin; acetylcholine; adrenaline; noradrenalin; endorphins; serotonin; opioids; oxytocin; endocannabinoids, amphetamines and dopamine. All are fundamental to the experience of satisfaction and pleasure – including sexual orgasm, which most people find pleasurable. Dopamine, a monoamine neurotransmitter and precursor of adrenaline is responsible for reward-based learning and may account for the effects of drugs of addiction.

We all have different proportions of chemicals, different speeds of transmission, experience different patterns and will have different thoughts. Some of these thoughts might be comparable to a significant number of other members of our culture or society. They may be regarded as 'rational,' and conclusions based on them as representing the closest we can get at this moment in time to the science of truth – and the truth of science. Other patterns may be experienced by people whose neuro-biochemistry is so relatively unusual that their thought processes are regarded as highly irrational, disturbed, pathological and an illness. They are worthy of care certainly, and treatment if possible. Some people experience patterns and have thoughts in which they firmly believe, but if there are no clear, plausible, rational explanations for those thoughts, they are termed as being due to faith – no matter how real they are to those who experience them. They may have been first experienced in a moment of sudden realisation and even attributed as the epiphany of divine revelation with deep emotional resonance. Many of those who have promoted healthcare systems we now describe as alternative have claimed such origins for their beliefs. Whether their feelings were truly epiphanic or they simply decided to quack and defraud is not easy to determine.

We all try to care for one another, and particularly for those patients suffering from dis-ease or injury of mind, body or spirit. To show compassion, to offer consolation, hope and love. We are constantly trying to devise new and better methods to achieve those tasks with ever-greater efficiency and effectiveness in a system we call 'medicine'. Our collective experiences of the world, studied by observations, analysed and refined by the most sophisticated methods available, provide knowledge which offers the greatest chance of success in achieving our aims. To provide succour, to cure, to care, to heal and to provide the benefit of satisfaction. Some patients have emotions, experiences, feelings and imaginations that allow them to identify alternatives to this scientific based approach. Some practitioners may intend taking advantage of that mindset.

Conventional orthodox medicine sets out its stall, warts and all. Any claims of benefit from new treatments are subject to rigorous review of evidence gained by using scientific methods and properly published. Claims are subject to challenge.[3] Conventional medicine is not infallible and is often wrong, but it changes when there are good reasons.

Faced with patients' demands for alternative systems, orthodox practitioners may be obliged to offer them – or arrange referral to a camist. Such acquiescence should not be taken as an endorsement of CAM but simply reflects the practitioner's desire to satisfy their patient. It is for politicians and policymakers to decide whether this approach is economically viable and fair to the rest of the community. It is for the orthodox professions to decide whether such practice is ethical, intellectually honest and demonstrates adequate standards of probity and integrity. Hence the value of thinking critically about the *Real Secrets of Alternative Medicine.*

Over the years, a number of registered medical practitioners, including those of high repute, have shown an interest in supporting the use of medical systems alternative to those they have conventionally employed. At one time, the GMC's standard was that professional association with a practitioner who was not registered was unethical. That standard has slipped but doctors are judged by the standards of those with whom they associate. Camists may be genuinely beholden to a faith and believe that 'energies', spirits and vital forces are capable of manipulation and that wellbeing can be achieved by esoteric, thaumatugical and magical means. On the other hand, they may be quacks, scamists and charlatans seeking deliberately to defraud the susceptible. How to tell the difference is of concern to not only camees but also to doctors and healthcare professionals who might wish to associate with them.

Clarity and integrity is essential. There is no plausible evidence water has 'memory' of the energies to which it has been subjected, nor that homeopathic remedies contain any therapeutically active principle. Massage may be pleasurable, but there is no plausible evidence that general illness or diseases of non-musculoskeletal tissues and organs may be assisted by manipulation of musculoskeletal tissue. There is no plausible evidence that subluxations of vertebrae can be adjusted and 'innate spirit' thereby allowed to pass more freely and affect distant tissues or organs. There is no plausible evidence for clinically relevant *meridians, chakras, chi* or other mediation of 'energy' that may be affected by needles. There is no credible evidence that unrefined molecules obtained from plants have 'spirits' of unidentified quality. Much less, that a whole plant can possess these powers. There is no evidence a human hand can transmit healing 'energy'. These considerations are all a matter of the esoteric, occult, if not bizarre. They are faiths – beliefs with no plausible base. They should be accepted for what they are – faith in nothingness – *wu*. They need to be understood in their historical, political and commercial context and their plausibility needs assessment in the context of modern healthcare and wellbeing. Plausible truth is established on the basis of objective scientific reasoning, not religious or metaphysical opinion (Latin: *plaudere*, to applaud – meaning 'having the appearance of truth').[4]

Given the lack of plausible objective evidence that CAM systems can affect specific pathological processes to any significant extent, it is inevitable that whilst many were once conventional, over time they have become alternatives. The advent of progressively effective scientific methods of study during the seventeenth century Enlightenment and rejection of the supernatural and mystical has led to science based systems now being regarded as the conventional with other methods becoming anachronistic and left behind. Yet many patients remain dissatisfied that not all their desires are being met. They want more attention and more time and trouble spent on compassion, care and comfort – they need the Cloak of Consolation. Conventional medicine all too frequently does not comply.

Given the propensity for camistry to be based on non, pseudo, and even anti scientific precepts, their status as alternatives cannot be denied. Given the propensity for camists to satisfy the irrational beliefs and faiths of their adherents, it is inevitable that people who are more attached to science as a basis for truth, regard those beliefs with cynicism bordering on distain. Yet many patients report benefit from the ministrations of camists. Others simply gain pleasure from the condimentary effects.

Quite why some people have irrational beliefs has been studied by psychologists and should be considered by students of all health care professions.[5, 6] Nobel prize winner Daniel Kahneman feels that everyone's thinking is handicapped by their own mental equipment. Together with Amos Tversky he suggested humans are naturally less rational than commonly assumed. The really interesting question is why we think rationally at all. In *Thinking, Fast and Slow*, Kahneman describes two systems of thought. One is fast, intuitive and emotional, dealing with issues requiring snap judgements – such as when driving a car or having a first impression about people. However, the thinker may have a misleading impression of their situation and be misled. The second system is slower and more judgemental. It is more logical but is lazy and may not undertake the full scrutiny that the situation demands. Again, the thinker may be misled. *Prospect Theory* considers how people weigh up alternatives and make decisions and suggests that pleasure depends more on subjective experience of benefits than objective, scientifically ascertained, reality.[7] Thinking is hard work. Critical thinking more so.

Secrets, Revelation and Exposure

Revealing the secrets of how CAMs work is likely to engender the same antipathy, opposition and disapproval from camists as evidenced by magicians when their secrets are exposed. Many CAMs originated in the Mysterious Orient, or were developed by practitioners who were occultists, claimed possession of secret hermetic knowledge and who advanced medical systems based on faith in spirits and vital forces. Critical examination exposes the irrationality of their practices, but by enveloping them in a miasma of obfuscation, a cloak of confusion, ill-defined jargon and misuse of scientific terms, patients and the public are deliberately misled. 'Deliberately' because there is no other reason camists would not be more forthcoming and demonstrate a higher degree of openness and intellectual honesty if that were not their intention. Many camists have ideas and concepts they would rather have kept secret. They argue that 'I believe it works and at least it does no harm'. But they have no evidence to support either contention, are in denial, and fail to properly inform their patients about the lack of demonstrable effectiveness of proposed treatments (unless they are highly selective about research they choose). Patients cannot give fully informed consent. That is unethical practice.

Since time immemorial, magicians have relied upon their effects being mysterious, esoteric, and secret. In ancient times, there was little difference between religion, medicine and magic – between priests, physicians and magi. Today we have to consider how the revelation of magical medical techniques affects the art and practice of both conventional and alternative medicine.

The motto of The Magic Circle, *Indocilis Privata Loqui*, captures the ethical obligations of its members and to which all members must assent – 'Not inclined to speak of secrets.' When joining the Circle, members solemnly promise and undertake: 'Not in any way knowingly, or intentionally, to disclose any secret of magic to anyone unless they be a magician and to confine the discussion of effects and secrets originated within the society to Members of The Magic Circle or affiliated societies.' Hippocrates' oath required physicians to 'keep secret and never reveal all that may come to my knowledge in the exercise of my profession or in daily commerce, which ought not to be spread abroad.' Today's doctors are still bound by a duty of confidentiality about patient's secrets.

Limited revelation of magical secrets to fellow magicians is acceptable in order to advance the Art of Magic, but not to the lay public.[8] Fortunately, purchasing a book devoted to magic makes you a magician. Conversely, the practice of medicine requires that the patient must give fully informed consent and all treatments, practices and outcomes should be honestly and transparently explained. Those with something to hide, who rely on their practices having thaumaturgical, magical, metaphysical elements, may wish to keep their secrets. They may even sue or denigrate those who expose them.

The revelation of secrets has a long history. In the twentieth century BC, tales were told about the skills of priests and magicians at the court of the Pharaoh Cheops. The oldest record of a magical effect is the account of court magician Dedi being able to decapitate animals and then restore them. Heron of Alexandria (10-70 AD) revealed how priests at temples in Delphi and Thebes used magic tricks to impress religious devotees. 1584 saw the publication of the earliest two books specifically written to expose the methods of magicians – by Scot in London and Jean Prévost in Paris.

Reginald Scot

Scot's *The Discoverie of Witchcraft* (1584) had two laudable aims. Firstly to help the public protect themselves against charlatans, quacks and mountebanks, by explaining that their amazing 'magic' was in fact sleight of hand and jugglery. Secondly, to save the poor women under death sentence as witches by showing that any 'magic' that might have been ascribed to them was mere trickery and there was no association with the supernatural or the Devil. Many of these women were practicing a style of shamanistic medicine. Scot even raised the possibility that the illusion of witchcraft was due to the mental state of the observers.

When James VI of Scotland acceded to the English throne, he declared Scot's revelations about witchcraft as 'damnable' and directed that all copies of the book be burnt – but some survived. Shakespeare drew on *The Discoverie* for the witches in *Macbeth* (c.1606). Scot's descriptions of magic tricks were plagiarised and formed the basis of *The Art of Juggling* (1612) and *Hocus-Pocus Junior* (1634). The Church of England removed reference to the Devil from its liturgy in 2015. Progress.

Angelo John Lewis (1839-1919)

Born in London, Lewis qualified as a lawyer and practiced at the bar. He wrote a series of articles on puzzles and magical problems published as *Modern Magic in* 1876. Naturally he was concerned that his clients might have some chagrin at their lawyer being so capable of deception, so he indulged himself by appropriating the title of 'Professor' and the name of a suitably sounding foreign gentleman. These tricks of marketing are not unknown to camists and their institutions. As 'Professor Louis Hoffmann' he went on to publish a number of other books and translated Jean Robert-Houdin's *Secrets of Conjuring and Magic* in 1878, commenting: 'The more important secrets of the art have been known but to few, and those few have jealously guarded them, knowing that the more closely they concealed the clue to their mysteries, the more would those mysteries be valued.'[9]

That remains the approach of many camists who fail to explain how their practices work, and who fail to provide any plausible evidence of them working beyond the placebo effects.

S.W. Erdnase

The Expert at the Card Table, first published in 1902 claimed S. W Erdnase as author. Although initially sold through magic shops, the wider public soon became aware of his exposé of methods used by card cheats. The author's name was probably an anagram for one Milton Andrews. When suspected of a murder in 1905 he shot himself, but Erdnase had set out his motives for writing *The Expert* in its preface:

> In offering this book to the public the writer uses no sophistry as an excuse

for its existence. It may caution the unwary who are innocent of guile and it may inspire the crafty by enlightenment on artifice. If it sells it will accomplish the primary motive of the author, as he needs the money.

Totday the camee has to consider the extent to which financial gain or personal advantage is the underlying motive for any camist they may consider.

David Wighton (1868-1941)
Undoubtedly the foremost magician of his day, as David Devant, Wighton was the obvious choice to be first President of The Magic Circle in 1905. Its Council was dismayed when in 1909 Devant authored a number of articles describing *Tricks for Everyone* in *The Royal Magazine*. When challenged, he suggested such publication was beneficial to the art of magic. Devant's status was not sufficient to prevent him being expelled by The Circle.

The impact of exposure of magical secrets, particularly since the advent of the Internet, has led to a greater degree of cynicism about the skills performed, yet with shrewd presentation the public is as intrigued as ever. The key issues are whether exposure spoils the benefit an audience gets from a magic presentation – and whether magicians' professional reputations and incomes are affected.

So it is with camistry. CAMs do work. We need to consider to what extent, and why the experience of a visit to a camist works. Camists understand placebo effects well, but prefer to continue with the tradition of invoking spirits, occult forces, ephemeral fluencies, imagined energy fields, implausible anatomical, physiological and physical constructs – that is, nothingness, *wu*. *Wudoka* who follow *wu* and camees who use CAM but are less adherent to *wu* as a philosophy, have to consider whether camists hold these beliefs with sincerity, integrity and honesty, or whether they are quacks, charlatans – even frauds. There will be no hard evidence to assist. Judgement will be called for – you must be the judge.

There are many reasons why people have faith and believe in alternatives to conventional medical systems. There are many reasons why patients and practitioners report benefit from any system of medicine, whether conventional or alternative. What matters is the extent to which any of the factors listed below apply to the camee who has the beneficial experience and to the medical system utilised.

CAMs work through type I effects of a constructive therapeutic relationship with an empathic practitioner. Conventional medicine likewise, but additionally by a direct type II effects on specific diseases. Setting aside quacks and frauds who understand perfectly well that CAMs have no type II effects on a specific disease, and those who feel they have the personal experience of an epiphany, the mindset of having faith in camistry can become entrenched and bolstered by factors which often overlap. Many apparently rational people, even with scientific training such as some doctors, do believe CAM has a worthwhile clinical value. By definition, there are no objective plausible reasons to believe that CAM pills, puncturing, pushing,

RICHARD RAWLINS

prodding, potions or paranormal preternatural powers provide a benefit greater than a placebo in the context of a therapeutic relationship. Nevertheless, if patients are to make wise choices and give properly informed consent, the reasons that belief in camistry persists have to be critically considered.

In addition to placebo effects, camees must understand that any perceived benefits of treatment may result from the natural history of the condition (many recover in any event); regression to the mean value (a statistical but natural phenomenon); and other treatments (which they took but did not declare). Anecdotes from other patients are unhelpful for all these reasons and because other camees may desire to please their camist.

The principle reasons camees turn to camistry are on account of disillusionment (with conventional care), deception (in manifest forms), denial (that their beliefs are irrational), dissonance (believing both conventional science and commercially promoted pseudo-science at the same time), delusion (with thinking gone awry), deferral (a preference to avoid convention), and being duped (in respect of all the above). All can be analysed further:

Secret 1. Disillusionment with conventional orthodox medicine

Conventional medicine does not have all the answers and practitioners are not always able to satisfy their patients. Patients may say 'Doctor's tell me they can do no more,' but although it may be the case medicine can do nothing about the disease process, healthcare practitioners most certainly can and should do much about patients' feelings, emotions, sense of self and mastery of the situation. Nevertheless, some patients will turn elsewhere. Some will want an alternative *to* Medicine.

There may be much unmet demand. Patients may have had poor outcomes from conventional treatment, adverse side effects from pharmaceutical drugs and negative experiences of the doctor/patient relationship. High costs are of importance especially parts of the world without a national health system. Regular medicine has fragmented into specialities and critics find the medical profession to be elitist, self-serving and insensitive to the needs of patients. Time constraints and bureaucracy are major issues, but patients want a personal approach, comprehensive examination, effective intervention and to be involved. They may have views on health and wellbeing not in line with the conventional medical model. They are beguiled by the imaginative claims of alternative practitioners.

Many camists who devised alternative systems did so because they had become disillusioned with the conventional medicine and science of their day. Some were unable or unwilling to train and qualify as orthodox doctors. They preferred to devise novel systems of practice, to style themselves as 'doctors' and to practice without a regulated licence. Some practitioners had originally qualified in the orthodox way, but instead of researching and developing contemporary practices to overcome their faults and problems, they grafted on bizarre concepts and occult precepts that simply had no basis in scientific understanding. Many were seen as nothing more than quacks.

In 1796 Dr Samuel Hahnemann wrote to a friend 'I renounced the practice of medicine that I might no longer incur the risk of doing injury, and I engaged in chemistry exclusively and in literary occupations.'[10] Hahnemann developed a system of remedies containing no active principle whatsoever. Many colleagues shared his disillusionment with the contemporary therapeutic armamentarium and Hahnemann's system of homeopathy expanded. Mainstream medicine did slowly put its house in order (giving up bloodletting was a start), but Hahnemann was not to return to the fold – he was more satisfied with his alternative. Edward Bach was another medically qualified homeopath who became 'somewhat disillusioned with the medicine of his day' and as a result devised a simple healing system based on flower essences.[11]

Disillusionment with the slow progress of modern medical science and practice continues and is shared to some extent by most of us. These feelings may have provided the motivation for some doctors to associate with the 'College of Medicine' which brings together 'a scientific perspective, albeit a slightly new scientific perspective with 'healing' and 'integration with patients' beliefs and wishes.'[12] Some of these beliefs and wishes are for non-scientific alternative medical systems. Whether such doctors are lost souls, deluded as well as disillusioned; knowing quacks; or insightful and progressive practitioners must be left to the judgement of patients – and those who fund such systems.

Contemporary problems of developing, researching, manufacturing and marketing drugs have resulted in dangers and difficulties. Ben Goldacre has reported these problems in *Bad Pharma*, which should be on every doctor's bookshelf. Missing data, flawed trials, suppression of unfavourable results and regulatory failure has all led to many doctors feeling decidedly disillusioned with the pharmaceutical industry and its products. Government interference with clinical decisions, target setting, and intrusive management has had a similar effect. Since 1948 UK doctors worked either directly for the patient, as doctors in the public service, or both.

Since the 1990s most doctors have been obliged to work as public servants who just happen to be medically qualified. Now doctors are to be employees of commercial companies which are required to generate a profit for their shareholders and whose 'product' just happens to be healthcare. A President of the Royal College of Surgeons of England has expressed concern at being told which patients to operate on by managers. Most surgeons share the same concerns.[13]

But this professional disillusionment can be assuaged. A free press survives and amongst others, we have Goldacre, Singh, Ernst, Lewis, Henness, Pemberton and Godlee to report and comment for our edification. And the scientific methods by which we can assess drugs, treatments and practices are improving – that is no illusion.

Secret 2. CAM systems work – but not as camists would have you believe

All medicine, whether conventional or alternative, can 'work' and patients may report they have 'benefited'. Patients gain pleasure and comfort from the therapies. To reiterate: those effects occur, to a greater or lesser extent, in one, or both, of two ways:

Type I effect: As the result of a non-specific constructive therapeutic relationship with an empathic practitioner. With emphasis on compassion, consolation, solace, hope and love. Patients receive Tender Loving Care, TLC. That works. That takes time. The patient is given meanings and interpretations about their health which is more coherent with their beliefs than hard science. The more expectations are reinforced, the greater the perceived benefit. Evidence is subjective.

Type II effect: As a result of identified therapeutic chemical or physical effects on specific biochemical, physiological and pathological processes which have been established, to the greatest extent possible, by scientific methods. They may work. Evidence is objective.

But are Alternative Medical Systems effective and efficacious? Do they have any Type II effects? Are there any effects aside from those due to the attentions of an empathic caring practitioner?

In assessing any CAM the question is whether it has a useful therapeutic effect and the extent to which it is efficacious or effective. Taxpayers, insurance companies, politicians and other funders will need to consider whether financial investment is worthwhile. Those who use any medical system have to consider whether they might be wasting their time and whether an alternative to an alternative system might be better. And if a condimentary, complementary or alternative system is being considered, which one and to what extent benefit is probable.

The House of Commons Science and Technology Committee's *Report on the Evidence Base for Homeopathy* (2009) inquired 'Should NHS spending on any treatments be based on evidence of efficacy or effectiveness?' James Thallon, Medical Director, NHS West Kent replied 'Absolutely; I think it should be an organising principle of our system of provision of healthcare.' He was then asked 'What is your understanding of the difference between efficacy and effectiveness?' He replied: 'I do not know if I have one.'[14]

Peter Fisher, Medical Director of the Royal London Homoeopathic Hospital commented: 'It useful to draw a distinction between efficacy and effectiveness...In simple terms the distinction is between ideal conditions and real world conditions – efficacy being ideal conditions and effectiveness being real world conditions.'[15] Edzard Ernst, Director of Complementary Medicine at the University of Exeter and Peninsula Medical School gave the following example: 'Efficacy tests whether treatment works under ideal conditions – and then will not work in the real world because people experience side-effects.'[16] Those 'ideal conditions' being established in laboratory tests and clinical trials.

Robert Mathie, Research Development Adviser, British Homoeopathic Association answered: 'It is indeed a fundamental point. Efficacy is judged in placebo-controlled trials of a very specific medicine or intervention. So it is very specific – a very specific drug and a very specific dose; treating a very specific type of patient. So efficacy is almost a laboratory experiment, if you like. Effectiveness is something that usually non-placebo-controlled trials are designed to do – in which the real world effect of a system of care is judged against what is usual at that point.' The reader must judge if that explains the difference.

Ernst added: 'Without efficacy, effectiveness can be quite meaningless.... If you understand what homeopathy entails, one hour of empathy and understanding towards the patient, it is predictable such a trial would generate a positive result simply because of its non-specific effect – its placebo effects – and therefore because it is predictable, such a trial should not be done because you know the result before the trial, and arguably such a trial is even unethical.' Paragraph 29 of the Science and Technology Committee's Report states: 'The answer to why a medicine can be effective without being efficacious lies with a phenomenon known as the placebo effect.' Ernst further explores this theme in *Trick or Treatment?* [17]

The Shorter Oxford English Dictionary defines 'efficacy' as: 'Capacity to produce effects; power to effect the object intended. A mode of effecting a result (John Locke).' 'Effectiveness' is: 'the quality of being effective.' 'Effective' is defined as: 'That is concerned in the production of effects; having the power of acting upon objects. Concerned with, or having the function of, effecting. That has an effect.' New Collins Thesaurus has an alternative word for 'efficacy' namely 'effectiveness.' Also a synonym for 'effectiveness' namely 'efficacy.' It is difficult to differentiate between the meaning of either word.

Regulations require that pharmaceutical companies producing new drugs must demonstrate their products are efficacious and safe. Generally, comparison with a group of patients given placebos will be required, but if not, results have to be compared with existing therapies – establishing 'comparative efficacy.'

The regulatory authorities need to judge whether the evidence on comparative risks and benefits of a new product places the public at undue risk. This subtle and semantic distinction between efficacy and effectiveness is really only of value for the regulators and pharmaceutical industry. Since homeopathy is not regulated in the same way as orthodox medicine and since homoeopathic and herbal remedies, supplements and other CAM products are not pharmacological medicines, it is disingenuous to use technical pharmaceutical terminology when assessing their value. There is no need to create a spurious distinction. Any attempt to suggest the words have different meanings is an attempt to set up a false dichotomy. There is either good evidence that a treatment or remedy has type II effects on a specific disease, or not.

There is no credible evidence that homoeopathic remedies have a beneficial effect in 'ideal conditions' – the pillules have no therapeutic effect. There is evidence that patients describe the experience of homoeopathic consultations and even self-prescribing in the 'real world' as being beneficial. In that sense, the practice of 'homeopathy' is effective – a type I effect, but that does not mean the remedy or pillule is effective. So why contemplate wasting resources on them, or on funding further research into them?

Camists must answer: 'Do patients derive any benefit from using your modality as the result of what you do or the way that you do it – which is simply the result of your patient's experience of a constructive therapeutic relationship with you?'

The House of Lords Select Committee on Science and Technology report on Allergy treatment considered the effectiveness of Homeopathy (2007). Question 538 was from Lord Broers: 'I have a simple technical question about homeopathy and drugs. Is it possible to distinguish between homeopathic drugs after they have been diluted? Is there any means of distinguishing one from the other?' Kate Chatfield from the Homeopaths Research and Ethics Committee at the Society of Homeopaths replied: 'Only by the label.'[18]

Is there any useful distinction between the terms 'efficacy' and 'effectiveness' as used in day to day healthcare? You must be the judge.

Secret 3. The Delight of Magic and Sex

CAMs work. The psychological wonders of sex result from the myriad of chemicals and neurotransmitters; released during any animal's sexual encounters. Many are indistinguishable from those released at other times, such as with pain or demonstrations of entertaining magic. There are comparable sensations, emotions, feelings of transcendence and spiritual dimensions – experiences of pleasure or otherwise, perhaps of the earth moving. Generally, we can distinguish between the various activities which give rise to such powerful feelings. The Marquis de Sade and Christian Grey may have had difficulty at times. These chemicals are easily synthesised from simple pre-cursors and over fifty have now been identified including opioids, endorphins, dopamine and cannabinoids (Sanskrit: *ananda,* bliss). Morphine, named for the Greek god of dreams, is an exogenous natural opioid but acts similarly. Dia-morphine is synthetic, makes the recipient feel heroic and is known as *heroin*. All these chemicals are acting in the brain and creating a sense of heightened reality and focussed imagination. Modern scanning techniques of the limbic system and nucleus accumbens, where neurons produce gamma-aminobutyric acid, have shown comparable activity when experiencing sexual ecstasy and when listening to a favourite piece of music. It is likely all pleasurable experiences work in a similar way. Conversely, other molecules such as corticotrophin releasing factor 1, a protein found in the pituitary gland, trigger feelings of stress, anxiety and depression.

From the first century AD the term 'thaumaturgy' was used to describe 'magic' (*thauma*: marvel, wonder). Medieval magicians conjured up spirits by spells – today's camists claim they can engage spirits, innate intelligence or vital forces by sugar pills, manipulation, waving their hands, or accessing occult forces within plants. The sight, sound, situation and circumstance of a therapeutic encounter are all important in creating the expectation that healing and benefit will ensue – to which the subject may respond if suitable techniques are used. Each CAM has its own technique. How CAM remedies and treatments work is easy to answer. In isolation, beyond the placebo, they do not. If they did, they would become conventional medicine. It is the Type I effect of being in a constructive therapeutic relationship with a caring practitioner which works. A visit to a camist works because such an encounter handled with empathy and sincerity, will engender feelings of pleasure. If you can fake sincerity, you can get away with anything.[19]

Secret 4. Traditional Magic

The challenges of an increasingly technological and scientific age have led many to value traditional magical thinking based on sympathetic causality and similarity. From ancient times man has believed that connections between similar things can cause effects; that contact between things can retain 'connection' even after separation; that symbols have significance; and that 'vital forces' such as *prana* and *brahma* (Indian); *psi* and *aura* (American); *qi* (Chinese); *kramat* (Malay); *ashé* (Yoruba); *wakan* (Sioux); *the Force* (Star Wars) mediate the effects of sympathetic magic.

Sometimes referred to as 'imitative magic', neuroscientists are exploring the importance of imitative cognition for learning amongst higher primates as well as humans. Use of 'magic' in this sense can help individuals retain a sense of control over their lives and improve self-confidence. Magic works, but not as camists would have you believe.

The term 'magic' can mean the performance of tricks and entertaining illusions; the creation of something from nothing; the wonders of alchemy; new age mysticism, astrology, Kabbalah and sorcery. Camists not infrequently claim to be able to access nature's 'forces', 'energies', 'powers' or 'innate intelligence' – unavailable to the uninitiated.

Samuel Hahnemann himself recognised that people might assume he was promoting magic and did what he could to test his theories and align them with contemporary ideas. He studied Mesmer's animal magnetism and absorbed Schelling's concept

279

that 'the more unsubstantial the matter became by dilution, the purer and more effective could be its spirit like function.' The fact that the water had once been in contact with an active compound was enough. Schelling had also proposed that the 'potency' of a remedy increased by succusing constituents together. Hahnemann's experiments satisfied him that was so and 'homeopathy' resulted. The scientific medical community awaits plausible evidence. Placebo effects can seem like magic to the hard of thinking who lack insight.

Secret 5. The Charisma of Camistry

Many camists are sincere and honestly believe they possess special powers or abilities which enable them to diagnose and treat medical conditions without the necessity of first qualifying in conventional medicine. Some who are regularly qualified believe they have additional insights which enable them to utilise alternatives effectively. They are prepared to set aside the challenges and requirements of the scientific method and embrace CAM systems. Some camists may know their methods cannot be rationally supported – they are quacks and charlatans. They will not want this recognised and may even be in denial themselves. Still others know the scams perfectly well but are prepared to take advantage of the vulnerable and gullible for pecuniary advantage. They are frauds.

Patients have an interest not just in illness but in wellness – as do conventional practitioners. Often that is not made clear – it is easier and quicker for doctors to concentrate on the disease – diagnosing by investigation, suppressing or curing illness with drugs or surgery and hoping to avoid complications or side effects. Camistry allows time and deeper consideration of natural restorative processes, within a balanced, harmonic, holistic framework. Camist consultations may place greater emphasis on lifestyle, diet, environment, emotions and feelings than on symptoms and process of disease. Camists emphasise the importance of patients' own active involvement in their wellbeing. History taking and examination may be more comprehensive. The conventional clinician may be too clinical and not have enough time for those who seek consolation and condimentary care.

Interest in camistry, as practitioner and patient, often runs in families. For some, camistry accords with their views on health and wellbeing and encourages their active participation in treatment to a greater extent than many conventional practitioners allow. Patients can feel more in control and able to make choices. The impression that doctors are only interested in symptoms, not the causes, may be as a result of pressure of time but still represents a negative doctor-patient relationship. CAM offers a more personal approach, quality time, is relatively free of side-effects and gives pleasure. In a wider context, camistry diversifies the conceptual framework of medicine. Orthodox practitioners have much to learn from camistry.

Secret 6. The Lure of *Wudo*

Twenty years after the deprivations, restrictions and melancholy of the Second

World War, the baby boom generation were ready to rock. Initially we *Rocked Around the Clock* with Bill Haley, then stayed in *Heartbreak Hotel* with Elvis, got no *Satisfaction* from Mick and saw in the dawn of the *Age of Aquarius* with our *Hair*, and much else, let down.

An amalgam of esoteric philosophy, self-help psychology, parapsychology, astrology, holistic wellbeing, spiritualism, theosophy, and even quantum mechanics was stirred in the pot of Western and Eastern spiritual traditions and came to reflect the 'New Age' in which the mind, body and spirit are to be integrated. If the pot reflected 'ancient wisdom' or was of oriental origin, it appeared 'authentic'.

Stimulated by the writings of Emanuel Swedenborg, Anton Mesmer, George Gurdjieff, Helena Blavatsky, and other occultists, a *New Age* dawned. William Blake first used the phrase in 1809 in his preface of *To Milton, a poem*. Madame Blavatsky then used it in *The Secret Doctrine* (1888). Much of the philosophical approach of New Age shaped the Modernist movement in the arts of the early twentieth century. Psychologist Carl Jung supported the concept of an Age of Aquarius and Rudolf Steiner's Anthroposophy became a major influence with its concepts of reincarnation and karmic destiny. A New Age Movement based on these ideas was established in California in the 1960s, particularly at Big Sur's Esalen Institute, before spreading to the Findhorn Ecovillage in Scotland and then world-wide. Alternative medicines are particularly prevalent at New Age stores and festivals. As are accoutrements for Kapnismatic Medicine.

Since the 1960s some astrologers claim we have now entered the Age of Aquarius. Using different calculations, others suggest the transition between Pisces and Aquarius as being anywhere from 1400 to 4000 AD. The logo of The Magic Circle, devised in 1906, also has the signs of the Zodiac – in a clockwise order for good luck.

Ruldolf Steiner predicted the advent of the Age of Aquarius will be in 3573 AD. Steiner also foretold the return of Christ in the Ethereal World and the incarnation of Ahriman – a destructive spirit first identified by Zoroaster that will try to prevent humankind's development. He could be right.

The concept that life is due to a vital spark or force, attributed by some to a deity – 'vitalism' – is integral to ancient wisdom and found particular resonance with Paracelcus. However, Erwin Schrödinger described how can chemistry and physics can account for the processes that turn a single cell into something as complex as a human being in 1943 – an aperiodic crystal contains enough information within its covalent bonds to create a wealth of complexity, and can be contained in a tiny cell. Schrödinger left vitalism nowhere scientific to hide, but science and cultures change. Some people have become sceptical of modern scientific medicine as it has evolved from Traditional European or Western Medicine – and prefer to commune with innate spirits, energies, or even 'nothingness' in homeopathy, herbs, TCM, TIM – anything but Western medicine. William Deresiewicz has pointed out: 'The problem is, there is no such thing as Western medicine. There's scientific medicine, and then there's everything else. Scientific medicine isn't Western, because science isn't Western. Science transcends culture. It is the same everywhere – there is no such a thing as Western mathematics.' [20]

The founder of Homeopathy was intimately involved with the occult and esoteric. Osteopathy and Chiropractic were founded by magnetic healers who claimed divine inspiration. Acupuncture relies on hermetic channels of indeterminate identity. Herbalism is part and parcel of a naturalist and vitalist philosophy. Other CAMs depend on energies and forces quite unknown to modern science. All give pleasure to their adherents, often at a deeply spiritual level. They all have value but they should not be confused with modern medicine.

Fringe beliefs in vitalism will perpetuate for much the same reason the theory existed in the first place: it serves as a counter to reductionist philosophies, compliments other supernatural beliefs and eases the discomfort and cognitive dissonance caused by not understanding modern hypotheses. Wudoka who value, appreciate and follow paths which have no material existence should recognise that way for what it is, the way of material nothingness – *Wudo*. (Chinese: *wu*, nothingness; Japanese: *dō*, way or path).

Secret 7. Sycophancy and the Lure of Celebrity

Mystical explanations are easier for some people than scientific. Science is hard work and requires intellectual robustness, preparedness to admit ideas are wrong, application and integrity. If someone a camee recognises as a 'celebrity' or as a figure in authority seems to use, support or endorse a CAM (or fails to question claims made by camists) – then camees will assume 'there must be something in it.' Wrong. If there is evidence of 'something' the CAM will become conventional. It is a CAM precisely because it is an alternative and appeals to people who like to feel they are responsive to 'nature', are behaving 'holistically' and are party to hermetic or secret knowledge available only to those with particular sensitivities and insights. Camees like to feel they have a sense of identification with the celebrity or even enjoy the *schadenfreude* of finding that the celebrity also suffers.

Sycophancy is an extension of the Lure of Celebrity. Camees, camists and journalists like to curry the favour of influential people by flattering them. That is, they are sycophants (possibly from 'informer', possibly from 'fig').[21] This may reinforce the celebrity's ego and feelings of self worth – which has the effect of 'proving' to them that their beliefs in camistry are not misplaced but are respectable and rational. This encourages more endorsement, patronage, circular reinforcement and homeostatic hogwash. 'Toadyism' is a synonym. In the middle ages, quacks often had an assistant who would pretend to eat a poisonous toad. The quack declared the remedy being peddled had protected his assistant from harm and that the sooner the audience availed themselves of the nostrum, the better they would be. The illusion of eating the toad was a magic trick but handling them was still unpleasant and the job for a toadying sycophant.

Charles II initially endorsed Valentine Greatrickes' claim that he could heal by touch. More perspicaciously, Charles Saint-Denis de Évremond commented on the psychology of his victims : 'The public opinion, timid and enslaved, respected this imperious and apparently well-authenticated error. Those who saw through the delusion kept their opinion to themselves, knowing how useless it was to declare their disbelief to a people filled with prejudice and admiration.'[22] It took Sir Robert Boyle, President of the Royal Society, to eventually stand up and expose the nonsense – whereupon Greatrickes left the Court and returned to Ireland. Charles was chastened.

Those who wish to express their charitable inclinations are to be applauded, but are sometimes misguided and misled. Charities are not always informed by good science and may endorse camistry without having any evidence there will be effect on the disease of interest. The status of the charity may lull patients and those who fund them into cognitive biases and lure them into wasting time and money on treatments that have no effects on disease or illness. Examples include some dyslexia charities (which recommend the use of coloured lenses), the Royal Marines Children's Fund (which recommends cranio-sacral therapy for post traumatic stress) and cancer charities which offer a smorgasbord of CAMs. Moreover, charities themselves frequently use celebrities to draw attention to their altruistic endeavours. The problem for today's celebrities is that they may be duped, lured into becoming *wudoka* and come to follow nothing substantial at all.[23]

Secret 8. Convincers

Fraudsters plying Find the Lady will 'inadvertently' and apparently unknowingly crease the corner of the Queen. 'Aha!' says the mark, 'I know now which card is the Queen.' But on flipping the card over it is a simple spot card. The bet is lost. The crease was removed from the Queen and put in another card by the card sharp, or even a 'spectator' who is in reality an assistant or shill. The mark will never win. Crooked gambling convincers rely on the greed of the mark.

Likewise, the camee will have to assess the integrity of the CAM practitioner. The appearance of the consulting room, claims of professional status, association with reputable medical institutions, titles, dress, use of 'medical equipment', anatomical charts, baffling jargon, hyper-imaginative and hyperbolic language all serve to convince the camee they are in the presence of an honest professional acting with integrity. But are they? How is the camee to judge whether or not they are a quack and charlatan out to hoax and defraud? Membership of a professional register which is regulated under the oversight of the UK Professional Standards Authority is of no assistance. All that PSA accreditation assures is that an accredited register exists. The practices and practitioners themselves are not regulated by the PSA.

These considerations apply not only to camists but also to conventional practitioners.

The issue is the extent to which any practitioner is genuine and acting with intellectual integrity and probity.[24] One test is to assess whether: (i) they provide patients with comprehensive and comprehensible information about their practices, (ii) they explain how many patients have benefitted, but also how many have not, (iii) they explain the lack of plausible evidence of their CAM's efficaciousness, (iv) they explain that they offer alternatives to conventional medicine, (v) they explain that their remedies or techniques act as condiments, providing pleasure, but which do not provide benefit beyond the placebo.

The camee needs to assess whether there is any intention to mislead. Politicians, government and regulatory agencies must judge whether there is fraud.

Secret 9. Iatrogenic endorsement

Camees seek endorsement of their chosen CAM from friends, relatives, celebrities, journalists and particularly from doctors (*iatros:* a doctor). Most orthodox doctors know little of camistry. Few actively oppose any patient obtaining such relief from their suffering as they can, from whatever source – but their lack of objection should not be taken as endorsement. Feelings associated with illness are complex and include pain, emotions, fears, desires and hopes. The intervention of an artful caring therapist with appropriate ceremony and ritual can profoundly affect these complexes. Patients may feel better but not be better in terms of pathology. Improved mood may be interpreted as improvement in the disease. Conventional practitioners themselves may have many motives for endorsing and supporting patients' use of camistry, not all of them entirely altruistic. Practitioners too have feelings and emotions that need to be satisfied. The problem is that practitioners' apparent endorsement may mislead patients as to the value of the specific CAM and of camistry in general.

Doctors and nurses can be at their wits end. They may simply have nothing more to offer, yet they do care and want patients to know they care. A referral or endorsement of a patient's self-referral to a camist might at least help maintain the doctor-patient relationship. If the doctor makes the referral, the GMC requires they retain responsibility for the work of the camist. The patient should have full information about the intended CAM. In order they can enhance understanding and better advise patients, doctors might find a place on their book shelves for guidance on placebos and placedo techniques.

A number of doctors are content to have difficult patients see a camist – that enables transfer of care and convenient disposal of the case. Any guilt because of failure of their own ministrations is assuaged and the doctor's own stress is reduced. They may feel they have offered their patients 'the best of both worlds.' They conveniently overlook the fact that there is only one world and we live in it. The days of superstition and reliance on the supernatural have passed from quotidian medical practice. Those of religious faith may also engage the spiritual dimension, but that will not be further considered in this book.

Another issue arises when doctors are approached by patients who expresses a faith that a particular CAM will help them and request funding by the NHS. The doctor's rationale for referral may then be: 'If I do not support their belief, wrong though it is, they will become depressed and that will adversely affect their condition.' Camistry assists patients in coming to terms with their situation and mitigating their worries. Doctors and health professionals do care and wish to meet their patients' needs for solace. Compliant with patient demands, with critical faculties repressed, referral to a camist may seem an easy option for a conventional doctor.

Nevertheless, patients, doctors and above all, the doctors' regulatory authorities have to consider whether this approach is ethical and maintains intellectual integrity and probity. To date, regulators have been dilatory in considering the delusion and deception involved in iatrogenic endorsement of CAM and are themselves complicit in a miasma of mystery – even to the extent of requiring that a doctor does not challenge patients' beliefs, no matter how bizarre. Doctors professional integrity may be compromised, but to date the GMC has failed to advise how to deal with this elephant in the room. The regulators must judge their own consciences.

Self-reinforcement can bolster a practitioner's own confidence in their methods. If patients improve, the doctor gets the credit. Likewise, many patients will want to reciprocate their doctors care of them and willingly report the benefit of camistry, even to the extent of unjustified exaggeration.

Anton Chekhov, a doctor and also a playwright and novelist, wrote in *The Malingerers* of a homeopath deceived by patients who wanted her to feel that her ministrations were doing good. This reinforced the homeopath's belief and confidence in her methods and enabled her to overlook issues of quackery.

Medical and health care practitioners must examine their own consciences and judge their own behaviour. They need to consider how the patient is to give informed consent and whether it is ethical to avoid explaining that there is no plausible evidence the CAM in question has any effect on the patient's specific condition other than the benefit of attention from an empathic practitioner. And if public funding is requested, whether referral for camistry is fraudulent.

Secret 10. Communal reinforcement

As Robert Carroll suggests in *The Skeptic's Dictionary*, CAM practitioners network and those in the network feed off each other's enthusiasm in a climate of mutual support. So of course do conventional practitioners. Camists may come to believe each other's hype and that they have 'the secret, the powers, the gift'. They note each other's patient testimonials of benefit – the CAM 'worked'. The camist feels revitalised and empowered. Testimonials are not followed up to check that what may be a patient's temporary lift in mood due to expectation actually lasts. The regressive fallacy is overlooked. There is no monitoring of patients who do not return to the camist and may not have benefitted. There is no credible scientific evidence. Camists are complacent about this lack of attention to detail, but given others in the network who accept this stance, the community simply reinforces its faith.[25]

Secret 11. Deferral and delay

Some patients simply like to put off orthodox attention. Of major concern are patients who use camistry but fail to use conventional diagnosis and treatments and frequently do not tell their doctor when they do. Sadly, this can mean that effective treatments are given too late or not at all. It can be hard to prove delay causes harm as outcomes are rarely established in black and white. The issue of MMR vaccination and measles epidemics has been made more problematic by parents following advice of some camists and ignoring that of conventional medical authorities. Would Steve Jobs be alive today had his neuro-endocrine pancreatic tumour been treated by conventional means and had he not initially resorted to camistry and diets? Statistics suggest he probably would – but statistics apply to populations not individuals and we will never know. The camee must beware.

Secret 12. Deception

Deception is the stock in trade of magicians, the basis of many CAM practices and the secret of the success of both. There is no therapeutically active substance in sugar pills, no innate intelligence susceptible to manipulation, no channels through which supernatural forces may pass – and those who suggest otherwise may be deceiving their patients. The critical analysis that camees should apply is reduced by techniques of standard magical misdirection.[26]

Camists generally offer no immediate quick cures, but they do give camees time – to talk, reflect, discuss personal matters – and time to return for further 'maintenance'. Camistry seems to provide meanings and interpretations which are more congruent with the beliefs of the camee. Camists take time to lure the camee and when the switch to non-scientific, un-scientific or pseudo-scientific constructs occurs, it goes unnoticed. The switch may be metaphysical, mystical or metaphorical and may be overlooked unless the camee has learned to be cautious. Many patients have returned home from a consultation and only then wondered how they were suckered into purchasing a supplement, remedy, orthotic foot support or therapeutic manoeuvre.

Could attempts at cynical deception be why the language is mangled, novel terminology used, names of institutions, styles of address and expositions of status are employed which can so easily mislead the unwary? The Royal London Homeopathic Hospital used that trick when it erased the word Homeopathic and inserted 'for Integrated Medicine' – as if the practices it offers can be integrated meaningfully with conventional medicine. The practices can be condimentary but as they are based on fundamentally different and implausible metaphysical constructs, are not complementary and cannot be integrated with any intellectual integrity. Is deception intended? You must be the judge.

The use of deception and fraud is to be deprecated. Today's practitioners who wish to help patients by enhancing the placebo effects of a therapeutic encounter must be open and honest about their practice and its placebo nature. To deceive by pretending placebos are not placebos is unethical and may be fraudulent. Endorsement of that approach, seen all too often in 'quackademic medicine', is unacceptable. Camees must beware.

Secret 13. Delusion

'An idiosyncratic belief or impression maintained despite being contradicted by reality or rational argument.' (Oxford English Dictionary). For whatever reasons, a number of people do come to have faith and belief in systems regarded as alternative to science-based medicine. Some simply lack insight. Some may have psychological problems, even paranoia. This is not a new phenomenon. In 1842 the eminent American physician Oliver Wendell Holmes explored the issue in *Homeopathy and its Kindred Delusions*, lectures to the Boston Society for the Diffusion of Useful Knowledge. These are essential reading for the serious student of camistry. Holmes recognised that as the course of diseases fluctuated there could be fallacies of observation and commented on 'the emptiness of pretension.'

From the latter half of the nineteenth century, as conventional orthodox medicine continued its evolution from the era of the supernatural, set aside the foolishness of 'heroic treatments' and demanded a base in scientifically acquired knowledge and understanding, doctors were encouraged to rethink the issues involved in alternative systems of medicine. Holmes wrote:

> When a physician attempts to convince the person, who has fallen into the Homœopathic delusion, of the emptiness of its pretensions, he is often answered by a statement of cases in which its practitioners are thought to have effected wonderful cures... Such statements made by persons unacquainted with the fluctuations of disease and the fallacies of observation, are to be considered in general as of little or no value in establishing the truth of a medical doctor and all the utility or method of practice.
>
> Those kind friends who suggest to a person suffering from a tedious complaint, that he "had better try Homœopathy," are apt to enforce their suggestion by adding, that "at any rate it can do no harm." This may or may not be true as regards the individual. But it always does very great harm to the community to encourage ignorance, error, or deception in a profession which deals with the life and health of our fellow creatures. Whether or not those who countenance Homœopathy are guilty of this injustice towards others has to be considered.
>
> To deny that some patients may have actually benefited through the influence exerted upon their imaginations, would be to refuse to Homœopathy what all are willing to concede to everyone of those numerous modes of practice known to all intelligent persons by an opprobrious title. So long as the body is affected through the mind, no audacious device, even of the most manifestly dishonest character, can fail of producing occasional good to those who yield it an implicit or even a partial faith. The argument founded on this occasional good would be as applicable

in justifying the counterfeiter and giving circulation to his base coin, on the ground that a spurious dollar had often relieved a poor man's necessities. [27, 28]

As patients' relative 'wants' become more important than absolute 'needs', an interesting parallel can be drawn between their attitudes and the views of Philip Mirowski on neo-liberal economics: 'There are no limits to imagination and a desire for conspicuous consumption – no limit to how much you want. And here advertising and marketing have a part to play. Yet a lot is delusion – people are not satisfied and are no happier.' [29]

Some delusions are clearly part of a definable mental disorder but there is no definitive dividing line between delusions and more general irrational fixed beliefs. Delusions are defined in the Diagnostic and Statistical Manual of Mental Disorders as 'fixed beliefs that are not amenable to change in light of conflicting evidence.' Other irrational beliefs are more generally prevalent in the general population. The tendency of people with such beliefs to continue to hold them despite being confronted with incontrovertible evidence to the contrary results in the psychological process of cognitive dissonance, and can be very stressful.

Notwithstanding that the ancient Greeks knew the earth was a globe, religious fundamentalist Samuel Birley Rowbotham carried out observations on East Anglia's Bedford Canal and convinced himself the earth was flat. *Zetetic Astronomy* and *Earth Not a Globe* explained all. After his death in 1884, followers founded the Universal Zetetic Society which slowly dissipated until reactivated as the Flat Earth Society in 1956 (*zetein*, to inquire into).

After his community in East Anglia failed, Rowbotham moved to London, styled himself as 'Dr Samuel Birley', sold quack 'Phosphoric Acid Nerve Tonic' and became rich. John Hampden was a devoted follower – for him, claims that the earth was a globe were a 'a huge sham' and Hampden issued a wager on the matter worth a year's wage for a working man. Most people regarded 'paradoxers' like Hampden as crackpots, but eminent scientist Alfred Russell Wallace (who had contributed to the theory of evolution) took him up in 1870. When Hampden lost, he became obsessed with the 'Bedford Canal Swindle' and harassed and libelled Wallace for fifteen years, culminating with a year in prison. The judge remonstrated with Wallace for having disputed with a man 'plainly not right in the mind.' Similar considerations may need to be applied today when dealing with irrational opinions about medicine. To this day people with delusions about scientific matters are often referred to as 'flat-earthers'.

Clearly, some people are much more suggestible and credulous than others. Critical thinking skills do not come naturally to most people but do need to be encouraged if the gullible are to avoid being duped. Camists themselves are deluded if they genuinely believe in 'meridians', 'energy fields' and the like. Charging patients to utilise such 'fields' may be fraudulent.

Secret 14. Cognitive dissonance, wishful thinking and misplaced optimism.

The term *cognitive dissonance* describes how humans strive for internal consistency. If two or more contradictory beliefs have to be faced at the same time, inconsistency becomes psychologically uncomfortable and mentally stressful. Leon Festinger described what happens in *When Prophecy Fails*: 'A man with conviction is a hard man to change. Tell him you disagree and he turns away. Show him facts or figures and he questions your sources. Appeal to logic and he fails to see your point.'

Those who have faith in camistry find it hard to set aside their beliefs and admit they may have been wrong – they find it easier to convince themselves they have benefited in some way. Healthcare outcomes are multi-factorial. If experiences contradict expectations, recollections may be distorted – particularly if they involved core beliefs. Patients may be in denial of the reality of the situation and continue to express belief in the CAM they have chosen. Patients are more comfortable, more consoled, by having their chosen CAM defended rather than contradicted. Conventional medicine and the challenges of science can simply be too demanding for some patients' taste. They have greater pleasure from condimentary medicine and *wudo*. Camists themselves can suffer from cognitive dissonance coupled with financial conflict of interest and mistaken professional vanity.

Patients want life to be nicer, for there to be harmony, balance, cooperation, peace and love. We all want that – but is such a mindset realistic? Wishful thinking and misplaced optimism may reduce stress from cognitive dissonance, but without insight, wishful thinking can be a logical fallacy and give rise to poor decisions on account of cognitive bias. The Law of Unintended Consequences will eventually gain sway. Martin Luther King declared 'I have a dream...' but that dream was based on possibilities now being realised, not impossible fantasies. We are alive, we dream – but basing decisions about healthcare on how things 'seem' is no substitute for having rational opinions based on evidence.

Secret 15. Confirmation Bias and Procrustination

Confirmation bias is a close relation of Delusion – reflecting partiality that results from camees remembering outcomes selectively and recalling only those which confirm their beliefs. The more strongly attached to the belief, the greater the potential for such bias. As Francis Bacon pointed out: 'The human understanding when it has once adopted an opinion, either as being the received opinion or as being agreeable to itself, draws all things else to support and agree with it.'

Emotions are powerful and may deeply entrench confidence in one or more CAM systems, even when scientifically acquired evidence would suggest that is unwise. Uncertainty is uncomfortable. Related to 'wishful thinking', such bias can lead to misplaced overconfidence and poor decision making. It is a long held criticism of the research methodologies employed by camists that they will look for results which support their theories rather than critically examining all the results. For them, the important scientific principle of falsification is a foreign field. Confirmation bias accounts for persistence of belief. Francis Bacon advised this was the cause of 'all superstitions, whether in astrology, dreams, omens, divine judgments or the like.'[30]

Lee Ross and colleagues suggest: 'Beliefs can survive potent logical or empirical challenges. They can survive and even be bolstered by evidence that most uncommitted observers would agree logically demands some weakening of such beliefs. They can even survive the total destruction of their original evidential bases.' [31] Confirmation bias is also a critical cause of poor decision making in the fields of finance, economics and state security. As Daniel Kahneman has advised: 'If we think we have reasons for what we believe, that is often a mistake. Our beliefs, wishes, hopes are not always anchored in reasons but in something else within us.'[32]

In healthcare, biases are best reduced, if not entirely avoided, by randomised controlled trials and systematic peer review wherever possible. Camists tend to be too wedded to anecdotes as a source of the 'evidence' of the benefit of their practices and selectively quote anecdotes which confirm their beliefs. They rarely report how many patients found no benefit from their attention.

A variety of confirmation bias is procrustination – making facts fit a pet theory and ignoring facts which do not fit. Procrustes was a mythical Greek villain who had the charming habit of making his captives fit his bed – by stretching them if they were too small or cutting off their legs if too tall. Do not try this at home.

Secret 16. Cognitive Bias

Normal people think normally. There is a range and objective assessment is not easy, but reasonable expectations can be identified. Some people, at some times, are outside the norm. Sometimes to the extent of being highly creative artistic and intellectual geniuses. Sometimes to the other, irrational side of 'normal'. Irrespective of how they may arise, illogical interpretations and distorted perceptions represent patterns of thought and bias which are described as 'cognitive.' The job of the magician is to help you on your way. That is how magical entertainment works. In healthcare there can be problems if these biases lead to logical fallacies and irrational judgements. It has been suggested that these biases can hinder public acceptance of non-intuitive scientific knowledge.[33]

The Dunning-Kruger effect describes a particular form of cognitive bias in which individuals rate their own ability higher than average and fail to recognise their own inadequacy: 'Miscalibration of the incompetent stems from an error about the self, whereas the miscalibration of the highly competent stems from an error about others.' [34]

Attribution Bias is variant of cognitive bias which explains why and how we create meaning about behaviour and how an observer uses information to create a causal explanation for events. Attribution theory provides explanations for why different people can interpret the same event in different ways. Patients may experience a general improvement over time, yet, without any reason, attribute their experience to the CAM they use. This may be how coloured lenses seem to help patients with dyslexia and the so-called 'Irlen syndrome'.

Not all camists and camees are open minded and prepared to change their opinion in the light of evidence. Proverbs had: 'The way of a fool seems right to him but a wise man listens to advice' and; 'In everything the prudent acts with knowledge but a fool flaunts his folly.' Touchstone in Shakespeare's *As You Like It* recalled an old saying: 'The fool doth think he is wise but the wise man knows himself to be a fool'; and Charles Darwin: 'Ignorance more frequently begets confidence than does knowledge.'

Camees will have to consider whether any belief they have in the value of their chosen CAM may be due to fraud by the camist; trickery by magicians; cold reading; subjective validation; selective thinking; confirmation bias; attribution bias; a poor grasp of probability; lure of celebrity; influence of well meaning charities; gullibility; deception; wishful thinking or the way they think – cognitive bias.

Secret 17. The Wrong Diagnosis and Prognosis

Doctors and other conventional practitioners are not infallible. Mistakes happen – no diagnosis is ever 'correct', simply the most likely and probable at the time. In the light of further and better information, a diagnosis may have to be changed.

In the field of joint reconstruction patients often say they have heard an artificial joint 'will last ten tears and then need revision.' They have simply misunderstood. There is a spectrum, a range of outcomes. Some joints fail almost at once. Most never do at all. Statistics apply to populations of patients, not an individual patient and are difficult to explain in any event. The ten year mark is a convenient device. Experience shows that for most cancers, survival at ten years is tantamount to a cure – though no guarantee. For joint replacements, by ten years up to ten per cent might reasonably be expected to have failed. In a lifetime, the majority of patients will have no trouble whatsoever but so often that is not what the patient understands. Doctors are responsible for good communication – *nostra culpa.*

Secret 18. Spontaneous remission and coincidence

Even the most chronic and intractable condition can recover, for no apparent reason. But without further evidence, it would be unwise to ascribe such a recovery to camistry rather than to Mother Nature herself. Diseases run their natural courses. Cures happen, and even should illness return, that may simply be part of the cyclical natural history of that particular condition. Patients will tend to seek help when they are at their worst, so when remission occurs they make the false assumption that the treatment caused the recovery. This is the classic logical fallacy of *post hoc ergo c.*

    an event will cause a response. In health care and wellbeing, we need to know whether any good outcome or perceived benefit is the result of treatment and care, or a mere coincidence. This requires analysis not blind acceptance. Just because the patient feels better after a treatment or remedy does not mean the benefit was caused by the treatment. Correlation does not imply causation.

Coincidences happen. For example, try rearranging the letters of the following statement: 'In one of the Bard's best-thought-of tragedies, our insistent hero, Hamlet, queries on two fronts about how life turns rotten.' And what do you get? 'To be or not to be, that is the question, whether 'tis nobler in the mind to suffer the slings and arrows of outrageous fortune.' [35]

Is that a coincidence – or what?

Secret 19. Regression to the Mean

Statistics are the basis of scientific inquiries into health and well being. Many individual patients genuinely believe 'It worked for me.' But how can a patient know it was the specifics of the treatment which had an effect and not simply the empathic encounter with an attentive practitioner? Patients rarely make this distinction. An individual patient might not be too concerned – if they believe it 'worked' that is good enough for them. But those with responsibility for the care of patients more generally, in a family practice, for a community or a nation, have to consider effects established by statistics – or patients cannot be properly informed, resources will be wasted and patients may be misled into delaying conventional care. Taking results overall, over time and for different patients will demonstrate 'regression to the mean'. First termed 'regression to mediocrity' by Sir Francis Galton, psychologist, mathematician and Charles Darwin's cousin – regression is an important consideration in the design of experiments and investigation of the benefit of drug treatment. So too for the benefits of alternative medicine.[36]

Regression is the 'tincture of time'. In the field of healthcare, regression accounts for the fact that many illnesses do seem to get better in due course. Even chronic conditions will provide patients with 'good days and bad days'. If a CAM is used just before the improvement was likely in any event, when the patient was feeling particularly low, the CAM may be credited with that improvement. The patient using a CAM at the same time as conventional treatment will declare the CAM 'worked for me.' And so it will seem, but that may be a false association. Unless camists understand these statistical subtleties, they too may be fooled. Unless there is rigorous follow up, and reporting of all the cases, including those which found no benefit, we all may be fooled. So the questions to put to a camist is not: 'How many patients has your treatment benefited,' but rather: 'How many patients have you treated altogether? To what extent did they benefit? How many reported no significant benefit?'

Randomised placebo controlled trials counter the effects of regression. They help ensure that good outcomes of a remedy, treatment or drug are not attributed to wrong causes. This possibility has to be considered when considering research of all kinds, but research in CAM often takes inadequate account of the effects of regression. The individual patient may be lulled into a false assumption that the treatment worked for them, whereas they have simply experienced a normal phenomenon of nature together with the benefits of care and placebo effects. The only answer is to study large groups of patients and to repeat the studies. Patients' anecdotes about their experience are not acceptable as statistical data.

Secret 20. The Fallacy of Causation

Post hoc, ergo propter hoc. To think 'after this, therefore because of this,' is a common logical fallacy – correlation does not imply causation. The false attribution of causality where none exists requires regular challenge from us all – otherwise we will only have ourselves to blame if we are misled.

Philosophers have spent centuries on the question of how the mere association of events might reveal their causal links and what it means to say that one thing can ever *cause* another. The ambiguity of correlations has been long recognised in health care. In 1870 Alexander Bain warned his readers of the 'fallacy of causation, whereby we might assume that the healthy effect of residence at a medicinal spa is attributed exclusively to the operation of the waters, as opposed to being caused by the whole circumstances and situation. The confusion between correlation and causation prevails in all the complicated sciences, as Politics and Medicine.' This is precisely why Type I and II effects need to be distinguished.

The concept of 'association of ideas' is found in sympathetic magic practised by the ancients and expressed in the 'laws of similarity'. The use of voodoo dolls to target and harm another person relies on these magical precepts, and Hahnemann based his suggestions for homeopathic remedies on similar ideas.

In his book *Introduction to Quality Control* (1990) Kaoru Ishikawa set out techniques for Cause and Effect Analysis which have become well known in business and industrial management and have also been applied to quality improvement in healthcare. Together with techniques of 'brainstorming' and 'mind mapping', many possible causes of a problem or outcome are analysed – not just the intuitively most obvious ones. 'It works for me...' is a common claim of contented camees. But did it? Or were there other possible causes of the benefits they perceived? The camee must be the judge, but unless a degree of scepticism is exercised, the camee may be fraudulently deprived of valuable time and finance.

Secret 21. Forer and Barnum Effects

Magicians place great reliance on misdirecting their audience from elements which might reveal the trickery. Sleight of mind creating dual reality is regularly invoked.

Psychologist Bertram Forer (1914-2000) gave a personality test to each student in his class. The students were then asked to give their opinion as to the accuracy of the test result as it applied to them personally. Using a scale of 1 to 5, where 5 represented 'highly accurate', the average score was 4.2. In fact, Forer had supplied each student with exactly the same vague and non-discriminatory analysis culled from newspaper astrology columns: 'You have a great need for other people to like and admire you...at times you are extroverted, affable and sociable, whilst at other times you are introverted, wary, reserved.'

The statements could apply equally to anyone. This experiment has been repeated by many observers with the same results. This technique of vagueness is used by astrologers, horoscopists, fortune tellers, personality testers, magicians, mentalists, mediums and spiritualists who undertake cold readings. People fall for results they like. Vagueness can create the initial confidence on which the dishonourable practitioner can then build with more personal and accurate information.

The famous showman and psychological manipulator P.T. Barnum claimed he offered 'something for everyone' and his name is also given to the Forer effect. In the field of camistry we see patients respond to non-specific treatments in a positive way, especially if they feel the treatment was individualised for them personally and that the remedy is unique for them, but camees need to take care they are not experiencing Forer/Barnum effects.

Secret 22. Hawthorne Effect

In 1924 Harvard University researchers studied the productivity of workers at the Hawthorne Works of the Western Electric Company in Illinois. These studies have become classic and well-known to students of psychology, management and organisational behaviour. Initially the study was commissioned to determine whether altering intensity of factory illumination improved productivity. It did. At first the illumination was increased, and so did productivity. The light intensity was then reduced – and a further increase in productivity was recorded.

Small subtle changes in factory illumination may have had an effect – as did having sympathetic supervisors paying attention to the workers and encouragement to work as a group. With so many variables there is no consensus as to the real meaning of the Hawthorne Effect but these studies remain a stimulus to ongoing research, and may account for perceived effects of homeopathy on children and animals. The very act of observing a situation can change the situation observed – the 'beneficial effects of attention'.

Stories of animals of all descriptions being successfully treated by 'homeopathy' abound. These cases are comparable to those involving human babies who cannot respond to suggestions. However there is no good scientific evidence that homeopathic remedies provide benefit to any extent greater than placebos. Diseases of animals of all species do demonstrate remission – they do recover. The care and attention of their owners/parents does have an effect, as did a change in lighting at the Hawthorne Works. That is how biology works. Placebo effects by proxy. Supernatural physics is not called for. Homeopathy, chiropractic and other CAMs work on animals for all the reasons they work in humans – type I effects from a caring relationship. Given the emphasis homeopaths place on the importance of individualisation and specificity of their remedies in accordance with the personalities and polycrests of their patients – how could their remedies possibly affect a group of animals? There is a Nobel Prize awaiting the scientist who can show any Type II effect on a specific disease plausibly attributable to homeopathic remedies or manual adjustment of subluxations. It would be easy to hold trials with controls – giving half a herd suffering mastitis placebo sugar pills and half the same pills prepared by the homeopathic method. The animals owners and those judging outcomes would be blinded as to the pills given to each group. This research has not been done.

John Haygarth devised placebo control experiments to expose the quackery of Perkins' Tractors and also considered how quack remedies affected innocent children and animals: 'In these cases it is not the patient, but the observer, who is deceived by his own imagination.' A thorough review of the issues involved in using homeopathy in veterinary practice can be found in a paper prepared for a debate at the 2013 meeting of the American Veterinary Medical Association.[37]

Secret 23. Tea Pots and Pastafarianism

Science is falsifiable. Non-science makes no such demands. Calls to 'prove it doesn't work…' have to be put in the context of reality and probability, not imaginative speculation.

Lord Bertrand Russell OM FRS (1872-1970), mathematician and social commentator suggested that were he to claim that a teapot orbits the Sun between Earth and Mars, it would be nonsensical for him to expect others to believe him – simply on the grounds they cannot prove him wrong. 'Prove there is no teapot in space' would be a nonsense request and rightly ignored.

In 2005 Bobby Henderson wrote an open letter of protest at the Kansas State Board of Education permitting the teaching of creationism in science classes. He wanted equal billing for *Pastafarianism*. Its deity, 'The Flying Spaghetti Monster', is regarded as being no less credible than belief in intelligent design. 'We can all look forward to a time when these theories are given equal time in science classrooms…' Pastafarians claim to believe pirates are divine beings. Henderson demonstrated a mathematical association between a world decline in piracy since the 1800s and rise in global warming – thus 'proving' pirates are of value in ecological metrics.[38] Henderson emphasised the principle that the philosophic burden of proof lies with those who make unfalsifiable (and therefore unscientific) claims, not on those who reject them. He emphasised that correlation does not imply causation.[39] Henderson is regarded as a satirist; Earl Russell as a founder of analytic philosophy.

Henderson was not the only critic to show the foolishness of believing correlation necessarily implies causation. In the 1950s the statistician Sir Ronald Fisher took issue with Doll and Hill's suggestion that smoking caused cancer of the lung and pointed out there was a good statistical correlation between the importation of apples and the divorce rate. It took further work to confirm the validity of Doll and Hill's conclusions.

Armstrong left a camera on the Moon; the manned space station may yet leave a teapot in solar orbit. As J.B.S. Haldane said in *Possible Worlds and Other Papers* (1927): 'The Universe is not only queerer than we suppose, but queerer than we can suppose.' There is plenty of proof of that.

Secret 24. Gullibility and Vulnerability

Gullibility is defined in Wikipedia as a 'failure of social intelligence in which a person is easily tricked or manipulated into an ill-advised course of action.' From Latin: *coleus*, sack. Hence Spanish: *cojones* or Old French: *couillon* and thence *cullion*, a base fellow, and English slang: *cull*, a dupe or sucker. Many CAM products and practices are indeed Round Objects.[40]

Related to *credulity* – 'the tendency to believe unlikely propositions that are unsupported by evidence', many gullible people are highly intelligent and the tricks required to fool them are subtle. Doctors and healthcare professionals have a particular responsibility for children, the elderly, and other vulnerable people. The emotions associated with serious life threatening or chronic disease can make any reasonable person drop their guard, set scepticism aside and become vulnerable. *Real Secrets* provides information to balance the books and encourage greater insight and circumspection. Whether politicians accept the responsibility for protecting the vulnerable and the public purse as they should has to be considered. You must be the judge.

Secret 25. Fear

In the UK many CAMs are used by patients with chronic conditions that have not responded satisfactorily to conventional care. The biggest fear is cancer. Many cancers are now very well treated by conventional medicine, but given success is not guaranteed, it is inevitable that some patients are prepared to go to the ends of the earth and take any steps to ensure reasonable survival. One can hardly blame them, or their caring relatives. The cold light of the rational clinical approach of conventional medicine may not assuage the fear of dying. More natural, gentler approaches may be preferred and orthodox medicine may even be rejected. Camists may provide more compassion, solace and hope – falsely based though that may be. In a fearful state, any rational person might become vulnerable and set aside precepts of wise critical thinking. Buyers must beware and consider the opinion of statistician R. Barker Bausell, Research Director of a Complementary and Alternative Medicine Specialised Research Center at the University of Maryland:

'There is no compelling, credible scientific evidence to suggest that any CAM therapy benefits any medical condition or reduces any medical symptom (pain or otherwise) better than a placebo.'[41]

In which case, why not take advantage of the placebo effects provided by conventional practitioners, counsellors, carers and placebists, providing the issues are explained and the patient gives fully informed consent? The US National Cancer Institute has warned camees to be careful of people or companies that: 'make claims they have a "cure"; do not give specific information about how, and how well, their product works; say they have clinical studies, but fail to provide references...If it sounds too good to be true, it probably is.'[42]

Secret 26. Intuition

Many camists claim or imply that they are able to use 'intuition' to diagnose and identify treatments for their patients (Latin: *in*, in; *tueri*, to look, contemplate. Wikipedia has: 'the ability to acquire knowledge without inference and/or the use of reason'). Carl Jung suggested intuition is perception via the unconscious. The OED definition is: 'the ability to understand something immediately without the need for conscious reasoning.'

From Archimedes and his heuristic insight, through virtually every philosopher and developer of CAM – the Yellow Emperor, Hahnemann, Smith, Palmer, Usui – all have claimed 'intuition'. Some describe it as a 'gift'. Some, such as Swedenborg who influenced many others, claimed divine and angelic intercession. Philosophers from the Dogmatics to Goethe put intuition down to their own intellectual powers. The prevalence of 'intuition' in intellectual life was precisely why the scientific method developed.

'Intuition' is the staple of quacks, charlatans, shams and fraudsters. Often with claims they are able to intuitively read the client's 'body language' and 'non-verbal means of communication' such as mannerisms, demeanour, gestures and facial expression. That is also how magicians claim to be able to demonstrate their powers of clairsentience, clairvoyance, clairaudience, mediumship and mentalism. Some practitioners claim they are able to provide meaningful personal information for a client or patient by intuition, rather than through the normal human senses. They are termed 'psychics' and may brazenly profess their vocation and commercial success. They may of course use methods well known to magicians such as 'cold reading'. This involves fishing for clues, demographic profiling, and acting.[43] They will almost certainly use buzz words or 'wonder words' as part of their sleight of tongue in order to engage and illuminate their clients' emotions and subconscious.[44] Quite how to distinguish psychics from camists in general, from quacks that lack insight, from quacks who are frauds, is beyond the scope of this book. Virtually all trustworthy magicians who demonstrate mentalism will deny any occult abilities or assistance from vital forces. Magicians ride the fine line between intuition and illusion, using our understanding of the law of averages, probabilities, powers of persuasion, memory techniques and reading of body language to create our effects. You must be the judge of camists, but a methodological scientific approach will assist you.

Secret 27. Psychology, Psychics and Parapsychology

Sincere camists and camees may come to their core beliefs for a very wide variety of reasons. In addition to all the above, some may actually experience altered states of their own psychology and neuro-physiology. Of interest are:

Synaesthesia (*syn*, together; *aesthesis*, sensation) is a neurological condition in which additional nerve cells connect areas of the brain not normally associated. This can give rise to a range of perceptions and sensations such as perceiving letters and numbers to have colours. More than sixty different types of synaesthesia have been identified but research is at an early stage and given the total subjectivity involved, scientific clarification is difficult. Recent work by Emilio Milan from Granada University, Spain, suggests that the intermingling of sensations could be the reason some people see 'auras' as coloured halos around others. This may give them cause to feel they have special powers or gifts and to develop careers as healers. Dr Milan has commented this is actually a case of self deception as synaesthesia is not an extrasensory power, but 'a subjective and adorned perception of reality.'[45] Number synaesthesia was described by psychologist Sir Francis Galton as *'The Visions of Sane Persons.'*[46]

Pareidolia (*para*, alongside, instead; *eidolon*, image, form, shape) allows the doors of perception to open and blow in the wind. Psychologists have described a phenomenon in which vague, even random images or sounds are perceived by an individual as being clear, distinct and significant. Senses are fallible but by this means religious significance is given to abstract patterns, deities are 'seen' in the clouds, shadows or landscape, the moon has its man, a face appears on a Devon cliff and a lion has been reported running free in Essex. Subjective experience is then determined as scientific fact. The Rorschach inkblot test utilises pareidolia to help psychologists unravel thoughts or feelings.

Dr Max Pemberton suggests: 'Someone's assertion that they are correct does not necessarily mean they are...the brain is hard wired to try and make sense of what we perceive and if we don't perceive something fully – if we don't see all of it or hear something clearly – then our brain tries to fill in the gaps. It's very open to suggestions when it does this and will often provide the individual with what they are expecting.'[47]

Suggestions and expectations: that is how hypnosis may work – and placebo effects as well. William Blake's doors of perception opened to reveal that: 'Energy is the only life and is from the Body – and Reason is the bound or outward circumference of Energy. Energy is Eternal Delight....If the doors of perception were cleansed everything would appear to man as it is, infinite. For man has closed himself up, till he sees all things thro' narrow chinks of his cavern.'[48]

'Science' represents the knowledge of what is – in the world and universe in which we live. In so far as it is possible, explanations are based on observations – scientists have learned how to learn. Those who experience and sense a transcendental supernatural quality, beyond normal experience, consider explanations ranging from religious to psychic. The Society for Psychical Research was founded in London in 1882 and continues to this day.[49]

Magician Louis Hoffman was initially a member of the society's research committee but left when he decided the psychic phenomena investigated could be achieved by contemporary magical methods. [50] Another magician, Joseph Rinn, joined the American Society for Psychical Research (founded 1885) but then left when it failed to expose fake psychics. In 1888, Rinn was present when the Fox sisters confessed to the *New York Herald* that their demonstrations of spiritualism had been hoaxes. In 1905 Rinn founded the Metropolitan Psychical Society. Rinn was a friend of Houdini and sponsored his magic shows and exposés of fraudulent mediums. Rinn offered rich rewards for any who could demonstrate psychic phenomena and he was particularly scathing of scientists who set aside scepticism and became involved with parapsychology – emphasising that: 'wonderful phenomena need wonderful evidence in their support to be of any value so far its truth is concerned, otherwise they are valueless.'[51]

Psychic phenomena occurring as a result of 'energies', 'aura' and paranormal agencies are usually distinguished from those due to spirits and evidenced by spiritualists. In 1889 the psychologist Max Dessoir termed the study of phenomena which are unexplained by science as 'parapsychology'.

Professor Joseph Banks Rhine (1895-1980) Director of the Parapsychology Department at Duke University coined the term 'Extra Sensory Perception' (ESP) to refer to clairvoyance – the ability to perceive and 'see' spirits, objects or events, even in the future, without the agency of the five recognised senses. Clairvoyance is synonymous with precognition, second sight, and telepathy. The repertoire has been expanded by psychic mediums who have added clairaudience (hearing a spirit), clairsentience (sensing a spirit) and psychokinesis (PK – moving inanimate objects by thought alone). Study of such phenomena continue to provide psychologists with careers, but plausible evidence for *psi* in the material world has not been established. To date, magicians have been able to replicate all the effects demonstrated by spiritualists and parapsychologists.[52] Rhine wrote:

> Science has discovered a new world – a region within what we call the mind, a world that has throughout the past been shrouded in dark mystery and superstition ... the great discovering human mind has never yet thoroughly explored its own puzzling complex nature. It now looks very much as though here and there a few pioneer explorers have broken through to a truly new world within man, a world of distinctively mental reality...As far back as the time of Franz Mesmer and his

followers, phenomena such as are now included under extrasensory perception were not uncommonly encountered incidentally during healing practices – in the eighteenth century they were simply taken to be part of the mesmeric state itself. Now in the twentieth century, purged completely of the association with hypnosis, telepathy has found a place in the new psychiatry of the psychoanalytic schools. [53]

Rhine initially used playing cards to demonstrate a 'transmitting' researcher could signify the value and suit of an observed card to a 'receiving' colleague by thought alone. Fifty two playing cards resulted in too many confounding variables for meaningful statistical analysis and Rhine went on to use cards designed by his colleague Karl Zener, with five more simple geometric symbols. Rhine was familiar with the methods of magicians who offered mind-reading as entertainment and he took care to avoid fraud, but his own research was later shown to have involved significant publication bias – he simply failed to report results which contradicted his beliefs. In the twenty-first century, telepathy has been rejected by regular science but its influence remains on those camists who claim to be able to move energies with their minds. There have been no demonstrations of ESP which cannot be duplicated by a magician competent in mentalism.

A series of remarkable demonstrations of telepathy were offered by Australian entertainers Sydney and Lesley Piddington in the early 1950s. Many stage performances were carried out throughout Britain, but they are best remembered for demonstrations carried out on radio with Sydney transmitting to Lesley whilst she was in a diving bell, prison or aeroplane. A committee of impartial observers ensured no confederates were used, the test texts were selected at random and use of secret radio devices was excluded. Magicians have since suggested how the effects could have been achieved using the regular tools of misdirection, dual reality and illusion. These are techniques also used by camists as they try to convince their patients that they can manipulate energies in one way or another.

Psychology's sub-field of anomalistic psychology rejects the paranormal claims of parapsychology. Speaking to the European Skeptics Congress in 2015, Goldsmith College's Professor Chris French advised: 'The difference between anomalistic psychology and parapsychology is in terms of the aims of what each discipline is about. Parapsychologists typically are actually searching for evidence to prove the reality of paranormal forces, to prove they really do exist. Whereas anomalistic psychologists tend to start from the position that paranormal forces probably do not exist and that therefore we should be looking for other kinds of explanations.' This parallels the respective positions of camists who claim to conduct 'research' and health claim sceptics.

Secret 28. Agnotology

(*A*, not; *gnos*, knowing, therefore: ignorance).This word was coined by Iain Boal in 1992 at the request of Robert N. Proctor whose book *Agnotology: A Missing Term to Describe the Cultural Production of Ignorance (and its Study)* considers that whilst there are academics studying what it is to have 'knowledge' – *episteme* (hence epistemology), there has not been a comparable focus on 'ignorance.'

Proctor suggests: 'Ignorance has many interesting surrogates and overlaps in myriad ways with and is generated by – secrecy, stupidity, apathy, censorship, disinformation, faith, and forgetfulness, all of which are science-twitched.' [54] He points out: 'Johannes Kepler in the sixteenth century had a rather brutal way of putting it – ignorance was: "the mother who must die for science to be born."'

Mark Crislip's commentary is also pertinent, suggesting that the most harmful domain for healthcare is 'ignorance as strategic ploy, or active construct.'[55] Proctor suggests: 'The focus here is on ignorance, doubt or uncertainty as something that is made, maintained and manipulated by means of certain arts and sciences – to suit their proponents' purposes, and not for enlightenment. Certain people don't want you to know certain things, or will actively work to organize doubt or uncertainty or misinformation to help maintain (your) ignorance. They know, and may or may not want you to know they know, but you are not to be privy to the secret.'[56]

Secret 29. Denialism

It is inevitable that much discussion about the relationship between science, evidence-based medicine, pseudoscience and alternative medicine is couched in language designed to prick consciences and arouse emotions. It cannot be denied however that camees and camists appear to be in denial in respect of undisputed scientific consensus about their CAM. Their rejection of overwhelming evidence contrary to their beliefs and attempts to deny scientific consensus and reality helps avoid uncomfortable truths. The term 'denialism' is more usually invoked in relation to the Holocaust, AIDS, climate change and politics but can certainly be applied in healthcare. Denialism is identified when rhetorical arguments are used to mislead and give the appearance of legitimate debate, where there is none. This is the basis of a classic magical illusion as applied to philosophy.

Many patients, perceiving conventional medicine has failed to deal with serious conditions as they hope and wish, turn to camistry in desperation. Others feel they need support for emotional issues but are concerned not to be stigmatised and find it more acceptable to announce publically that they have benefited from a CAM remedy, manipulation, or 'energy'. Some find it hard to admit the underlying psychological nature of their distress and more comfortable to be in denial.

In the opinion of Chris Hoofnagle of the Berkeley Centre for Law, University of California, 'There are those who engaged in denialist tactics because they are protecting some 'overvalued idea' which is critical to their identity. Since legitimate dialogue is not a valid option for those who are interested in protecting bigoted or unreasonable ideas from scientific facts, their only recourse is to use these types of rhetorical tactics.'[57]

Chris Hoofnagle's brother Mark is a doctor of philosophy and a surgeon who has expressed concern at strategies which confuse public understanding of scientific knowledge. He has emphasised particular tactics used to give apparent legitimacy to controversy, including: Conspiracy theories (suggesting opponents are involved in 'a conspiracy to suppress the truth'); moving the goalposts; dismissing critical evidence; and the oft heard suggestion that 'more research is called for'.[58] The truth or otherwise of the basic premise is not addressed – only the consequences. This is exemplified when the camee declares 'it works for me.' [59]

Michael Specter expresses concern that the 'antipathy toward the ideas of progress and scientific discovery represents a fundamental shift in the way we approach the world in the twenty-first century. More than at any time since Francis Bacon invented what we have come to regard as the scientific method (and Galileo began to put it to use), Americans fear science at least as fully as we embrace it.' In *Denialism* he further explores how irrational thinking prevents progress and threatens our lives and how irrational pseudoscience and scare-mongering has got in the way of truth and good decision-making.[60]

Denialism is the refuge of scoundrels. In the words of American author Upton Sinclair: 'It is difficult to get a man to understand something, when his salary depends upon his not understanding it.'

Secret 30. Care, Compassion and Consolation

Talking to the students of the Harvard Medical School on *The Care of the Patient* in 1927, Dr Francis Peabody advised: 'One of the essential qualities of the clinician is interest in humanity, for the secret of the care of the patient is in caring for the patient.' The Prince of Wales emphasised in 2012: 'There is much more that can be done to foster and enhance those age-old qualities of human kindness and compassion' and asked 'Should we not, perhaps, be doing more to enhance the length of contact and continuity, when it comes to relationships between professionals and patients?' [61] Most of us agree.

A fundamental reason for patients turning to camistry is a need for consolation (Latin: with; solace, comfort, cheer), and for their practitioners to demonstrate compassion (Latin: together; suffering). Michael Shermer employs the term *credo consolans* and suggests people believe in CAM because they want to and it gives them pleasure.[62] Such a belief is comforting and consoling. Hope springs eternal – 'salve our souls' the motto.

All patients seek consolation. We all have emotional needs which at times may be 'spiritual', though not necessarily religious. These need articulating and although conventional practitioners and systems should attend to these needs, camists are often better at the task. In 2014 Kesheta and Simehaib carried out a literature review of sociological and anthropological articles in order to study why women in particular use and practice CAM and engage more than men with 'holistic new age spiritualities':

> Although CAM practices are neither inherently feminine nor masculine, they are constructed in CAM discourse and conceptualized by practitioners as 'soft' and 'feminine' alternatives to the 'hard' scientific practices of biomedicine...the main characteristics of the realm of CAM and holistic spirituality readily tap into femininity: notions of normative caring, communication, gentleness, 'natural' remedies, touch, and release of emotions are generally associated with, represented by, and even experienced through purportedly 'feminine' qualities.
>
> Many CAM modalities are characterized by individualizing treatment by means of obtaining diverse information from each patient regarding diet, lifestyle, and social and personal relationships. This contextualizes healthcare within the patient's life, and allows patients to feel like an expert and an active partner in their treatment. Studies demonstrate the importance to women patients of being listened to, spending more time with the practitioner than in biomedical consultations, and enjoying the emotional support offered by women practitioners. Thus, CAM practitioners relinquish a degree of control and recognize patients' authority, which potentially reduces power asymmetries.'[63]

Caring takes time. Time is not cheap. It is poor excuse, but a truism that the pressures and demands of current healthcare systems are inimical to the highest standards of compassionate care. Camists have found ways of delivering condimentary care which engages many patients – which offers excuses to administer socially acceptable placebos. CAM does not have type II effects on the course of clinical conditions, but camists' compassionate approaches are worthy of emulation. Camists must of course be sincere, practice with integrity in a framework of fully informed consent and provide patients with any evidence they may have as to the genuine effectiveness of their interventions. Encouraging patients to indulge in wishful thinking must be avoided. Here, camists' integrity, ethics and scruples must be engaged. You must be the judge as to whether that is the case.

Camists do seem better at attending to these needs. Orthodox practitioners can learn much from CAM and conventional medicine and healthcare clearly ought to put its house in order. The opportunity costs are likely to be high but some placebists may have the time and be prepared to take the trouble to have a role here.

Secret 31. Hypnosis and Placebo Effects

These are the ultimate secrets and have the next chapter to themselves.

Decisions, decisions.

This chapter has considered how CAM works in the context of modern culture. That requires governance. There are many criticisms of political systems and of politicians who have devised and benefit from them. The field of medicine, healthcare and wellbeing is ultimately a matter for the individual. There are choices and decisions to make, resources to ration. Personal faith and experience will be taken into account by individuals but society at large and governments have to accept responsibility for ensuring those who suffer from disease and need support and consolation are properly and fully informed about options, are given truthful accounts of the practices and procedures they are considering, and are not quacked, rooked, gulled and cheated by those who seek to take advantage of them by dishonest fraudulent claims and bogus practices.

It is no secret that cost is an issue, and decisions have to be made about rationing healthcare. In counties which have no national health systems, many patients turn to CAM because they cannot afford conventional treatments or medicines. That may be a consideration for individual patients, but should not be. Spending any money at all, let alone time and trouble, on futile remedies and practices which have no plausible evidence for effectiveness is money wasted, no matter what the treatment is. Any funds available could have been saved for effective treatments or spent on practitioners offering consolation, hope and love without dishonest claims to be able to summon or conjure 'vital forces' and the like. Wasted money represents a loss of the opportunity to have spent more wisely – significant 'opportunity costs'.

Lastly, medical scientists and practitioners have to be sure to avoid the Tomato Effect. Doctors James and Jean Goodwin have pointed out that the South American plant *Lycopersicon esculentum*, the tomato, arrived with potatoes, corn and cocoa from the New World in the sixteenth century and became regularly seen on European dining tables thereafter. In North America, because tomatoes are in the same *Solanaceae* plant family as deadly nightshade, they were for long regarded as poisonous and were not eaten until the early nineteenth century – after some brave souls went ahead, did the experiment and ate basket loads with no ill effect. The Goodwins wrote: 'The tomato effect in medicine occurs when an efficacious treatment for a certain disease is ignored or rejected because it does not 'make sense' in light of the accepted theories of disease mechanism and drug interaction...Recognition of the reality of the tomato effect, while not preventing future errors, may at least help us better understand our mistakes... However, we can reduce the detriment by asking certain questions. Before we accept a treatment we should ask "Is this a placebo?" and before we reject a treatment we should ask "Is this a tomato?"'[64] The answer is to demand good plausible evidence of efficacy, and to distinguish the specifics of a treatment, remedy or practice from the placebo ministrations of the practitioner.

'Science' does not provide any ultimate truth, but the methods which science and conventional medicine use help us to get as close as possible. Science continues on that path against a backdrop of laws and regulations. Those are the responsibility of politicians. May their consciences be constantly pricked.[65]

Endnotes to Chapter 17

1. William Shakespeare, *Hamlet*. Act 1. Scene 3. 78-82. c.1600. This injunction is inscribed on the proscenium arch of the lecture hall at the South Place Ethical Society in London. A thematic variant of 'Know thyself' – the maxim was used in ancient Egypt and later inscribed on Apollo's Temple at Delphi.

2. Michael Shermer. *The Believing Brain*. Constable and Robinson. London, 2012.

3. Claims are challenged by many – Dr Fiona Godlee, Editor of the British Medical Journal and its Open Data Campaign, Tracey Brown of Sense About Science, Dr Sarah Wollaston MP and Dr Ben Goldacre are notably active.

4. When checking the truth of the beliefs underpinning these various practices, make sure you judge the integrity of the practitioners as well. Some like to style themselves as 'Dr' when they have no widely recognised doctorate degree and are not on the medical register. Why do they do that? And why do others associate with such practitioners? Why not ask them?

5. Michael Shermer. *Why People believe Weird Things*. Souvenir Press, London, 2007.

6. Matthew Hudson. *The 7 Laws of Magical Thinking*. Oneworld Publications, Oxford, 2012.

7. Daniel Kahneman, *Thinking, Fast and Slow*, Allen Lane, London 2011.

8. Richard Rawlins. *Exposure of Magical Secrets*. The Magic Circular Issue 1156, Volume 106, November 2012.

9. George Knight, *Professor Hoffmann and Conjuring*. The Windsor Magazine, Ward Lock October 1896. Personal communication, Will Houstoun, Editor of the *Magic Circular,* 2012.

10. Peter Finegan in *Neal's Yard Natural Therapies*, Thorsons. London 1994

11. Ibid.

12. According to Dr Michael Dixon, GP and founder of the College of Medicine, talking on its website. For a discussion of Dr Dixon's fallacious reasoning see: http://www. sciencebasedmedicine.org/dr-michael-dixon-a-pyromaniac-in-a-field-of-integrative-straw-men/#begincomments.

13. Prof. Sir Norman Williams PRCS. *Daily Telegraph*. 26th January 2013.

14. Graham Stringer MP, House of Commons, Science & Technology Committee Report. Stationery Office. London. Question 113. 2009.

15. Ibid, paragraph 26.

16. Ibid, paragraph 27.

17. Simon Singh, Edzard Ernst. *Trick or Treatment?* Bantam Press, 2008

18. www.publications.parliament.uk/pa/ld200607/ldselect/ldsctech/166/7022105.htm.

19. George Burns.

20. *William Deresiewicz.* www.theamericanscholar.org/eye-of-newt-2/

21. See www.billcasselman.com/unpub3/fig.htm for etymology of *sycophant*, but not if you are a maiden aunt. In drafting this paragraph I inadvertently typed 'sycophant' as 'sychophant'. In many cases the latter might be apposite.

22. James Randi in *The Faith Healers*, Prometheus Books, New York, 1987.

23. www.quackwatch.org/01Quackeryrelatedtopics/holmes.

24. Stethoscopes are seen draped round the necks of chiropodists, some of whom describe themselves as being a 'consultant surgeon'. In the UK, there is no legal requirement for a practitioner who carries out surgery to be qualified or registered as a doctor. Chiropodists/podiatrists are not. A survey by the British Orthopaedic Trainees Association suggests 98% of patients do not know this, are misled and so do not give fully informed consent to their treatment. The government has taken no action to correct this anomaly.

25. Robert Todd Carroll. *The Skeptic's Dictionary.* John Wiley & Sons. Hoboken, New Jersey 2003.

26. Not only magicians use the method. In 1967 at Monterey, Jimi Hendrix apparently set fire to his valuable iconic Fender Stratocaster. In fact, he had switched to a cheap copy earlier but allowed enough time for disassociation of this action from the subsequent performance, and so pass unnoticed by the audience. A trick he repeated in 1969. The original guitar has now been sold for $175,000.

27. Michael Specter. *Denialism.* Duckworth Overlook, London, 2010.

28. Oliver Wendell Holmes. *Homœopathy and Its Kindred Delusions.* www.ebooks.adelaide.edu.au/h/holmes.

29. Philip Mirowski. *Thinking Allowed.* BBC Radio 4 13.11.13: http://www.bbc.co.uk/programmes/b03h428y.

30. Francis Bacon, *Novum Organum Scientiarum* 1620, reprinted in Burtt, E.A., ed. (1939), *The English philosophers from Bacon to Mill*, New York: Random House via Nickerson 1998.

31. Lee Ross, Lee; Craig A Anderson,. (1982), *Shortcomings in the attribution process: On the origins and maintenance of erroneous social assessments,* in Kahneman, Daniel; Slovic, Paul; Tversky, Amos, *Judgment under uncertainty: Heuristics and biases*, Cambridge University Press, ISBN 978-0-521-28414-1, OCLC 7578020.

32. Daniel Kahneman: *Horizon*, BBC 2, 24th February 2014.

33. Günter Radden, H. Cuyckens. *Motivation in language: studies in honour of Günter*

Radden. John Benjamins. 2003.

34. Justin Kruger, David Dunning. *Unskilled and Unaware of It: How Difficulties in Recognizing One's Own Incompetence Lead to Inflated Self-Assessments.* Journal of Personality and Social Psychology 1999 **77** (6): 1121–34. doi:10.1037/0022-3514.77.6.1121. PMID 10626367.

35. *Cory Calhoun.* www. fun-with-words.com/anag_short_long.html.

36. Francis Galton: *Regression towards mediocrity in hereditary stature.* The Journal of the Anthropological Institute of Great Britain and Ireland 15. 1886.

37.https://www.avma.org/About/Governance/Documents/Resolution3_2013_Homeopathy

38. www.en.wikipedia.org/wiki/Flying_Spaghetti_Monster.2012.

39. Also see www.invisiblepinkunicorn.com, and www.palmyria.co.uk/humour/ipu

40. Having read this annotation on a war plan, Churchill enquired 'Who is Round and to what does he object?'

41. R. Barker Bausell. *Snake Oil Science: The Truth about Complementary and Alternative Medicine.* Oxford University Press. Oxford. 2007.

42. www.cancer.gov/cancertopics/CAM/thinking-about-CAM/page9.

43. Ian Rowland. *The Full Facts Book of Cold Reading.* www.thecoldreadingbook.com. 2008.

44. Kenton Knepper. *Wonder Words.* www.wonderwizards.com.

45. *Daily Telegraph,* 8th May 2012.

46. Francis Galton. *The Visions of Sane Persons.*1881. Fortnightly Review 29.

47. Max Pemberton. *Health,* The Daily Telegraph. 3rd September 2012.

48. William Blake. The *Marriage of Heaven and Hell* (1789-1790).

49. The Society for Psychical Research's offices are at the address of J. H. Kenyon, Funeral Directors. The spirits do not have far to go to attend meetings.

50. Personal communication, Will Houstoun, Editor, *The Magic Circular.* 2012.

51. Joseph Rinn. *Topics of the Times,* New York Times. January 17, 1906. *Sixty Years of Psychical Research,* The Truth Seeker Company, New York, 1950.

52. I first encountered Rhine's work whilst I was at school and was intrigued to learn of the high regard in which his work on *'psi'* was initially held – until enthusiasm waned as it became clearer that Rhine had simply discarded data which did not support his beliefs –

egregious publication bias. I also discovered the branch of magic known as mentalism and that magicians were able to reproduce all of Rhine's findings. I had an attack of scepticaemia which has yet to enter remission.

53. J.B. Rhine. *New World of the Mind.* Faber and Faber, London 1954.

54. Robert N.Proctor. *Agnotology: A Missing Term to Describe the Cultural Production of Ignorance (and Its Study).* Stanford, CA: Stanford University Press, 2008. http://scholar. princeton.edu/rccu/files/Agnotology%20Intro%20Chapter,%20Robert%20Proctor.pdf.

55. Mark Crislip *Agnotology* in Science-Based Medicine: http://www.sciencebasedmedicine. org/agnotology-the-study-of-ignorance/#comment-203887

56. Another title I considered for this book was *'What Camists Don't Tell You.'*

57. Chris Hoofnagle in: Rick Stoff. *Denialism and Muddying the Waters.* St. Louis Journalism Review 37 (296): 21-33, June 2007.

58. Mark Hoofnagle. *Climate change deniers: Failsafe tips on how to spot them.* The Guardian, Manchester. 11th March 2009.

59. H.R.H. The Prince of Wales. *Integrated health and post modern medicine.* Journal of the Royal Society of Medicine. 2012: 105. In which he also expressed a wish to see the 'best of ancient wisdom' integrated with conventional practice. He did not explain what wisdom this might be. Also see responses to his injunction in letters from Richard Rawlins and from Nick Ross: J. R. Soc. Med. 2013.

60. Michael Shermer. *Why People believe Weird Things.* Souvenir Press, London, 2007.

61. H.R.H. The Prince of Wales. *Editorial, J. R. Soc. Med.* December 2012 in which he also advocated 'integration' of CAM with orthodox medicine – which is of course quite unnecessary for achieving his other laudable objectives and may be harmful.

62. Michael Shermer. *Why People believe Weird Things.* Souvenir Press, London, 2007.

63. Yael Kesheta , Dalit Simchaib. *The 'gender puzzle' of alternative medicine and holistic spirituality.* Social Science & Medicine. Volume 113, July 2014, Pages 77–86

64. James S. Goodwin, Jean M. Goodwin. *The Tomato Effect Rejection of Highly Efficacious Therapies.* JAMA. 1984;251(18):2387-2390. doi:10.1001/jama.1984.03340420053025.

65. Many politicians seem not to have made intellectual progress into the twentieth century, let alone the twenty-first, yet they are determining how our taxes are spent and some advocate expenditure on irrational precepts and non-evidence based healthcare. That is pandering, not wise policy making.

Chapter 18

The Inner Secrets of Alternative Medicine

I said that the cure itself is a certain leaf, but in addition to the drug there is a certain charm, which if someone chants when he makes use of it, the medicine altogether restores him to health, but without the charm there is no profit from the leaf.
Socrates as quoted by Plato 380 BC[1]

It is extraordinary what a hold the mystic and marvellous still have on many people; there seems to be in almost every one a vein of credulity and superstition against which argument is useless. The disposition to be humbugged preponderates in human nature over reason and common sense. Education apparently has no influence in depriving people of this quality. Men of education are the very ones who have been, and are now, duped by clever quacks. A man may be an able politician, distinguished in literature, of great shrewdness in the ordinary business of life, and yet believe in spiritualism, homoeopathy, Perkinism and tar- water. When he is ill he will probably, after taking in vain the various much vaunted and advertised panaceas, call in some quack who promises a cure in a certain time and in some uncommon manner.
Francis J. Shepherd 1883[2]

Any sufficiently advanced technology is indistinguishable from magic.
Arthur C. Clarke 1962

The history of medicine is largely the history of placebo effects.
Arthur Shapiro 1997[3]

Academics of alternative medicine present themselves as scientists but they are all using science as a drunk man uses a lamp post: for support and not for enlightenment.
Edzard Ernst 2011

I like magicians, because they are honest men. They tell you they are going to fool you – and then they proceed to do it.
Will Rogers

Magic and Thaumaturgic Medicine

Camistry is a strange country. Many camists are well meaning and intend acting with integrity but they travel perilously close to the chasm of deception. Most would very much prefer that the spotlight of scientific inquiry is not shined too brightly upon their esoteric and arcane practices. All healthcare practitioners use just a touch of charm and charisma akin to magic, but are they open about this or do they envelop themselves in the Cloak of Thaumaturgy and seek to preserve their secrets? Over time, change of style and emphasis has led to a wide variety of terms being applied to non-orthodox medical systems. The major grouping is as 'supplementary, complementary and alternative medicine' – CAM, but as discussed, other terms such as magical, integrated, integrative, integral, holistic, tandem, paranormal, natural, pleuriform, functional and interactive medicine have also been used.

The spiritual dimension is significant. 'Concomitant with the spiritual decay of the Vietnam War, the redeeming influence of the humanistic psychology movement was born. It was followed by the transpersonal psychology movement, and then the holistic health and medicine movement. Humanistic psychology emphasises the importance of the individual, of feeling, of self-actualisation. The transpersonal psychology movement emphasises a connectedness with spirit, soul and god. The holistic health movement emphasises the importance of the spiritual aspects of life in overall wellbeing.'[4]

It all helps marketing. My preferred description of non-orthodox systems of medicine which add a soupçon of flavour to the mix but which have no discernible effects on specific underlying disease processes is *Condimentary Medicine*. For those CAM systems which make particular use of theatrical and 'magical' techniques, *Thaumaturgic Medicine* is apposite (*thauma*, marvel, wonder; *ergon*, work).

During the first century AD, *thaumaturgy* was the term used to describe events thought to be miraculous. In sixteenth century England the word referred to magical powers more generally. John Dee (1527-1608) was a renowned scholar and adviser to Elizabeth I. Although reputed to have the ability of conjuring up spirits, he was open about the mechanical devices he used to present his magical effects. As an astrologer, mathematician and hermetic philosopher, Dee recognised the cold rationality of techniques used by magicians to deceive an audience. Nevertheless he spent years trying to commune with angels and 'pure verities' and claimed he could divine the future.

Dee became dissatisfied with developing scientific methods and returned to magic and the supernatural. The angels dictated books in their own 'Enochian' language, named for the great-grandfather of Noah. Ancient texts told that Enoch described how 'the angel Michael seized me by my right hand and showed me all the secrets of the heaven.' (Book of Enoch 71:3). Mystical experiences were oft recorded in ancient times – Dee may have been deluded. Terry Pratchett's *Discworld* tells us that a 'thaum' is a unit of magic, and equals the amount of mystical energy required to conjure up one small white pigeon, or three normal-sized billiard balls. Such energies are measured with a thaumometer.

Techniques used by modern magicians are designed solely to entertain, not to conjure spirits and occult forces. Nevertheless, magic today has derived its historical context from shamans, priests and 'white magicians' who sought to do good, and even a few naughty ones who practised 'black magic'. Today the aim of 'magic' is to please an audience, but the techniques used by magicians are also used by camists and quacks to create illusions which seem to offer cures and benefits. Misdirection by sleight of hand, tongue and mind is basic. Magic works because memories of events are less than perfect, even within the time frame of a moment. 'The quickness of the hand deceives the eye' – but misdirection is the key. In the nineteenth century a number of quack chiropodists were arraigned for duping their patients by claiming they had removed a large number of corns. More perspicacious observers identified the materials 'excised' were parings from horses' hooves. The most extreme example of the sleight, particularly popular in the Far East, is 'psychic surgery' by which the practitioner is able to remove 'harmful tissue' from a patient's abdomen with his bare hands. The method is well known to students of the magic arts.

Today's Reiki practitioners claim they conjure energies to influence spirits, holding their hands in mysterious ways and employing symbols and magical charms to assist the process, much as do magicians. A wide variety of 'energy medicine' systems seek to move forces, spirits and innate intelligences in ways that are indistinguishable from the practice and arts of modern magic. Manipulation, magic hand passes, magic spells and magic remedies are invoked. Most camists deny they are using magic of any kind, and prefer to suggest there are underlying scientific principles they are able to engage. They use wonder words designed to misdirect. Their practices and advertising abounds with magician-like patter, which is deliberately designed to deceive. If these energies and forces were in any sense real, practitioners would have to comply with health and safety regulations, because clearly their power would have the capability of doing much harm. A lecture note for a course in homeopathy states: 'It is illegal to treat cancer, so treat patients who happen to have cancer.'[5] This is the slippery semantics of a charlatan. Dishonest or what? You must be the judge.

The magic arts of modern magicians provide mysteries, challenges to the intellect, engagement of emotions and stimuli to the imagination. Magician Harlan Tarbell enlisted in the US army as a food chemist, but as he was a qualified naprapathist and styled himself 'doctor' he was inevitably taken for a medical man. He recounts being asked to help with an influenza epidemic ravaging Clermont Ferrand in France in 1918. He was summoned to a village where an elderly woman lay dying. 'Fear not' he declaimed, 'for no one else will die of this epidemic. See, I make the sign of the Magi. Now none will die.' He recounts that 'I prepared magic potions from lemon juice, a magic mark with chalk on a bed – anything to restore confidence. Then I went from house to house with my magic potions, lemon juice, and good cheer. Now, you can believe this or not, but not one further person died in that epidemic. Then more than ever what *faith* could do in an emotional emergency. Today, ...ugists and psychiatrists are awakening to the value of magic in reducing emotional strain.'[6] He was to all extents, a placebist. Tarbell went on to create a well known instructional course in contemporary magic and did much to encourage performances of magic to boost morale in hospitals, institutions and rehabilitation facilities.

Penn Jillette has described techniques used by magicians to alter perceptions: pattern recognition; exaggeration; humour; misdirection; confusion, plus 'one of the darkest of all psychological secrets – if you are given a choice, you'll believe you have acted freely.'[7] It is not beneath the camists' dignity to use the tools and techniques of the magician's art; to engage the camee, patient, spectator, audience with empathic conversation and enquiry; to open the doors of imagination by well crafted phraseology and language which may itself be designed to deceive the unwary. Even to the extent of suggesting the camist possesses special powers and should be regarded as every bit an equal of practitioners who have trained, qualified and are regulated by orthodox mainstream healthcare systems. Clinical surroundings with impressive certificates and anatomical diagrams on the wall, may induce an atmosphere of confidence and therapeutic legitimacy – the trap is baited. The camist may then switch and claim that by the means of their special powers or remedies, a magical experience is created from which the camee will benefit. The magician will dress for the part. The camist likewise. Flowing robes or white coats – whatever best suits the situation and therapeutic ritual.

Claims may be made that 'energies' or 'intelligences' can be engaged by purchasing pills, potions, pins, pushing, pummelling and preternatural powers of camistry. The magician will use these energies to move objects by vanishing them or producing them – by transposition, levitation, penetration, or metamorphosis. The camist may claim to use energies at a cellular level where disease or injury benefits from the stimulus. The outcome is the same – by these mysteries the patient feels better; they will be pleased; they will declare the experience of being with the camist has 'worked'; they will declare they have benefited.

Expectation and heightened imagination may be used to beneficial effect, but may also be enlisted by fraudulent camists who play on the emotions of vulnerable patients causing imaginary perceptions of that which did not occur, inaccurate observations, hallucinations, irrational conviction, and logically fallacious reasoning.

Magic and camistry engage the fast, emotional, intuitive thinking processes – more deliberative and harder critical thinking is conveniently avoided. Eminent physicist Nils Bohr was asked about the horseshoe hung above his door: 'I don't believe in it, but I'm told it works even if you don't.'[8] Camistry is theatrical thaumaturgy.

312

Harnessing the Imagination: Hypnotic and Placebo Effects

Expectances and the power of Suggestion

Henry Beecher famously suggested 'To array a man's will against his sickness is the supreme art of medicine.'[9] It is now recognised that 'The effects of suggestion are wider and often more surprising than many people might otherwise think.'[10] When we expect a particular outcome, we automatically set in motion a chain of cognitions and behaviours which produce that outcome – and we may misattribute its cause. Our performance in tests and even in response to drugs is affected by our *response expectancies* – the myriad ways in which we anticipate responding automatically to various situations. This can be critical when researchers are assessing the value of a new drug. 'If a "real" treatment and a "suggestion" leads to a similar outcome, what differentiates the two? If we can harness the power of suggestion, we can improve people's lives.'[11]

It is not enough simply to have an imagination, what matters is harnessing it. This can be achieved through the expectancies generated by shamanism, ritual, hypnosis, suggestion, camistry and placebo. Conversely, magic works by confounding expectancies – drawing the audience into a web of wonder and unexpected experiences and by confounding them, creating mystery and awe. The final common pathway of neurochemical activity is the same for all these experiences. It can be nothing else.

All the factors discussed in earlier chapters may have a part to play in offering the camee the benefit and satisfaction they so earnestly seek. The final common pathway for the beneficial effects of CAM is through the constructive engagement of the patients' imaginations against a background of expectations. Those mechanisms can reasonably be termed 'hypnosis' and may also be induced by dummy pills and sham therapeutic manoeuvrings – by placebos. If there was plausible evidence that the pills, potions, pricking, pummelling or prestidigitation of preternatural powers did affect pathological processes, they would be taken up into conventional practice overtly, not smuggled in covertly by misleading marketing and policies promoting 'integration'.

Patient expectations provide a wide variation in the effects of placebos themselves: placebo injections have more effect than oral remedies; capsules are perceived as being stronger than tablets; bright coloured placebos are more effective than dull; larger than smaller; multiple more than single; branded more than un-branded. For depression, red are better than blue; for anxiety, green better than orange. It has even been shown that placebos which appear to be expensive are perceived as being more effective than cheaper versions. The placebos in all cases are inert with respect to their effects on disease, they are dummies – but not all have the same effects. That depends on patients' expectations – and this may account for the variation in placebo response observed for the same condition amongst different patients; in the same patient at different times; and amongst different CAMs. Some are more theatrical than others and have greater thaumaturgic impact. Patient preference is all. This may account for the fact that many camists use multiple techniques.

Placebo effects may be related to, but are not entirely identical with the outcome of classic Pavlovian conditioning. Ader and Cohen have suggested conditioning can account for some immuno-suppression, and that placebos can have a direct effect on the physiology of immunity, and therefore disease.[12] Generally, expectation involves the patients' socio-cultural framework and environment and is different from a simple evoked conditioned response.

The answer as to how CAM works lies within us. And 'we' are our minds, thoughts, imagination – and the neuro-physiological goings on of our brains. As the Buddhist scripture *Dhammapada* has it: 'Our life is the creation of our mind.'

Hypnosis

We left off the traditional account of animal magnetism and magnetic medicine after considering Mesmer and Braid and how two 'magnetic healers', Still and Palmer, founded their own systems of therapeutic manipulation – osteopathy and chiropractic. Given neither system has been shown to have any substantial type II effects on specific organ or tissue pathology, other than that on local musculo-skeletal tissue (which can be provided by any trained manipulator) – any wider benefits experienced by patients are as a result of placebo effects. They are mediated by the same 'magnetic' mechanisms used by Still and Palmer in their original practices – central psychological mechanisms.

The 'state of hypnosis' continues to be analysed, though the jury is out as to what exactly that may be. Today, hypnotic techniques are practised in four principal ways: firstly, by lay and orthodox medical or healthcare practitioners as part of a therapeutic programme; secondly by doctors and clinical psychologists as part of academic research; thirdly, for the purposes of entertainment by magicians or 'stage hypnotists'. Fourthly, techniques of hypnosis are used by orthodox practitioners and camists alike as part of their respective medical systems in order to induce patients to accept suggestions about their wellbeing. 'This will make you better...'. That amounts to placebo – and why not? We want patients to have hope, and feel better for it. Practitioners may not be altogether aware of the effect they have by making such suggestions and may not use fully developed methods of hypnosis and engagement of response expectancies, but that is a matter of semantics, not science.

In his book *Tricks of the Mind* Derren Brown suggests 'It seems to me that hypnosis is best understood as a process by which the subject allows herself to become highly responsive to the hypnotist, in a way similar to the responsiveness that we tend to exhibit when we go to a doctor or interact with most authority figures.' All magicians use the force of their personalities to induce an element of entrancement and wonder, mentalists and mind readers to a greater extent than others. Some 'spiritualist mediums' use methods hardly distinguishable from those of hypnosis – and here we

314

stray into the world of frank quackery, charlatanism and fraud.[13] 'Psychic readings' which utilise cold reading techniques of word play and disassembly are easily incorporated into a thaumaturgic encounter barely distinguishable from sessions of genuine hypnosis.

Hypnosis enables people to turn on their own placebo effects, release their own endogenous neurochemicals and moderate pain and pleasure. That is how camistry works.

In its 2000 Report the House of Lords Select Committee on Science and Technology classified *hypnotherapy* as a 'complementary' medical system – because establishing outcomes on a scientific basis with randomised controlled trials is difficult. It may be 'complementary' if it is used by unqualified practitioners and couched in the irrational terms so often used by camists, with reference to 'fields of energy' and 'vital forces', but the underlying techniques are also used by orthodox practitioners. Providing hypnotists are honest, ignore pseudo-science, retain the dash of scepticism necessary in scientists, are prepared to set aside theories which do not stand the test of observation and experiment, some patients will genuinely feel benefit from their ministrations. Whether hypnosis can have a lasting effect on pathological conditions remains to be established.

In the American Psychological Association's *Essentials of Clinical Hypnosis* (2006) Steven Lynn and Irving Kirsch described hypnosis as an ethical use of placebo. It is not expected that hypnosis will cure a physical condition but it can manage expectations, assist pain control and aid relaxation. The causes of the pain must be treated by conventional medicine to the greatest extent possible, before the subjective experience of pain and emotions can be modified by hypnosis,. The patient should be fully informed that hypnosis works by suggestion and their own heightened imagination. The patient or subject is an active participant.

Professor Irving Kirsch, formerly Professor of Psychology in Plymouth and Hull Universities in the UK is now Director of the Program in Placebo Studies at Harvard Medical School. In a presentation at the Inaugural Meeting of the Pain Medicine Section of the Royal Society of Medicine in November 2011, he advised ethical hypnotists to be non-deceptive and obtain informed consent, even if that weakens the placebo effects. Ethics trumps effectiveness, and in any event, placebo effects are not entirely negated by patients' knowledge they are being used.

Hypnosis has been successfully used for a range of conditions from pain relief in surgery and childbirth to hysterical paralysis (now termed a motor conversion disorder). Establishing the effectiveness of these techniques on a scientific basis is not easy and may be controversial but orthodox medical professionals and psychologists do have sufficient grounds for continuing scientific research. Anecdotes will not do – 'the plural of anecdote is not data'.[14]

Some magicians have incorporated hypnotic techniques into programmes of entertainment. With that experience, some entertainers have developed careers helping clients with issues of wellbeing. Some healthcare practitioners have developed a wide variety of methods to take advantage of their patients' heightened expectations and imaginative experiences. In a modern context, focussed communication between practitioner and patient involving significant suggestion may be thought of as a form of hypnosis. There are no supernatural influences or occult forces involved.

Clinicians may use different definitions of 'hypnosis' but for the purposes of a simple explanation appropriate here, the suggestion of *The Oxford Handbook of Hypnosis* suffices: The 'process' or procedure of hypnosis begins with the hypnotist making an *introduction*, followed by *suggestion* to which there is a *response*.[15] Some authorities distinguish this from the 'product' of hypnosis, which can involve apparent *trance*. Physiologically this is not 'sleep', but is sometimes referred to as such for convenience. The concept of trance may be unhelpful and is avoided by many contemporary hypnotists who prefer 'focussed concentration'. Other dimensions beneath the umbrella of hypnosis include: challenges preventing the subject defeating suggestions ('try to lift your hand'); ideomotor responses resulting in apparently involuntary physical movements (entertainers will invite their subjects to behave in outlandish ways); cognitive suggestions involving emotion and even hallucinations; amnesia (rare); analgesia; and post-hypnotic suggestions. A distinction can be drawn between instructions – 'raise your hand,' and suggestions – 'your hand is beginning to feel light and to rise.' At the end of the day, only the subject will know if they have been under any influence. Only the subject will experience a change in their sense of reality. Although there is no substantial evidence that hypnosis can make people do anything they would not wish to, some subjects do have a latent wish for outrageous, even immoral behaviour, so care has to be exercised.

Nash and Barnier suggest a hypnotic procedure has two components: firstly, an *introduction*: the subject is told that what is to follow involves suggestions for imaginative experiences. Secondly, *suggestion*, operating as an induction and enhancing expectations. In the *Oxford Handbook*, John F. Kihlstrom explains the basis of the 'consensus' definition offered by the American Psychological Association and defines hypnosis as being 'a process in which one person, designated the hypnotist, offers suggestions to another person, designated the subject, for imaginative experiences entailing alterations in perception, memory and action.' At the end of the day, all hypnosis is self-hypnosis.

American psychologist Clark Hull advise: 'hypnosis is not sleep...there is no special relationship to sleep, and the whole concept of sleep when applied to hypnosis obscures the situation.' Hull considers hypnosis is not a distinct state, but the result of motivation and suggestion.[16] Hypnotists and magicians Anthony Jacquin and Kevin Sheldrake regard their subjects not as 'sleeping' but rather 'dreaming', with the hypnotist suggesting the dreams they might experience.[17]

In Hartland's Medical and Dental Hypnosis, Psychologists Michael Heap and K. K. Aravind have defined a suggestion as: 'A communication, conveyed verbally by the hypnotist, that directs the subject's imagination in such a way as to elicit intended alterations in sensations, perceptions, feelings, thoughts and behaviour.'

The practical magician and camist may study the wide variety of models of hypnosis available in textbooks, but the practical placebist will be more interested in what motivates patients. Placebists will try to understand why healthcare choices are made as well as the effects of those choices. There is considerable overlap between the effects of hypnotic techniques and placebo effects resulting from constructive therapeutic relationships with an empathic practitioner.

How a hypnotist differs from a camist, and from a placebist, has to be considered. A hypnotist facilitates disinhibition and makes suggestions to a subject that they will experience different and heightened imaginative experiences. A camist might suggest to a patient that inert sugar pills, the release of blocked innate intelligence and vital forces by spinal adjustment, the insertion of needles, or the manipulation of occult energies will give the patient the benefit of 'feeling better'. The key difference is that the hypnotist explains in the introduction to the act of hypnosis that the patient's own imagination will be engaged. Modern ethical hypnotists do not suggest they possess occult supernatural powers. Conversely, some camists maintain they are able to manipulate 'energies' and 'vital forces', open 'occult channels' and engage the preternatural. Some claim their remedies utilise forms of energy fields unknown to science. Indeed, if they are not doing these things, what are they doing? Why have they not qualified conventionally in one of the orthodox professions? Or if they have, on what basis do they believe they have these additional powers? There is no evidence that 'energies' are engaged, for if they were, the ministrations would be part of conventional medicine.

Conventional practitioners also use hypnotic techniques to a greater or lesser extent but are expected to be open and honest about all methods they use and to secure fully informed consent. This principle applies also to the placebist who pays particular attention to methods of heightening the effects of placebos. All need to consider their patients' own reason for desiring, wanting and needing to engage in a healthcare process.

Psychologist Abraham Maslow (1908-1970) studied the complexities of motivation and positive qualities of successful people. He preferred not to consider people as a 'collection of symptoms' and he became regarded as a humanistic psychologist. His theories of self actualisation established a *hierarchy of needs* which resonate even today in institutions as diverse as military officers' training colleges and schools of business management.

Maslow also described short lived peaks of profound *transcendent happiness* or even rapture experienced by some individuals. His work was not as scientific as many would like but it pushed the envelope and still gives significant stimulus to further studies of motivation and psychological needs – and how desires differ from wants and from needs. Where public funding is concerned, needs have to be established on a consensus agreement of what is really and actually necessary for health and wellbeing. Desires and wants have to be left to the individual.

The needs of an individual for psychological and emotional security, to receive attention, to have a sense of autonomy and control, and for life to have meaning and purpose are all significant. To achieve this we have evolved emotions and instincts as well as a more objective conscious rational mind. At the same time, a dreaming brain retains the integrity of ancient instincts, defusing expectations held in the autonomic arousal system.

Joe Griffin and Ivan Tyrell are psychologists who continue research along these lines, and have styled their approach as being that of *Human Givens*. Their system is said to identify where a person's life is not working well and 'helps tailor solutions for each individual by a combination of effective psychological interventions and direct practical help.' [18]

The principle that patients or subjects can be assisted in engaging their imaginations and achieving a heightened sense of wellbeing and satisfaction has been the basis of 'medicine' provided from ancient shamans' tents to today's shining clinics. Just the thought of a glass of wine can help relaxation – even without taking one.[19] Running parallel to the process and product of 'hypnosis' is another diverticulum of the mind and the world of imaginative experience – the effects of placebos.[20]

Placebo Effects

Physicians have always known that much they had to offer was useless. Purgatives certainly purged, emetics caused emesis, bleeding let out the harmful humours. Apothecaries made up the recipes prescribed by physicians – but scientific evidence for effectiveness and consequent benefit of any of these nostrums was hard to come by. Yet doctors felt they needed to have something to prescribe – and sell. It was recognised that by using ineffective dummy pills made of bread or simple sugar, many patients would report benefit and be tolerably satisfied – particularly if there was no other drug or procedure which could help a patient's suffering. These were simply attempts to appease and please the patient.

Using the term which described medieval singers who tried to placate mourners at funerals, the pills themselves are described as *placebos*. Today, doctors are not supposed to fool patients in this way but the practice continues. Anti-biotics have no effect whatsoever on the viruses which cause colds and influenza but some patients think they will and make demands of doctors, to which many acquiesce. To all intents and purposes, the antibiotic in these cases creates only *placebo effects*. Ironically, using interferons to treat a common cold would be regarded as outrageous and unethical, even though they are effective antiviral agents. In camistry, suggesting that benefit will accrue and intimating that therapeutic manoeuvres such as pointless

318

pillules, pushing, pricking, potions and preternatural powers may provide benefit can also be thought of as *placebo*. It is usual to describe the effects of placebos or placebo treatment as being that of *placebo effects* or *responses*. Note the plural. These effects have no discernible reproducible objective effects on any specific pathological process or disease but may have a self-generated effect on physiology. Placebos 'work'. Researchers are now finding that inert pills may cause the release of neuro-chemicals such as endogenous opioids which give rise to pleasure, reduce stress and which will be reported as 'benefit'. This is why placebos are needed as controls in drug research. The base line for comparison in such research is not against 'zero effects', but against 'effects which can be produced by placebos.'

Some definitions of *placebo* and *placebo effects* are:

'A medicine given more to please than to benefit a patient.' OED.[21]

'A means of reinforcing a patient's confidence is in his recovery, when the diagnosis is undoubted and no more effective treatment is possible. For some unintelligent or inadequate patients, life is made easier by a bottle of medicine to comfort the ego; that to refuse a placebo to a dying incurable patient may simply be crueller; and that to decline to humour an elderly 'chronic' brought up on the bottle is hardly within the bounds of possibility.' The Lancet, 1954.[22]

'A placebo is something which is intended to act through a psychological mechanism. It is an aid to therapeutic suggestion, but the effect which it produces may be either psychological or physical....Dummy tablets have two real functions, one of which is to distinguish pharmacological effects from the effects of suggestion, and the other is to obtain an unbiased assessment of the results of experiment.' J.H. Gaddum, 1954.[23]

'The placebo cannot possibly enter into any process by virtue of its chemical composition. It has neither the reactivity nor the physical dimensions required of an 'effective' drug. It does not matter in the least which the placebo is made of or how much is used, so long as it is not detected as a placebo by the subject or the observer.' Henry Beecher, 1955.[24]

Subsequent research has suggested that the size, shape, colour, quantity, and even perceived price of placebos does in fact affect responses achieved. Also, although responses may be diminished if the patient has knowledge that placebos are being used, responses are not entirely negated.

'Reasons for use of a placebo: as a psychological instrument in the therapy of certain ailments arising out of mental illness; as a resource for the harassed doctor in dealing with the neurotic patient; to determine the true effect of drugs apart from suggestion in experimental work; as a device for eliminating bias not only on the part of the patient but also, when used as an unknown, of the observer; and, finally, as a tool of importance in the study of the mechanisms of drug action...It is important to distinguish the very respectable, conscious use of placebos. The effect of placebos has been shown by randomised controlled trials to be very large. Their use in the correct place is to be encouraged ...' Archie Cochrane, 1972.[25]

'We define the placebo effect as the nonspecific, psychological, or psychophysiologic therapeutic effect produced by a placebo...the placebo may be an inert sugar pill, an active drug, or any treatment no matter how potentially specific or by whom administered.' Arthur and Elaine Shapiro, 1997.[26]

'The placebo effect is where the patient's belief that they are receiving treatment makes them behave as if they had actually received it, and therefore they persuade themselves that they feel better.' Bob Lloyd, 2009.[27]

'The placebo effect is any health effect measured after an intervention that is something other than a physiological response to a biologically active treatment ... it is not a single effect but the net result of many possible factors ... subjective outcomes like pain, fatigue, and an overall sense of well-being, are subject to a host of psychological factors... A common belief is that the placebo effect is largely a 'mind-over-matter' effect, but this is a misconception. There is no compelling evidence that the mind can create healing simply through will or belief. However, mood and belief can have a significant effect on the subjective perception of pain. There is no method to directly measure pain, and studies of pain are dependent upon the subjective report of subjects. There is therefore a large potential for perception and reporting bias in pain trials.' Steve Novella, 2008.[28]

'When the effect of administering a drug is found to be independent of its specific ingredients (i.e. when an inert preparation produces the same effect), the drug is deemed to be a placebo. Similarly, hypnotic inductions must be expectancy manipulations, akin to placebos, because their effects on suggestibility are independent of any specific component or ingredient. In fact, it is possible to produce all of the suggested effects of hypnosis by giving subjects a placebo and telling them that it produces a hypnotic state.' Irving Kirsch, 2008.[30]

'The most interesting, and perhaps most coherent, approach to understanding placebo effects suggests that they should be conceived of as the result of a range of context-specific psychological and social factors, operating through specific physiological mechanisms.' Andrew Turner, quoting Beecher.[31]

'Physicians and patients may gradually learn that the placebo effect is an integral and inevitable component of the practice of medicine, that it constitutes its art and augments its science.' Jay Katz, 1984.[32]

'The placebo effect itself is poorly understood and almost certainly contains elements of the doctor's approach to the patient, the natural resolution of the underlying illness, the effects of receiving treatment for an illness, and the belief system of both the patient and the consulting physician.' George Lewith, 1994. [33]

In summary: Placebo effects and healing result from the practitioner-patient relationship, medical ritual and context, the power of the imagination, responses to expectances, compassion, hope and trust. The more caring, compassionate, empathic and supportive the practitioner is, the more 'pleasure' the patient is likely to experience. Analysts such as Ernst and Resch distinguish between 'true' placebo effects which are real psychological phenomena and 'perceived' effects which are multi-factorial but may include the natural course of disease, statistical regression to the mean and parallel interventions.[34] It is hardly possible to distinguish the effects achieved by placebos from those achieved by hypnosis.

In the early twentieth century placebos had been thought of as useless drugs given by unscrupulous physicians to fool patients. Clinical pharmacologist Harry Gold of Cornell University in New York wanted to improve the methodology of clinical drug trials. In 1937, Gold's report on the use of placebos to improve double-blind trials saw a change in approach. Gold went on to found the *Cornell Conferences* which considered *The Use of Placebos in Therapy*. In 1946, 'Du Bois commented that although scarcely mentioned in the literature, placebos are more used than any other class of drugs. He objected to the definition of a placebo as an agent designed to pacify rather than to benefit and held, reasonably enough that to pacify is to benefit....Diethelm suggested that that the person reacts to suggestion because what is suggested becomes to him reality. In believing, the expected reaction takes place. Gold made a strong plea for 'pure' placebos that do not contain any element that could conceivably have a direct effect on the body's cells; otherwise the physician is likely to deceive himself. He comes to believe that these unlikely agents are effective, when really all the power they have is as a placebo.'[35]

'The power of the placebo should not be underestimated'. So advised US Army anaesthetist Dr Henry Beecher whose 1955 paper *The Powerful Placebo* is seminal. 25% of seriously wounded soldiers reported little or no pain, and Beecher surmised this was a consequence of the 'power of the mind'. For soldiers, a wound could be perceived as being a 'benefit' as they were repatriated from theatres of war. It has been suggested that when tending wounded soldiers Beecher had run out of anaesthetic and used sterile water injections instead – with comparable results. This may be apocryphal but certainly Beecher carried out a meta-analysis on over twenty published reports and concluded that in about one third of cases the beneficial outcomes were due to non-specific placebo effects. Placebos were already being used as dummy pill controls in research, but Beecher emphasised their value in clinical practice.[36]

More recent analysis of Beecher's data suggest he did not take sufficient account of spontaneous improvement, regression to the mean, scaling bias, irrelevant response variables, acquiescence of patients, conditioned responses, neuroses or psychosomatic phenomena. Nevertheless research has continued and placebo effects are now receiving closer attention with full scientific scrutiny. Beecher originally suggested that only about a third of patients are placebo responders. Probably the response rate in patent populations varies between zero and 100%, with significant responses being at the 33% mark.[37] And studies must take care to exclude outcomes due to the non-specific effects of 'natural healing'.[38]

Consensus has yet to be reached. The Quackometer's Andy Lewis warns: 'Placebo effects do not just mislead patients, but also practitioners...placebos can give rise to the appearance of effective treatments without any actual healing having taken place...it is a common misrepresentation to say that placebo effects are about mind-body interactions actually changing the course of an illness for the better.'[39] Ernst and Resch have advised the 'perceived placebo effects' resulting from 'natural healing' as a result of measurement errors, remission, regression, and the natural history of the disease must be excluded before outcomes can be considered as resulting from 'true placebo effects'.[40] The latter are referred to as 'contextual effects' by some authors.

It is conventional to consider pathological conditions as 'diseases', and to reserve the term 'illnesses' for how patients feels about them – the antonym of 'wellness.' On that basis patients report they have benefited from remedies or therapies – even when those benefits are solely due to placebo effects. Some commentators refer somewhat disparagingly to 'mere placebo' as if the effects are plain or meagre. They are not. Placebos can have powerful effects, as camistry demonstrates. Naturally, every practitioner should be offering the compassion, hope and love which are at the heart of all caring practice.

Placebo effects are generated by placebo pills. In addition, placebo effects can result from medically ineffectual treatments or interventions themselves. For research purposes, even significant interventions such as electro-convulsive therapy and knee arthroscopy have been carried out in sham.[41] Sham acupuncture with needling at non-acupuncture points, or using retractable sham needles akin to fake stage daggers has been shown to be just as effective as the real thing. Therefore the real thing is no better that a placebo – and *is* a placebo.

Patients' perceptions and expectations matter, and the practitioner can frame these by style, deportment and bedside manner. It makes a difference if the practitioner is calm, caring or curt. 'Framing' is an important element of both hypnosis and the performance of magic. The frame is the context through which we consider a situation; the references we use to measure ideas and statements in order to decide whether we agree or disagree with them. In medicine, caring may not cure disease, but it can make disease endurable, and schmaltz satisfies. In magic, the success of intentional deception is dependent on the frame in which it occurs.

Steven Jay, Irving Kirsch, and Michael Hallquist have reviewed Kirsch's *Response Expectancy Theory of Hypnosis:*

> A subject's expectancy for change in experience can affect the experience itself, and can cue automatic responses in the form of self-fulfilling prophecies. Kirsch

opines: "This is best documented by the ability of placebos to produce changes in pain, anxiety, depression, tension, sexual arousal and other subjective states as well is in the physiological substrates of the states. Similarly, hypnotic response expectancies can produce hypnotic experiences ... hypnotic inductions are expectancy modification procedures that produce placebo effects without the use of placebos... when the effect of administering a drug is found to be independent of its specific ingredients, the drug is deemed to be a placebo. Similarly, hypnotic inductions must be expectancy manipulations, akin to placebos, because their effects on suggestibility are independent of any specific component or ingredient. In fact, it is possible to produce all of the suggestive effects of hypnosis by giving subjects a placebo and telling them that it produces a hypnotic state." [42]

Alternatively, suggestions to patients in hypnosis can be that they will experience placebo effects. There is no difference for the practical placebist. If hypnotism is akin to a placebo and its effects cannot be distinguished from a placebo, its mechanism of action is surely that of a placebo. Given that, then placebos create an effect on patients in the same way as hypnosis does – by the final common pathway of heightened expectations and confident suggestion. Kirsch has described hypnosis as being a 'non-deceptive mega-placebo.' Most contemporary authorities regard hypnosis as 'self-hypnosis' and not as the result of some force or energy imparted by the hypnotist and certainly not magnetism. By various techniques, the hypnotist assists the subject in engaging their imagination. The camist and placebist will also use a patient's expectation of response and heightened imagination and may use imaginative methods to achieve this. It is for academic psychologists to determine if there is any substantial difference between hypnotic and placebo effects. Both are acting on the brain utilising the same neuro-chemicals. Camists use practices which are distinct alternatives to scientific evidence-based medical systems but they do not always explain this to their patients. Some may intend being deliberately deceptive to dupe the unwary. Placebists, hypnotists and physicians should be honest about their approach and obtain fully informed consent.

Some orthodox practitioners utilise CAMs without explaining their nature. Some have been castigated for giving worthless or unnecessary and illegitimate injections. No doubt this enhances the placebo effects but many regard this as dishonest, abusive, and fraudulent practice. Only occasionally have such medical quacks and charlatans had their licences to practice revoked.[43] Be warned.

Research at the Hawthorne electrical factory in the 1920s demonstrated how humans respond to changes in environment even when they are not conscious of any change. Other species likewise. The various mechanisms of placebo effects have been shown in many animals – the mere fact of perceived intervention can trigger physiological responses. In animals, a change in environment, lighting, feeding schedule or attention from the owner can invoke an immune response. Nicholas Humphrey has postulated that during evolution of a species, sustained immune responses to an initial insults drained physiological resources. Natural selection then favoured those animals which responded to disease only a little, before the animal had better indications that a full blown response was necessary.[44,45] He suggested the mechanisms of evolution sought the 'most cost effective way to manage the species' and so increase overall chances of survival.

Positive placebo effects may be inherited adaptive characteristics giving evolutionary advantage by enabling animals, including us, to cope better with life's vicissitudes. There is now evidence in support of Humphrey's contention from computer modelling – suggesting evolutionary benefit to having a system for switching the immune response on and off. That may account for the some of the effects described as placebo. Peter Trimmer of Bristol University suggests: 'A deeper understanding of why the placebo effect exists may allow it to be invoked more easily in the future.'[46] The precise case for this book.

Research by McGlashan and colleagues has suggested there is no intimate relationship between a subject's susceptibility to hypnosis and to placebo/nocebo responses.[47] But given the *modi operandi* are so similar (by introduction, suggestion and response), given the outcomes are so similar ('it works for me'), given placebo responses vary with expectations and desires and the underlying dis-ease for which help is sought – both hypnosis and placebo effects could still have a final common neurological pathway and comparable underlying mechanisms. That seems more probable than not and, being predicated on the scientific principles of probability, more research along these lines is indicated. Ancient wisdom has it that if it looks like a duck, flies like a duck and quacks – it's a duck. That insight applies to both hypnosis and placebo effects. They cannot be usefully distinguished, probably.

Placebo response
The antonym of placebo is nocebo – effects which are unpleasant, even harmful – induced by subjects' expectations and responses to inert substances or sham procedures (Latin: I will harm). The effects may be real, and reported as such by some subjects, but the same substance or procedure does not produce an unwanted effect in other subjects, nor in the same subject on other occasions. Nocebo effects are like placebo and represent the side effects of placebo. W.R. Houston had referred to harmful placebo effects in the 1930s and the term *nocebo responses* was first used by Walter Kennedy in 1961. At the extreme, voodoo deaths following unmitigated terror, responses to the 'evil eye', 'hex' and self-willed illness have been described as nocebo responses.[48]

These must be distinguished from psychosomatic or psychophysiological disorders which require the attention of specialists in those fields. Just as with hypnosis, the subjects' imaginations and expectations are critical. Placebos have been shown to affect a part of the brain that modulates pain perception. Nocebos likewise, but additionally, a slightly different area which is associated with memory and anxiety – the hippocampus.

'Expectations' themselves are hard to assess and measure, and therefore their contribution to placebo and nocebo effects is difficult to determine. There is a problem for researchers in judging negative expectations and at present evidence is piecemeal and ambiguous. As Robert Hahn advises: 'An understanding of these processes should illuminate the range and inevitability of these side effects of culture.'[49] It seems that therapeutic rituals, demonstrated in spades by camistry, stimulate the same molecules and neurochemical pathways as those activated by pharmacological drugs.

The House of Lords Science and Technology Committee Report on CAM, 2000

This extensive review of CAM is essential reading for all students of medicine and healthcare, whether CAM or conventional.[50] Few now refer to this work, and fewer still have acted upon it. The Lords' Report emphasises many of the themes developed in *Real Secrets*. The House of Lord's Report, Chapter 3 on *Placebo Effect* in précis:

3.19 Studies have shown that patient expectations concerning a treatment, patients' experience of the treatment and patients' attitudes towards their healthcare provider can all affect the impact a treatment has. Such factors as these can all be brought together under the term 'the placebo effect'...However, the placebo effect has often in the past had a negative stigma attached to it, and has often been considered either as a nuisance which hampers research, a sign of patient neuroticism, or a sign of clinical quackery.

3.21 The placebo effect is nothing new, nor are attempts to enhance its effect unconventional. The history of conventional medicine has largely been the history of the placebo effect. Most medicines used by doctors up until the twentieth century are now known to be inert, but they were often of exotic origin and thus were often perceived as having magical properties.

3.22 All treatments, physically active or otherwise, have a psychological impact when administered to a conscious patient. This psychological effect should not be considered as a nuisance or some kind of fraud, but an essential element of any holistic therapy. It could even be suggested that the placebo effect is a legitimate form of psychotherapy.

3.26 ...evidence shows that people who are placebo responders on one occasion may not be on the next. Awareness of the fact that any patient may benefit from the placebo effect might do much to de-stigmatise it as a sign of patient neuroticism.

3.27 Treatments that employ sophisticated technical equipment enhance the placebo effect. Research on therapist variables has shown that those therapists who exhibit greater interest in their patients, greater confidence in their treatments and higher professional status, whatever their background of training, all appear to promote stronger placebo responses in their patients. It is also possible that the almost 'magical' approach of some complicated and unusual therapies may have a similar effect to highly sophisticated technologies in inducing wonder in patients.

3.28 It is important to consider the possible modes of action through which the placebo effect may operate. Professor Patrick Bateson, Vice President of the Royal Society, explained how psychological factors might affect physical health: '... when somebody suffers chronic stress, bereavement or loses a job, under those conditions they are much more prone to disease and more likely to get cancer, and it is now believed that this is because of suppression of the immune system, which is constantly cleaning up bacteria and viruses and also cleaning up cells which are cancerous cells. So if you do the opposite of that and give a patient some reassurance, and if they are given a treatment which they believe in, then this will enhance the immune response – it will remove the stress which is causing the immune response to be suppressed – and so that may be one rather powerful mechanism by which the placebo effect works.'

3.29 Despite a lack of understanding of the exact mechanisms through which the placebo effect may operate, research clearly shows that the effect exists and can have a significant impact on health. This work has important implications for anyone who has identified a therapy which appears to be efficacious but which does not have a clearly identified mode of action and it is important that all research on such therapies takes account of the placebo effect.

3.30 Evidence we have heard suggests that it may be over-simplistic to ask whether the treatment is a placebo or not. The more pertinent question will often be: 'In what proportion may the effects of this treatment be accounted for by psychologically-mediated, as opposed to direct physically-mediated, changes?' In the absence of direct evidence from placebo-controlled double-blind trials it is proper to regard any new or unusual form of treatment as potentially a form of psychotherapy. This is the reason why the debate over the need for randomised controlled trials has become a central debate in the CAM world.

3.31 We have also considered the implications of finding that any particular CAM therapy relies largely on the placebo effect and has little or no treatment-specific effect. Several of our witnesses have suggested this is a very important question. Professor Tom Meade of the Royal Society summed up this sentiment: 'I think the important question is that if a CAM is claiming that it has a specific value for a particular condition, then it does have to be able to show that there is a treatment-specific effect over and above the placebo effect. I think that is important because, first of all, a lot of CAM is practised in private practice at the moment, and people are entitled to know how they are spending their money. I think it is also important from the health service's point of view, as various trusts and general practitioners take CAMs up in increasing numbers.'

3.32 If a treatment makes people feel better, whether that be through treatment specific effects or the placebo effect, then it could be considered as being worthwhile.

In fact, as the placebo effect is not just an imagined experience but can positively improve objective biological measures of health, then a treatment which enhanced such an effect could even be considered worth attaining in its own right. As well as stressing the need to prove treatment-specific effects, Professor Patrick Bateson, giving evidence with Professor Tom Meade for the Royal Society, acknowledged that sometimes the placebo effect may be worth attaining in its own right.

3.33 However, the idea that the placebo effect might be something worth using as a treatment was not a majority opinion, and Professor Timothy Shallice of the Academy of Medical Sciences suggested that there is probably little justification for supporting the wider advocacy of any technique that relies on the placebo effect within the NHS, '...since it depends so critically on the particular beliefs of that particular person at that particular time'.

As the Report suggests in paragraph 3.30 – the pertinent question to ask is 'In what proportion may effects of the treatment be accounted for by psychologically-mediated, as opposed to direct physically-mediated changes?' Given that no CAM studied demonstrates substantial plausible reproducible evidence of type II specific physical effects, then the benefits experienced by patients are due to non-specific type I effects, that is – they are indeed placebo. As Professor Meade pointed out, when it comes to CAM, 'people are entitled to know how they are spending their money.' This principle is especially important for commissioners of healthcare services which use public funds.

Some contributors to the Report recognised placebo effects can positively improve objective biological measures of health and could be considered as 'worth attaining in its own right'. Others suggested the use of placebo effects within the NHS would be hard to justify. That does not mean patients should not access camistry on their own account and at their own expense.

If a patient feels they benefit from camistry, well and good, on condition that they have been fully informed as to the nature of placebo effects. Only then can they trust their practitioner and give legitimate consent. And society does now actively forbid some remedies, such as rhinoceros horn for erectile dysfunction, even though some patients claim benefit. Horn, comprising the protein keratin, is biochemically equivalent to toe nails but for some reason toe-nail clippings are not used in traditional medicines, and the rhinoceros continues to suffer.

In January 2013 Arthritis Research UK reported on the effectiveness of CAMs commonly used for treating arthritis and other musculoskeletal conditions. There is 'lack of scientific evidence to support their use.'[51] Professor Alan Silman, the medical director, commented: 'the relationship between the patient and practitioner seems to be crucial in the effectiveness of the treatment...we wish to focus on how this relationship, which may be part of the placebo effect, can help to give the patient benefit.'

Arthritis Research UK 'interprets the term "placebo" with considerable caution.' As is often said – more work is needed. After studying the scientific evidence for CAM, R. Barker Bausell, the former Director of the Complementary and Alternative Medicine Specialised Research Center, reported in *Snake Oil Science* that: 'CAM therapies are nothing more than cleverly packaged placebos. And that is almost all there is to say about the science of CAM.'[52]

Ethical use of placebos

Medieval placebo singers intended to please and console the bereaved. Physicians have for long sold pills which had no therapeutic effect but which provided an element of cheer. In time, these became known as placebos – the deceit being justified on the grounds of 'doing our best for the patient…it's better than nothing… we might as well.' In the twentieth century, this patronising practice became too close to fraud for comfort and slowly declined. We now use placebos in two ways: as controls in drug trials and as treatments in their own right. As controls in research into drug effectiveness, different placebos have different effects dependent upon their size, shape, colour, number, dose regime, packaging and even perceived cost. Nevertheless, when sufficient numbers of patients are studied these biases are ironed out and researchers can be reasonably assured as to the extent their findings can be attributed to the specifics of the drug being studied.

Placebos in research
The academic and research community has regularly considered the ethical use of placebos in research. The World Medical Association developed a set of ethical principles regarding human experimentation in its 1964 Declaration of Helsinki: Patients should be 'assured of the best proven diagnostic and therapeutic method' – even if they are in the placebo control group. If a proven treatment exists, placebos should not be used as controls and reports using such methods should not be accepted for publication. Austin Bradford Hill pointed out that the question at issue is not whether the new treatment is better than nothing but better than an existing proven treatment.[53] Archie Cochrane stated no new treatment should be introduced until randomised controlled trials have shown it to be superior to existing treatments.[54] Commercial pressures should be resisted.

The Declaration of Helsinki states: 'Medical research involving human subjects must conform to generally accepted scientific principles, be based on a thorough knowledge of the scientific literature, other relevant sources of information, and adequate laboratory and, as appropriate, animal experimentation.' This implies that conducting randomised clinical trials into camistry (the domain in which CAMs function) is unethical because the practices do not conform to generally accepted scientific principles. The basic work to identify and demonstrate the existence of the 'healing energy', 'memory', 'subluxation', 'median', 'chakra', 'dosha', has simply not been done.

328

When there is no established 'proven' treatment, it is generally accepted that placebo-controlled trials are ethical and establish a benchmark. Mark Sullivan has suggested that such trials are what define modern medical practice and separates it from mystery, 'thus casting alternative medicines into shadowy byways.'[55] Laboratory research into placebo and nocebo effects continues apace, identifying specific neuro-modulators and associated brain areas. 'However, little progress has been made in translating this knowledge into improved patient care.'[56]

Placebos as therapy

Luana Colloca and Franklin Miller suggest strategies for how, when and why interventions promoting beneficial placebo responses might be administered therapeutically and integrated with physicians' expertise and patient attitudes. They emphasise that whilst the traditional use of the word 'placebo' has referred to inert substances and simulated interventions, research into placebos indicates there is an impact of expectations on brain-mind-body interactions. They suggest: 'What makes substances or interventions cast as placebos is the lack of specific efficacy in treating a specific patient's condition based on the inherent properties of the treatment. Clinician-patient interaction and communication is critical and reflect the "conditioning and meaningfulness" of Irving Kirsch's "response expectancies".'[57]

Colloca and Miller's analysis of empirical studies in twelve different countries found that between 70-80% of doctors and 50-100% of nurses used placebos therapeutically. Commonly, a physician would tell the patient they were using 'medicine not typically used for your condition, but which may benefit you.' [58]

Attempts to harness placebo benefits should take place within professional norms and ethical-legal requirements of informed consent. These must be consistent with professional integrity and offer a favourable risk-benefit ratio. Colloca and Miller have argued that if the placebo effect is a real phenomenon it may be legitimate to promote use of the effects within the contemporary medical paradigm.

Comments about 'mere' placebos or intimations that placebo effects cannot be of value are misplaced. All CAMs rely on them. Unless and until there is plausible evidence of meaningful specific effects on physiology or pathology, it should be accepted that is how camistry works. So, to a degree, does conventional medicine.

Some suggest that effective placebo effects will not occur without deception – which presents an ethical problem. Jean Robert-Houdin said: 'A magician is an actor playing the part of a magician.' Likewise, a camist is an actor playing the part of a camist. Magicians are honest and admit they use tricks and not supernatural forces – nevertheless, audiences still derive pleasure from their thaumaturgic performances. Likewise in medicine, patient expectations may still be engaged and beneficial effects achieved even when patients understand they are being given placebos.

Ted Kaptchuk reports finding significant improvement in patients with irritable bowel syndrome when using 'medicines' openly labelled as placebos and when compared with a no-treatment control group. Patients who knew they were taking placebos reported twice as much relief of irritable bowel symptoms as those in the no-treatment group.[59] Inevitably this work has been criticised, not least because of selection bias – recruits to the research were patients interested in 'mind-body medicine'. Kaptchuk countered that patient improvement came about because 'it's not something they're thinking about, it's something they're doing...this is the context in which the pill is administered.'

Nor is illness the only perception to be affected by expectations. Brain scans of the striatum, posterior insula and dorsal pre-frontal cortex have shown that neural responses to the taste of chocolate and milkshake were moderated according to expectancy and that cheap wines packaged as expensive were enjoyed as much as fine vintages. These expectancy responses are referred to as 'marketing placebo effects.'[59]

The ethical placebist and condimentary medicine

Most patients know there is no active principle in homeopathic remedies, no 'meridians' which respond to needling, no 'innate intelligence' which can be released by spinal adjustments, yet many report beneficial effects from appropriate ministrations. There is criticism of those who call for 'more research' into camistry but where the use of placebos is openly declared as a therapy, further research can be justified.

Edzard Ernst finds that placebo responses are 'unreliable, short lived, inevitably involve deception, might displace effective treatment, are not all entirely safe and their use promotes irrationality.'[60] He considers 'Research into all this is very important. But, even if one day we have a full understanding of placebo effects, this will not amount to a justification of placebo-therapies. There are several reasons for this, the most important being that we do not need a placebo to generate placebo effects: treatments with non-specific effects administered with compassion will do this too – and will produce specific effects in addition.'[61]

We are getting a tad semantic here. The term 'placebo' can include 'treatments with non-specific effects administered with compassion.' Ernst recognises 'placebo effects' may be beneficial but holds that use of 'placebos' is unethical. Some doctors are prepared to use placebos on the basis that anything that produces a placebo effect is beneficial. The use of placebos may indeed involve lying and physician deception which violates patient autonomy and the legitimacy of medical professionals. That need not be the case. The key is informed consent, honesty, intellectual integrity and candidness.

Conversely, the covert use of placebos may medicalise counterproductive illness behaviour. Patients may be given false hope that a solution is available and the distinctive benefits of science-based medicine may be lost. Camists (those who practice camistry) plough their own alternative furrow but an ethical placebist (one who studies or utilises placebo effects) should consider the original Colloca and Franklin paper. The practitioner should ensure the patient is honestly told what is intended, and that properly informed consent is obtained. Philosopher Janet Stemwedel offers a suggestion for obtaining consent and ensuring patient autonomy on an ethical basis:

> I am going to offer you a treatment that might do nothing, but that might help relieve your symptoms. We have no reason to believe that this treatment will make your symptoms worse, nor that it will cause other harm to you. Treatments of this sort have helped other patients, but we still aren't clear on the mechanism behind it. I am leaving the choice of whether to try this treatment up to you, and I'm happy to talk with you about the research we have now about the efficacy of this kind of treatment. If you feel you would like to try it, I am happy to provide it. If not, I will do my best to alleviate your symptoms and treat your condition with the other tools available to us. [62]

The ethical placebist must make sure all conventional avenues of treatment have been explored and that appropriate effective medical care is being given. Placebos must not delay or supplant conventional care, nor should the placebist undermine confidence in rational science-based medicine. Placebos are the basis of condimentary medicine – which is pleasurable and nice to have but is not expected to provide disease-specific treatment.

Irving Kirsch offers an elegant research design to avoid pitfalls of patient autonomy and informed consent: 'You're going to be in an experiment, some of the people in the experiment are going to get an active drug, some are going to be a control group and not get it.' Then that person is informed, 'You're getting the active drug,' or 'You are in the control group and are not getting the active drug.' Until de-briefed at the conclusion, for half the subjects that information is true, for half that information is deceptive. Honesty and integrity are satisfied as well as the maintenance of patient's autonomy. Howard Spiro suggests there is a swing of the pendulum over these ethical issues and that beneficence can now be more readily recognised.[63]

The clinical conundrum is whether doctors, in doing their 'best' for a patient, should offer placebos which might provide benefit (from the perspective of the patient) or whether that is trumped by the importance of doctors being honest and telling the truth. Dylan Evans comments:

> The existence of the placebo response makes the dilemma far more acute. For if beliefs can have a direct impact on the functioning of the immune system, then modifying those beliefs by imparting new information to the patient might help or hinder his chance of recovery. If hope itself can cure and there is little basis for such hope in reality, should the doctor lie to the patient?

Evans noted the medieval French surgeon Henri de Mondeville advised doctors to lie to keep patients cheerful, 'Even by telling him that he has been elected to a bishopric, if a churchman.' [64] Conversely, should patients mislead their doctors?

Some patients may prefer to be ill – to maintain welfare benefits, sympathy, or even get to the front of a queue. This is not a harsh judgement. Observe how many folks have 'disabled' stickers for their cars – not all are justified.

Evans goes on to suggest that just as cigarette packets have statutory health warnings attached, so too should alternative medicines:

> Homeopathic remedies should be sold with a label reading: "Warning: this product is a placebo. It will work only if you believe in homeopathy and only for certain conditions such as pain and depression. Even then, it is not likely to be as powerful as orthodox drugs. You may get fewer side effects from this treatment than from a drug but you will probably also get less benefit." As medical decision-making becomes an increasingly co-operative venture involving patients as equal partners in the prescription process, providing them with accurate information about the various remedies available becomes of the utmost importance. This applies just as much to alternative medicine and psychotherapy as it does to the various resources of orthodox medicine.

In order that patients can give fully informed consent to the proposed intervention and can make an intelligent choices, practitioners must be trusted to provide all relevant information. The UK General Medical Council requires that: 'Doctors should share with patients the information they want or need in order to make decisions...you should not make assumptions about the information a patient might want or need; the clinical or other factors a patient might consider significant, or a patient's level of knowledge or understanding of what is proposed.'

Medical paternalism has been consigned to history. Since the 1950s it is expected that patients not only give informed consent but are also fully involved in decision-making. Patients must have enough information to decide whether the risks of any proposed intervention is acceptable to them. That includes the risk of wasting their time and money on ineffective treatments. This means patients should be told what the evidence is that the proposed intervention will affect a specific pathological process. If there is no such plausible evidence, that is what patients should be told. A reasonable explanation of the proposed therapies should be given. This is a particular problem for camists who would much prefer to keep the placebo nature of their ministrations secret. Some homeopaths deny outright that their remedies are placebos and continue asserting that 'ultra-dilute remedies have biological activity.' [65] They persist in conflating the type I effects of the care they offer with type II effects of the remedies themselves – conflating the therapy with the therapist, the practitioner with the practice, style with substance. Discourses by homeopaths abound with logical fallacies, but alternative logic is no logic. Randomised placebo controlled clinical trials are difficult to apply in homeopathic research but when controls are used, results show remedies have no plausible effects beyond the placebo.

Patient autonomy and practitioner integrity

A recent survey showed most patients themselves find it acceptable for doctors to recommend placebo treatments providing there is transparency about benefits, risks and purposes.[66] A BMJ Editorial by Professor Vernon Oh discussed *The placebo effect: can we use it better?* He noted placebos do not work if the disease is hyper-acute (for example, cardiac arrest), when vital functions degenerate (as in metabolic acidosis) or with hereditary syndromes. Nor does CAM. Oh suggested: 'In appropriate patients doctors might consider giving a placebo when active treatment is both costly and likely to confer only marginal or transient benefit.'[67] There is nothing inherently or morally wrong with using camistry for the powerful placebo effects offered – as long as the patient gives fully informed consent.

Harvard Medical School's Program in Placebo Studies observes: 'Placebo effects are increasingly recognized as a central (if often invisible) element in the provision of care. Yet they remain mostly absent from clinical guidelines and from the decision-making process between provider and patient. This is currently being addressed by widening understanding through meetings and publications in an inter-disciplinary environment bridging science and the humanities.'

Ethically, practitioners must avoid deception. There may be an ethical place for a doctor to lie to a dying patient – but that compassion for an individual should be distinguished from lies about mechanisms of action and effectiveness for the panoply of CAM practices created for the population in general. The secret to the ethical use of placebos is to obtain fully informed consent based on the most probable mechanisms of action of CAM systems. Implausible suggestions of 'bio-energy fields', 'innate intelligence', 'holistic natural forces', 'quantum entanglements' and the like must be set aside – CAMs work by placebo effects. There is no other rational explanation.[68]

Patients deserve protection from deceptive and ineffective treatments that waste their time and may defraud them. Transparency and intellectual integrity are the bedrock of good healthcare practice and are essential if the interventions of heath care professionals are to provide honest pleasurable benefits.[69] Integrity is the enemy of quackery, which is where we turn next.

Endnotes to Chapter 18

1. Plato. *Charmides*, (Temperance), 155-6. In a Dialogue of 380 BC, the beautiful youth Charmides complains of an early morning headache and Socrates provides relief: '...the part can never be well unless the whole is well...you must begin by curing the soul. That is the first thing...Is not medicine the science of health?'

2. Francis J. Shepherd. *Medical Quacks and Quackeries*. The Popular Science Monthly, June 1883.

3. Arthur K. Shapiro: *The Placebo Response*. In Modern Perspectives in World Psychiatry.

Ed. John Howells. Oliver & Boyd. Edinburgh. 1968.

4. Norman Shealy MD. *Soul Medicine: Awakening Your Inner Blueprint for Abundant Health and Energy.* Elite Books. Santa Rose. 2006.

5. Andy Lewis. http://www.quackometer.net/blog/2009/11/can-we-trust-homeopaths-to-accredit.html.

6. Harlan Tarbell. *Tarbel Course in Magic.* D. Robbins and Co. Brooklyn, New York. Vol. 8. 1993.

7. www.smithsonianmag.com/arts-culture/Teller-reveals-His-Secrets. 2012.

8. Matthew Hutson, *The 7 Laws of Magical Thinking*, Oneworld Publications, Oxford, 2012.

9. Henry K. Beecher. *The Powerful Placebo.* Journal of the American Medical Association, December 24th 1955.

10. Robert B. Michael, Maryanne Garry, Irving Kirsch. *Suggestion, Cognition, and Behaviour.* Current Directions in Psychological Science. June, 2012. 21.

11. Press release for the Association of Psychological Science: www. psychologicalscience. org/index.php/news/releases/the-power-of-suggestion.June 6th 2012.

12. Ader, R.A.,and Cohen, N. 1975 *Behaviourally Conditioned Immuno-suppression.* Psychosomatic Medicine, 37.

13. Ludwig van Hoödwinke's *Charlatanic Suggestibility amongst Aphelics*, Journal of Speculative Thaumaturgy, 1 April 1890, is seminal.

14. Robert Park. *The Seven Warning Signs of Bogus Science: The Chronicle Review- Journal of Higher Education*, January 31, 2003. http://chronicle.com/free/v49/i21/21b02001.htm

15. Michael R. Nash and Amanda J. Barnier. *The Oxford Handbook of Hypnosis.* Oxford University Press 2008.

16. Clark L. Hull, *Hypnosis and Suggestibility.An Experimental Approach.* Crown House Publishing Bancyfelin, Wales and Williston 1933.

17. www.whatsonmybrain.com/head-hacking-free-your-mimd-part-1-pc.

18. www.hgi.co.uk. The Human Givens approach is now being used to assist recovery from Post Traumatic Stress Disorder.

19, Robert B. Michael, Maryanne Garry, Irving Kirsch. *Suggestion, Cognition, and Behaviour.* Current Directions in Psychological Science. June 2012.

20. Latin: *deverticulum*, a bypath. In this context, one in which reside a set of emotions and transcendental experiences which can affect physical physiology, and which please the patient.

334

21. Shorter Oxford English Dictionary, 1811. Presumably, 'benefit clinically' – the experience of pleasure is itself a benefit.

22. Anonymous. *Humble Humbug.* The Lancet, Vol 264, 6833, page 321 August 14th 1954.

23. Prof. J. H. Gaddum: *Clinical Pharmacology.* Walter Dennis Dixon Memorial Lecture: Proceedings of the Royal Society of Medicine. 47; 195-204, 1954.

24. Henry K. Beecher. *The Powerful Placebo.* Journal of the American Medical Association.

25. Professor Archie Cochrane. *Effectiveness and Efficiency: Random Reflections on Health Services.* The Nuffield Provincial Hospitals Trust, 1972.

26. Arthur Shapiro, Elaine Shapiro. *The Placebo, Is it Much Ado about Nothing?* In *The Placebo Effect.* Ed. Anne Harrington. Harvard University Press, Cambridge, MA. 1997.

27. Bob Lloyd. *Leaving the Land of Woo.* www.leavingthelandofwoo.com. 2009.

28. Steve Novella. *The Placebo Effect.* www.sciencebasedmedicine.org/index.php /the-placebo-effect. January 16, 2008.

29.www.en.wikipedia.org/wiki/Placebo. 2012.

30. Irving Kirsch in *The Oxford Handbook of Hypnosis.* Oxford University Press. 2008.

31. Andrew Turner. *Evidence Based Medicine, 'Placebos' and the Homeopathy Controversy; Dissertation for Ph.D.*, University of Nottingham, 2012. quoting Beecher 1955. http://etheses.nottingham.ac.uk/2577/1/AT-PhD-Thesis_FINAL-2012.pdf

32. Prof. Jay Katz. *The Silent World of Doctor and Patient.* The Free Press, Macmillan, New York, 1984.

33. Prof. George Lewith, in correspondence with Dr Rob Buckman. *What does homoeopathy do – and how?* BMJ 1994; 309 doi: http://dx.doi.org/10.1136/bmj.309.6947.103.

34. Edzard Ernst, K.L. Resch. *Concept of true and perceived placebo effects.* BMJ, 311,1995

35. Wolff, H.G.; Du Bois, E.F.; and Gold H. *Cornell Conferences on Therapy: Use of Placebos in Therapy.* New York J. Medicine. 46. 1946.

36. Henry K. Beecher. *The Powerful Placebo.* Journal of the American Medical Association. December 24, 1955.

37. Kienle G.S., Kiene H. *The powerful placebo effect: fact or fiction?* Journal of Clinical. Epidemiology. 1997 Dec; 50 (12).

38. Jean Brissonnet. *Placebo, es tu la?* Science et Pseudo sciences, 294,38-48 Jan 2011 and translated,: Harriet Hall, www.sciencebasedmedicine.org. Feb 24, 2015.

39. www.quackometer.net/blog/2012/09/chechov-homeopathy-and-the-placebo-effect.html

40. Ernst E. and Resch K.L. *Concept of True and Perceived Placebo Effects.*BMJ 311: 551-553.

41. Moseley J.B., et al. Personal communication and: *A controlled trial of arthroscopic surgery for osteoarthritis of the knee.* New England Journal of Medicine. 2002. July 11; 347(2):81-8. Also: Linde, K. et al. *Acupuncture for patients with migraine.* JAMA, 2005. 293.

42. *The Oxford Handbook of Hypnosis.*

43. Philip Alper. *Legitimate indications for Intramuscular Injections.* Archives of Internal medicine. 1978; 138(11).

44. Nicholas Humphrey. *Great Expectations: The Evolutionary Psychology of Faith Healing and the Placebo Effect.* In *The Mind Made Flesh*, Oxford University Press, 2002.

45. Arthur and Elaine Shapiro, *The Placebo Effect, is it much ado about nothing?* In Anne Harrington, ed: *The Placebo Effect.* Harvard University Press, Cambridge MA.

46. Pete C. Trimmer et al, *Understanding the placebo effect from an evolutionary perspective.* Evolution and Human Behaviour. On line 30th August 2012: www.ehbonline.org/article/S1090-5138(12)00070-0.

47. McGlashan T.H., Evans F.J. & Orne M.T. *The Nature of Hypnotic Analgesia and Placebo Response to Experimental Pain*, Psychomatic Medicine, Vol31, No 3, 1969.

48. Walter Cannon. *Voodoo Death.* American Anthropologist, 44 (2).

49. Robert Hahn.*The Nocebo Phenomenon.* In The Placebo Effect, Ed. Anne Harrington. Harvard University Press. 1997.

50.www.publications.parliament.uk/pa/ld199900/ldselect/ldsctech/123/12305.

51.http://www.arthritisresearchuk.org/news/press-releases/2013/january/new-report-on-complementary-therapies.

52. R. Barker Bausell. *Snake Oil Science. The Truth About Complementary and Alternative Medicine.* Oxford University Press. Oxford. 2007.

53. Austin Bradford Hill. *Medical ethics and controlled trials.* BMJ, i, 1963

54. Archie Cochrane. *Effectiveness and efficacy: random reflections on health services.* BMJ, 1989.

55. Sullivan M.D. 1993. *Placebo Controls and Epistemic Control in Orthodox Medicine.* Journal of Medicine and Philosophy, 18.

56. Hike Plassmann, Bernd Weber. *Individual Differences in Marketing Placebo Effects: Evidence from Brain Imaging and Behavioral Experiments.* Journal of Marketing Research.

doi: http://dx.doi.org/10.1509/jmr.13.0613, 2015.

57.Luana Colloca and Franklin G. Miller, *Harnessing the placebo effect, the need for translational research.* Philosophical Transactions of the Royal Society. June 2011 vol. 336.

58. Ibid. Note, Bedside Manor is not a residence in Gloucestershire.

59. Kaptchuk T.J., et al. 2010. *Placebos without deception: a randomized controlled trial in irritable bowel syndrome. PLoS ONE* 5, e15591. The Program in Placebo studies and Therapeutic Encounter (PiPS) at Harvard's Beth Israel Deaconess Medical Centre conducts training for researchers who wish to develop careers in placebo studies. See also: www.npr.org/blogs/health/2010/12/23/132281484/fake-pills-can-work-even-if-patients-know-it.

60. Prof. Edzard Ernst. Personal communication, speaking to the Secular Medical Forum, Edinburgh, June 3013.

61.http://edzardernst.com/2013/01/prince-charles-vision-of-a-post-modern-medicine. January 24 2013 at 09:23.

62. Janet D. Stemwedel. http://scienceblogs.com/ethicsandscience/2008/10/24/conditions-for-ethical-therapy/

63. Irving Kirsch and Howard Spiro: *Placebo: Conversations at the Disciplinary Borders* in *The Placebo Effect.* Edited by Anne Harrington. Harvard University Press. Massachusetts and London. 1997.

64. Dylan Evans. *Placebo: Mind over Matter in Modern Medicine.* Harper Collins London 2004.

65. Richard Moskowitz commenting on Kevin Smith: *Against Homeopathy – a Utilitarian Perspective.* Bioethics 26, 398-409,2012. http://onlinelibrary.wiley.com/doi/10.1111/j.1467-8519.2012.01949.x/abstract.

66. Sarah Hull et al, *Patients'attitudes about the use of placebo treatments: telephone survey.* BMJ 2013; 346:f3757 doi: 10.1136/bmj.f3757.

67. Vernon M.S. Oh. *The placebo effect: can we use it better?* Editorial, BMJ 1994; 309 doi: http://dx.doi.org/10.1136/bmj.309.6947.69

68. Richard Rawlins. *On the Ethical Use of Placebos.* Focus on Alternative and Complementary Therapies: An Evidenced-Based Approach. F.C.T. Wiley, London. February 2015.

69. Ibid.

Chapter 19

Quacks and Quackery

Creton secretly suborns this trick devising quack, this wily beggar who has only eyes for his own gains.
Oedipus Rex

There are no greater liars in the world than quacks – except for their patients.
Benjamin Franklin

A quack is a turdy-facy, nasty-paty, lousy, fartical rogue.
Ben Jonson, *Volpone,* 1606

A quack is a practitioner who takes no fee in specie, but makes the deluded patient pay very extravagant fees by the intolerable prices he puts on cheap medicines, and by passing upon him very many more doses than the disease requires
Robert Pitt, *The Crafts and Frauds of Physic exposed,* 1703.

Quack: A boastful pretender to an art he does not understand.
Samuel Johnson, *Dictionary,* 1755

Man is a dupable animal; quacks in medicine, quacks in religion, and quacks in politics know this, and act upon that knowledge. There is scarcely anyone who may not, like a trout, be taken by tickling
Robert Southey, *The Doctor,* 1799

If quackery, individual or gregarious, is ever to be eradicated, or even abated, in civilized society, it must be done by enlightening the public mind in regard to the true powers of medicine.
Jacob Bigelow, 1858

The physician is only allowed to think he knows it all, but the quack, ungoverned by conscience, is permitted to know he knows it all; and with a fertile mental field for humbuggery, truth can never successfully compete with untruth.

Albert Abrams. 1922
A quack is as a quack does.
W.F. Bynum. 1987[1]

CAM therapists thrive in a wider British culture that is curiously indifferent to the concept of truth.
Edzard Ernst. 2014

A chiz is a swiz or a swindle, as any fule kno.
Nigel Molesworth. 1953[2]

This book is about intellectual truth, honesty and integrity. People prepared to take advantage of the ignorant, gullible and vulnerable, particularly those suffering from chronic conditions such as cancer, have always challenged convention. Conventions have evolved. Through history, physicians who achieved a measure of learning and had taken the time and trouble to gain a formal education in the healing arts built their practices by reputation – but not all were so professional and many were regarded as 'quacks and wily beggars' as Oedipus had it in the fifth century BC.

Physicians have always competed for patients, but association with colleagues and the eventual establishment of colleges brought some order and regulation amongst those whose practice was conventional, orthodox, and mainstream for its time. The brightest stars pushed the boundaries, but were always expected to report to colleagues in lectures and books, and to give account of their innovations. Even William Harvey was cautious as to how his revolutionary ideas about the circulation might be received.

By the thirteenth century, away from towns the population was served by wise women, bonesetters, teeth pullers, corn cutters, wound chirurgeons, and medicine makers. Some found a living selling their own potions, pills, oils, liniments, drugs, and secret remedies containing 'remarkable spices from the Orient' often promoted and puffed as 'our remedies' or *nostra remedia* – 'nostrums'. Some of these nostrums contained compounds which had purgative or emetic results which certainly and sometimes dramatically proved their 'effectiveness'. Some included mercury and other heavy metals which were toxic. None were quality controlled, no trials had been carried out to determine their value, and the dose was decided upon by trial and error. Error could be fatal.

Fourteenth century itinerant peddlers were referred to as hawkers, and those who hawked medicines as *quacksalvers* (Middle Dutch: *kwacksalver* from *quacken*, to brag, boast; *salve*, Old English, *sealf*, healing ointment, *salbo*, oily substance). Quacks for short. The orthodox medical profession derided these swanking itinerant competitors and *quack* and *quackery* became terms of abuse along with *charlatan* (Italian: *ciarlatano* from *ciarlare*, to prattle, babble) and *mountebank* – mount on a bench in order to be seen. They were not the sort of shyster who was 'here today and gone tomorrow'. They were more risk adverse than that – and were usually here today and gone tonight!

Some regularly trained physicians pushed the envelope of professional propriety and practice and due to their boasting became regarded as quacks. In the sixteenth century Phillipus von Hohenheim, Professor of Medicine at Basel, had the bombast to style himself as 'Paracelcus' and equal to Celsus himself. He claimed to have discovered the vital principle of 'Azoth' – held to be the tincture of life with the power to imbue immortality. Paracelsus sold azoth as a nostrum, but died at forty-eight.

Robert Burton advised 'Empericks, Mountebanks, Quacksalvers, Paracelsians and Charlatans should be distinguished from rational physicians.'[3] Followers of Paracelcus were regarded as quacks because they claimed they could treat the 'soul' and 'vital spirit'. Regular physicians were not entirely adverse to quackery – which was seen in a spectrum and which is still practised by some conventional doctors, nurses and other practitioners today.

Modern medical science has moved on from the days of hide-bound dogmatic authority and simplistic trial and error – today understanding is based on the integration of reasoning and theory with observation based science. The important distinctions between quackery and good practice are the integrity of the practitioner; the honesty about the practice or remedy having any plausible science-based evidence of merit; the extent to which it relies on placebo effects; whether this is explained to patients; and whether patients give fully informed consent.

In the seventeenth century orthodox doctors began setting aside bloodletting, purging, and the use of secret patent medicines. By the eighteenth century alchemists had given way to apothecaries who prepared remedies based on progressive science. The Apothecaries Act of 1815 created a regulated profession. The professions of physician and then surgeon became statutorily regulated – the Medical Act founded the General Medical Council in 1858. The class-ridden intellectual snobbery of the seventeenth and eighteenth centuries when physicians were regarded as professionals, apothecaries as tradesmen and surgeons as mere manual workers, softened. Starting with herbs, the pharmaceutical industry applied ever more refined methods of chemistry to the preparation of potions and pills.

The America of the nineteenth century saw rapid increase in population which outgrew the number of trained doctors. Unqualified itinerant medicine men filled the vacuum – moving their shows from place to place, promoting snake oil derived from the recipes of the wise indigenous Indians. The term *snake oil salesman* is now synonymous with *quack*.

'Quackery' is not defined in black and white terms. Elements of quack practices and remedies may have a genuine plausible rationale. Certainly the 'care' element does, and that should be part of all healthcare practice – producing the type I effects from which patients benefit. But if a practitioner promotes irrational implausible practices and boasts, puffs and quacks about them, then what are we to call that practitioner?

Quack practices are based on meta-physical constructs which may be pseudo and often are anti scientific. 'Health fraud' is sometimes a term used as a synonym for quack, but not all quacks are frauds. Some quacks might be sincere, though how are we to tell? Frauds seek to gain pecuniary advantage from gullible people by deceit and deception. All health fraudsters, using treatments they know to be useless, are quacks. Assessing whether any individual is a fraud or is sincere is a matter for the courts, not a placebist. As George Burns advised: 'If you can fake sincerity, you've got it made.'

US courts have ruled that accusing someone of quackery is not the same as accusing them of medical fraud. Fraud refers to offering unproven treatments for financial advantage, abuse of position, false representation or prejudicing someone's rights for personal gain. Quacks may honestly believe the treatments they are offering are effective. As with the mainstream, their deportment, dress, demeanour, apparent qualifications, claims for the status of 'doctor', cloak of respectability and celebrity endorsements will all induce a sense of awe and wonderment. Their quacking, advertising and boasting of the remarkable effects of their ministrations may appeal to many, particularly if they have not had the benefit of reference to *Real Secrets of Alternative Medicine.* [4]

In seventeenth century Britain, diverse practitioners advertised endorsement of their remedies by declaring *litterae patentes* from royalty and governments. These were 'open letters' declaring the privilege of selling the particular commodity (Latin: *patere,* to lay open). In fact the remedies of *patent medicines* were usually secret and there was no way of telling what toxins they contained. Testimonials abounded, declaring how marvellous the treatments were – but there was no proper scientific analysis. Samuel Johnson's dictionary (1755) defined a quack as being 'a boastful pretender to arts which he does not understand – an artful tricking practitioner in Physic.'

Orthodox physicians had their recipes made up by apothecaries but patent remedies were sold directly to the public by hawkers, quacks and regulars alike. Patients could purchase Richard Stoughton's Elixir (the second medical compound to receive a royal patent, in 1712); Epsom Salts (magnesium sulphate, for which Dr Grew took out a patent); Morison's Vegetable Pills and even *eau de Cologne* as a 'panacea for all ills'. Daffy's True Elixir (rhubarb, aniseed, liquorice, fennel, senna, and brandy) was one of the first products to be widely recognised and promoted as a 'brand' – originally advertised in 1690 by Rev. Thomas Daffy as being 'Miraculous and found by the Providence of the Almighty'. By 1748 *The Gentleman's Magazine* listed 202 nostrums of various sorts.

In America, the first newspaper advertisement for a patent medicine was published in the *Boston News-Letter* of 1708 – for Daffy's. Advertisements were initially infrequent but as the eighteenth century wore on more were seen and criticism became levelled at the hyperbole of 'London Quack Bills'. The British government had originally imposed a tax on all importations into the colonies but by 1776 all these had been abolished – except for the one on tea...

The Philadelphia College of Pharmacy was established in 1821 and became concerned manufacturers were providing misleading information. It 'set forth boldly to strip these English nostrums of their extravagant pretensions.' Nevertheless, it was 1906 before Congress passed the first Pure Food and Drug Act.

Infamous quacks

Johann Dippel (1673-1734). Born in Castle Frankenstein near Darmstadt, Germany, Dippel distilled animal parts and declared he had an *elixir vitae* which could cure all ills. He experimented on transferring souls from corpse to corpse with a funnel and used his oil to exorcise demons. He may have been a template for Mary Shelly's *Frankenstein*.

Joanna Stephens swindled Parliament of 1739 into granting her £5000 to disclose her secret remedy for dissolving stones in the urinary tract. Stevens' remedy consisted of nothing more than powdered snails and egg shells, earwigs and soap. Parliamentarians are easily duped. Even in modern times Margaret Thatcher was the only member of her cabinet with a degree in science. Politicians' insight and integrity in dealing with quacks remains a contemporary concern.

Dr James Graham (1745-1794) became a prominent practitioner whose ingenuity in assisting those suffering from unmentionable diseases by his prescription of Imperial Electric Pills was matched only by his Grand State Celestial Bed to encourage the relevant activities. The apogee of his fame came in 1779 when he opened his Temple of Health where he sold his patent medicines.[5] Graham's arrogant self-promotion placed him in the camp of quacks, though some now regard Graham not so much as a quack but as the world's first sex therapist and fertility guru.

Gustavus Katterfelto (1743-1799) spent decades as an itinerant conjurer on the continent but on coming to England in 1781, devised an entertainment of magic combined with scientific lecturing. By his own admission he was 'The greatest philosopher since Sir Isaac Newton.' In 1782 London was ravaged by an influenza epidemic and Katterfelto promoted 'Dr Bato's medicines' which he claimed 'cured many thousands of persons.' James Graham became a great rival, calling Katterfelto 'a German Maggot Killer'. A satirical cartoon showed them both enjoined in a battle of quackery – Katterfelto holding a large magnetised column and Graham astride a vast priapic conductor rod – 'the largest in the world'.

James Morison (1770-1840), born in Scotland, declared he was a 'Hygeist, not a doctor.' He founded the British College of Health in London to promote his No.1 and No.2 pills – 'The more you take, the better you'll get. The old medical science is completely wrong, every one may now be his own doctor and surgeon with my pills at a cheap rate and enjoy a sound mind in a sound body.' Morison was of course correct that doctors who used bleeding and toxic drugs did no good – but there was no evidence his 'natural' pills were more effective.

The *Lancet* suggested many deaths had occurred due to excessive purging caused by Morison's pills and an editorial accused Morison of 'fraud and extortion.' An article of 1835 called him the 'King of Quacks' and suggested the formation of an Anti-Quackery Society. Morison was in court many times as the regular profession attempted to outlaw quackery. On one occasion the *Lancet* commented: 'What a spectacle has this trial exhibited in a civilised country! What a reflection it is upon the discernment of the public! What a stigma on the state of medicine! What a disgrace does it reflect upon the government!' A comment which would be apposite today.

The new headquarters of the Royal College of General Practitioners is not far from the site of the former College of Health, its rear being opposite the Centre for the Magic Arts, and headquarters of The Magic Circle.[6]

Blurred Boundaries

Roy Porter suggested that quacks were 'Less cheats than zealots. More fanatics than frauds.'[7] But how could anyone be sure to what extent any practitioner might be a quack and also intend fraud? This remains a contemporary problem. Ben Jonson had no difficulty – a quack was a 'Turdy-facy, nasty-paty, lousy, fartical rogue.'[8]

A number of ostensibly conventional doctors were accused of quackery. Regular practitioners also relied heavily on placebo responses, their recipes were often toxic and their methods did not stand scrutiny. Swathed in the fine robes of their colleges, orthodox practitioners clambered on their high horses to sling barbs at the competitors deemed beneath them – but sound rationale for such antipathy was sadly lacking.

Amongst the most eminent doctors charged as quacks were Dr Thomas Beddoes, who set up his Bristol Pneumatic Institution to treat patients with gases; Professor Louis Pasteur who proved the germ theory of disease; and Ignaz Semmelweis who worked on puerperal fever. Dr Thomas Allison was so strongly opposed to vaccination, advocating Hygienic Medicine and Naturopathy, that he was struck off by the GMC in 1892. His wholemeal bread is still available. Dr John Harvey Kellogg's enthusiastic promotion of cereals led to charges of quackery. Even today, Kellogg's Cocoa Krispies are promoted as 'helping to support your child's immunity.' You must judge if this is quackery.

Regular practitioners and quacks alike described their pills and practices in flowery language referencing connections with royalty, the Orient and mysterious secrets. The regulars were cloaked in the respectable garb of their royal colleges and societies – quacks employed more imaginative marketing techniques. And thereby hangs the tale – regulars objected to quacks because their puffery was effective in attracting custom. Even today some universities offer degrees, including doctorates in 'science' for studies of medical systems which are antithetical to science. The title 'doctor' should not be taken at face value and the claims of quackademia need critical examination.

Some patent medicine manufacturers and companies moved away from un-scientific quackery and embraced the science of chemistry. Chemistry applied to the manufacturing of medicines and drugs from herbs, plants or other natural substances is termed 'pharmacy'. Historically, pharmacy started with natural compounds and then removed molecules which had harmful side effects, adding other which enhanced efficacy. Today, drugs can be built up synthetically but all are likely to have some unwanted effects. The trick is to minimise these. All companies want to maximise their investments and drug research is expensive. There are now regulations and blatant fraud is generally prevented by rules on advertising, promotion and labelling – all of which must be lawful, honest, decent and truthful. Critical examination of claims continues, but the tendency for publication bias (the avoidance of reporting of unhelpful results) remains a problem. This issue is now under review by doctors, regulators, politicians, and journalists. The latter are likely to be the most effective in keeping practitioners honest.

Some chemists and entrepreneurs moved from the quackery of secret remedies to the pharmacy of legitimate businesses.

Peter Squire (1798-1884)
Born in Bedfordshire Squire came under the mentorship of the Warden of the Worshipful Society of Apothecaries and went on to study in London and Paris. He then set up in business as a druggist and was appointed Chemist in Ordinary to Queen Victoria's family. Squire was in charge of the committee which published the first standardised pharmacopoeia in Britain. Squire's formula was used for the anointing oil for Victoria's coronation and for those of subsequent monarchs. The recipe is secret, but may include hemp.

Squire's Extract relieved twitching, coughing and offered a degree of pain relief. It included *Cannabis indica* and Squire's company became 'the most renowned supplier of cannabis medicine in Europe and abroad.' Squire's son, Peter Wyatt Squire, continued with the business and was knighted for his role in the development of pharmacy as a modern profession.[9]

Thomas Holloway (1800-1883)
Holloway began making ointment in his mother's kitchen. At an early stage he recognised the value of advertising and by this means he rapidly built a substantial business selling patent medicines. None of which had any real medical value but which eventually provided the funds for an asylum in Epsom and the Royal Holloway College of the University of London. His advertisements consisted largely of testimonials from satisfied celebrities and persons of eminence, some of which may have been genuine. He remained prejudiced against doctors who were generally scathing of *Holloway's Pills and Ointment*. They knew the contents of aloe, myrrh, and saffron provided minimal clinical benefit, notwithstanding claims they were the 'best in the world' for virtually every disease.

Thomas Beecham (1820-1907)
Beecham started selling herbal remedies whilst working as a shepherd but then became a chemist. He developed his pills (aloes, ginger and soap) as laxatives and his *Powders* (aspirin and caffeine) are still available as a cold and flu remedy.

Beecham's company has become a major pharmaceutical enterprise, merging with others including Glaxo Wellcome to become GlaxoSmithKline (GSK). His grandson Thomas became a noted and knighted orchestral conductor.

Sir Henry Wellcome FRS (1853-1936)

Wellcome first marketed lemon juice as invisible ink when a boy in Wisconsin. He then studied pharmacy, worked as a salesman and founded Burroughs Wellcome & Company in 1880. Pills were generally prepared with pestle and mortar and doses were hard to standardise but the company developed the tablet form of medicines, trade marking 'Tabloid' in 1884. His initiative in giving free samples to doctors was regarded at the time as a brilliant marketing strategy but because of the potential for conflict of interest, that practice is now banned. Wellcome became a British subject in 1910 and was knighted in 1932. The Wellcome Trust was established on his death in 1936 and is now the U.K.'s largest funder of scientific research.

Freiedrich Bayer

Bayer AG was founded in Germany in 1863, initially as industrial chemists and dyestuff manufacturers. Inorganic chemistry enabled the synthetic manufacture of dyes superior to those obtained by natural extraction. For centuries wise folk had known that the bark of the willow tree could be used for pain relief. Bayer developed a synthetic form of the active principle, acetylsalicylic acid. Marketed as *aspirin,* this established Bayer as an international company. An opioid analgesic, diamorphine hydrochloride followed. Recognising it evoked 'heroic' qualities in those who indulged, it was marketed as *Heroin* and was initially available over-the-counter.

Quackery exposed

1858 saw the publication in Boston, MA, of *Quackery Unmasked* by Dr Dan King and the tide turned against medical dishonesty. The Dutch Society against Quackery was founded in 1880. The British Medical Association, concerned about the chloroform, morphia, tincture of hemp and prussic acid (cyanide) in *Dr Collis Browne's Chlorodyne,* soon followed with a campaign against secret remedies. In the US, disquiet about false claims, quack remedies and dangerous ingredients led to eleven articles about *The Great American Fraud* in Collier's Weekly during 1905. Written by investigative journalist and one of the first 'muckrakers', Samuel Hopkins Adams, these were a significant stimulus to better regulations. Following the American Medical Association's criticisms of patent medicines, the US Pure Food and Drugs Act was introduced in 1906.

In the UK, patent medicines continued to keep their recipes secret, in spite of a number containing opium. The BMA eventually exposed many formulae in *Secret Remedies* (1909) and *More Secret Remedies* (1912). The preface declared 'The quack takes advantage of the common foible of human nature to impress his customers. But secrecy has other uses; it enables him to make use of cheap drugs and to proclaim his product possesses virtues beyond the ken of the mere doctor.'

The AMA published *Nostrums and Quackery: Articles on the Nostrum Evil, Quackery and Allied Matters Affecting the Public Health* in 1912. Evan Yellon advised: 'There is not a Quack trading on the credulity of the public who has not at some period or other received testimonials – perfectly genuine documents and truthful in so far as the untrained mind is able to record facts without embroidering them. This is because even the most flagrant quacks have their happy flukes.' Many thousands of quack remedies were reviewed, and exposed, by the BMA and AMA.

Established in 1930, today the US Food and drug Administration protects consumers and promotes public health by preventing food adulteration and regulating food safety, dietary supplements and prescription pharmaceuticals. Approved drugs have to reach high standards of efficacy. As in the UK, a company may advertise a drug for specific medical use only if approved, and risks as well as benefits have to be explained.

White Coat Underground has noted 'quack Miranda warnings' put on many health and wellbeing websites and product labels such as: 'These statements/products have not been evaluated by the Food and drug Administration. This product is not intended to diagnose, treat, cure or prevent any disease.' Given the products have no evidence of any benefit beyond the placebo, such warnings are quack designed simply to deflect criticism that claims about the products are false. These glib warnings should serve as red flags to any who read them.[10]

A valuable review of concerns about the globalised pharmaceutical industry is offered by Professor David Colquhoun's *Improbable Science*[11] and in Ben Goldacre's *Bad Pharma.*[12] Be prepared to be amazed. Many companies fail to publish data which does not suit their purposes. The smoke and mirrors of the magician are enlisted and the charge of quackery might very well be applied, but at least Goldacre and other commentators are able to expose wrongdoings and regulators can be invoked.

A principle concern about CAM is that the research is either not done, or simply is not scientifically robust enough for meaningful critical analysis. The evidence provided is usually implausible and based on anecdotes – 'it worked for me'. The products and practices are therefore 'alternative'. Of great concern is that conventional research may be carried out but all outcomes are not reported because some are inconvenient, embarrassing, or commercially unhelpful to the sponsoring company.

Goldacre wisely said 'selectively withholding unflattering trial data is research misconduct, and the ultimate end product is a biased picture of the effectiveness of your intervention…that's why I think it's really disappointing that nobody has stood up and said: "selective non-publication of unflattering trial data is research misconduct, and if you do it you will be booted out."' Stimulated by Ben's challenge, in June 2013 the BMA's Representative Body established BMA policy about this misconduct and called for miscreants to have their fitness to practice considered by the GMC.[13] Press on.

There have been international calls for a boycott of products from drug firms which do not release all their research data and suggestions that governments should sue those companies. Fiona Godlee, editor of the BMJ has written an open letter in similar vein and she and others, including former GP Dr Sarah Wollaston, now an MP, have discussed with ministers the role of regulators in ensuring that all trial data is registered and published.[14]

Confirmation bias is seen in many areas of conventional medicine – people simply do not want to talk about results which do not confirm their pet theories or hypotheses. Such unethical behaviour moves up a few notches when unwanted results are ignored and even hidden – adding publication bias to the underlying confirmation bias. A notch further up when doctors or scientists who discover and expose this behaviour are threatened with libel or loss of their careers in order to silence them – fear bias. This is why caution is necessary when commenting on modern research claims. Quackery is alive and well, and evident in products near you.

Professor Lawrence Krauss of Arizona State University, has warned that health-related claims which invoke quantum mechanics should be regarded as pseudoscientific:

> Many things in quantum mechanics sound like magic but sounding like magic and being magical are two different things. When you hear about quantum mechanics and devices, you can say, "OK, that sounds reasonable." But when you hear about quantum mechanics and consciousness, you should assume the author is a crackpot unless proven otherwise. Moreover, assume that they want your money.[15]

We now have formal codes of practice for marketing, and Advertising Standards require honesty and plausible evidence that the practice or product is effective and does what is claimed. Meanwhile those who practice outside the mainstream have become ever more sophisticated at inventing products and procedures which not only avoid the stringencies of scientific evidence-based medicine but which take advantage of opportunities for misleading marketing. Quacks are continually reinventing themselves and finding new ways of creating illusions. Just like magicians. As to whether any particular present day camist should be regarded as a quack – that is for you to judge.

The Royal Touch

Quacks have come in all shapes and sizes and from all strata of society. In ancient Rome, emperors helped their subjects by the ceremonial donation of coins which were credited with alleviating a range of diseases. In the Middle Ages tuberculosis caused lymph nodes in the neck to discharge. Many believed that receiving a touch from the King would cure the scrofula. Edward the Confessor in England and Philip I of France seem to have started the practice in the eleventh century. Both proclaimed their success as healers confirmed that their regal rights and authority were divinely bestowed.

James I of England declared he would no longer touch for scrofula 'as the age of miracles is passed and God alone can work them.'[16] Nevertheless the practice continued and by the seventeenth century Henry IV of France was touching up to two thousand sufferers at a time. In the United Kingdom, Charles I was credited with touching ten thousand subjects during his reign. The practice ceased with George I in 1727 as being 'too Catholic.' In France, Charles X only desisted in 1825.

'Touch therapy' does not have to be 'Royal' – numerous healers, quacks and charlatans have claimed to be able to heal by touch down the centuries. *Reiki* and other systems of 'body work' are modern versions. In 1666, Sir Robert Boyle, President of the Royal Society, examined the practice of 'The Stroker' Valentine Greatrickes, who developed a lucrative practice by the method. Boyle interviewed a lame tinker who forswore he had been cured of sciatica by being stroked. Boyle found he could achieve the same results merely by stroking the afflicted part with one of Greatrickes' gloves. After failing to impress a sceptical Charles II, Greatrickes returned to Ireland, and obscurity.[17]

Why do conventional health professionals become involved in quackery?

Because they care. Although doctors are trained in the ways of science and are expected to base their practice on scientifically acquired evidence, clinicians who treat patients are not employed as scientists. Doctors recognise patients do not always have evidence based symptoms and may have irrational desires, whims and fancies – but if satisfying them with a CAM improves an individual patient's sense of wellbeing, some doctors argue: 'how can such patients be denied?' However modern doctors are not just responsible for the patient in front of them but also a population of patients – for commissioning care and using scarce financial resources responsibly. If quackery is funded – what will not be?

Science is undoubtedly exciting – the world of camistry can be more so. Some doctors 'are often taken by the novelty of quack systems and the feeling of insight and grandeur they provide.'[18] Some practitioners find themselves attracted to metaphysical constructs and practices. The danger is that such practices can distort regular scientific medicine, patients understanding and are patronising. The days of medical paternalism should have passed.

Magicians constantly discuss how to be intentionally deceptive. Quack doctors will usually be in denial as to the true nature of their practice. So often their own colleagues are too inhibited to challenge them. They envelop themselves in the cloak of respectability, playing up to *wudoka* who follow the path of *wu*, nothingness – all the time emphasising how patients will benefit not only from regular medicine but by having access to 'the best of both worlds' and the salving of their souls.

The doctrine that the functions of a living organism are due to a 'life force' or 'vital principle' is not simply unscientific but anti-scientific. Such philosophy ignores the processes of scientific analysis. Intuition is held in higher regard than reason and logic. Vitalism links to concepts of an immortal soul and religious ideology. This is seen especially as advancing age and the approach of life's final *dénouement* impinges on the consciousness and emotions. Feelings such as these are best assuaged by religion, not medicine. A study of why doctors had taken up 'holistic' practices showed that most were on account of 'spiritual or religious experiences.'[19]

Peter Canter has advised: 'Vitalistic rationales for unproven therapies are attractive to sufferers because they offer hope despite the lack of any feasible scientific mechanism and are attractive to practitioners because they provide the gobbledegook for a sales pitch. Although science doesn't support the existence of meridians, qi, or any other type of vital force, the more mysterious ancient, traditional, spiritual and holistic an explanation is, the more powerful and attractive it seems to be. The fact that vitalism is unscientific and posits the existence of an ethereal force beyond the powers of science to detect, may in itself, be attractive to those who can't live with the realities of the material world, are unable to deal with negative or uncertain diagnosis or prognosis, those who fear science and those who are unable to understand it.'[20]

Doctors are severely constrained in discussing issues of camistry and quackery with individual patients for whom they are responsible. Creating cognitive dissonance by challenging beliefs is stressful to the patient. Doctors must be 'neutral' and not upset a patient by suggesting their beliefs are bizarre or irrational. The GMC has set out its requirements for ethical practice in *Personal Beliefs and Medical Practice:* paragraph 19: You should not normally discuss your personal beliefs with patients unless those beliefs are directly relevant to the patient's care. Paragraph 20: Patients have a right to information about their condition and the options available to them. You must not withhold information about the existence of a procedure or treatment because carrying it out or giving advice about it conflicts with your religious or moral beliefs.'[21]

Given these requirements, it is hard for a doctor to discuss the implausibility of beliefs in CAM systems. We must not robustly challenge an individual patient's belief in a soul, a 'vital force', subluxations, innate intelligence, *chakras, yin, yang,* mystic energies, water with memory, novel occult forces and the like. It is difficult to counter any enthusiasm a patient may have for camistry. Even if a doctor believes it is unethical to invoke supernatural spirits or quackery to facilitate health and wellbeing, paragraph 20 implies doctors must give patients information about camistry. If a doctor has a conscientious objection to spending healthcare resources on referring patients for camistry, they must tell the patient of their right to see a doctor who does not!

Conversely, doctors must provide patients with all the information they need to make wise choices. That must include the information that CAMs are 'alternative', for the very good reason that they are pseudo, non and even anti-scientific. Information means not just bare facts, but facts presented in a manner that is comprehensible – and acceptable to patients who may not be pleased about having their beliefs challenged.

However, it is recognised that doctors have a living to earn, and quackery can be lucrative. William T. Jarvis comments on not only the profit motive, but also the prophet motive: 'Many quacks simply revel in the adulation and discipleship their pretence of superiority evokes.'[22] Patients must judge the motivation of their practitioner.

Egos need massaging and nice trips are arranged to conferences and meetings. If Big Charma (Complementary health and alternative remedy manufacturers) covers the expenses, so much the better.[23] Psychologist Robert Hare investigated health professionals and identified the traits of quacks: 'glibness, charm, manipulative behaviour, a lack of guilt, proneness to boredom and lack of empathy. Many seem to suffer from cognitive defects which prevent them from experiencing genuine sympathy or remorse.'[24] Stephen Barrett has suggested that 'the promotion of quackery involves deliberate deception, but many promoters sincerely believe in what they are doing.'[25] Rose Shapiro's standard of probity should be noted: 'Quackery is quackery regardless of the merits or otherwise of the practitioner's character.'[26] Andy Lewis has suggested that quackery can be measured in canard units and he provides the means at www.quackometer.net.

This leads us back to current trends for 'integrated medicine' – meaning integration of the standards, ethics, and practices of CAM into conventional medicine.[27] In 2003 Prince Charles called for 'NHS trusts to be given guidance on how to provide complementary healthcare, community schemes to be developed to provide therapies, funding integrated healthcare and encouraging medical schools to teach complementary medicine.' Dame Lesley Rees, then chairman of trustee's at his Foundation for Integrated Health, and a number of other eminent conventional doctors clearly felt such an insurgency was beneficial and supported the Prince. Quite why, they have never adequately explained. *Anintegrity medicine* might be a more apposite appellation (*an*, for 'without' – *integrity*).

There simply is no need for integration of any CAM with convention except for one thing – it pays. Many patients want to feel their chosen path of *wu* does have the approbation of conventional medicine – and that they are not naïve *wudoka* but have chosen wisely. Many patients want to patronise institutions where *wudo* is accorded the same status as evidence-based medicine and where 'tradition' authenticates *wu*. So, they pays their money and the medical profession respects their right to choose, if not their actual choice. Doctors seek to satisfy patients, not the demands of scientific truth. That is for others. Whether conventional doctors who endorse such an insurgency of camistry are really doing their best for patients has to be judged by camees, camists, health care professions, the public and politicians. But honesty and intellectual integrity should prevail and practitioners who associate with quacks must look to their own consciences.

Why do patients persist with quack products, practices and practitioners?

Because it pleases them. – against a background of disenchantment and disappointment with traditional consultations; distrust of science-based medicine; ignorance of the science and evidence; wishful thinking about nature; a sense it is important to work with 'nature'; a wish to engage with 'magic'; the lure of *wu*; lack of understanding of placebo effects; a hope that gentle natural panaceas can cure all; lack of trust in regulatory authorities; influence of celebrities; distorted journalism; duping by unscrupulous advertising; thinking 'gone awry'; the challenge of cognitive dissonance and failure to critically evaluate the evidence.

Investigating quackery in 1853 Dr Grafton Page counselled: 'The instant the idea of the superhuman gets possession of the mind, all fitness for investigation and power of analysis begins to vanish, and credulity swells to its utmost capacity. The most glaring inconsistencies and absurdities are not discerned and are swallowed whole.'[28]

Unless there really are proven worthwhile effects on disease, quackery is best avoided. It has to be recognised some patients are gullible and favour camistry even to the dangerous extent of foregoing or delaying conventional treatments which might help them. Please do not be one of them.

Endnotes to Chapter 19

1. W. F. Bynum. Author, with Roy Porter of *Medical Fringe and Medical Orthodoxy.* Croom Helm, London, 1987. Quoted by Roy Porter. *Quacks.* Tempus Publishing, Stroud. 2000.

2. Geoffrey Willans. *Down with Skool!* Max Parrish. London. 1953.

3. Robert Burton. *The Anatomy of Melancholy*, 1621. Edited by Thomas Faulkener *et al*, Clarendon Press/Oxford University Press. 1989 -1994

4. That boast is itself a quack!

5. Katie Carr, *Saints and Sinners*, Bulletin of the Royal College of Surgeons of England. No.1 Vol. 95, January 2013. Graham was assisted in his Temples of Health and Hymen by 'Goddesses' such as Amy Lyon, who displayed their physical perfection for the edification of patrons. When twenty six, she married sixty year old Sir William Hamilton. As Lady Emma Hamilton she became mistress of Admiral Lord Nelson.

6. The rear of the Royal College of General Practitioners in London faces the Centre for the Magic Arts and headquarters of The Magic Circle.

7. Roy Porter. *Quacks: Fakers and Charlatans in Medicine.* Tempus Publishing. Stroud Publishing, Gloucestershire. 2003.

8. Ben Jonson, *Volpone* (Sly Fox), 1606.

9. Diana Douglas, great-grand daughter of Sir Peter Wyatt Squire. Personal communication.

10. www.scienceblogs.com/denialism/2008/03/24/quack-miranda-warning.

11. David Colquhoun. www.dcscience.net/?p=5538.

12. Ben Goldacre. *Bad Pharma: How Drug Companies Mislead Doctors and Harm Patients.* Fourth Estate. London 2012.

13. BMA policy established by Annual Representative Meeting, Edinburgh, June 2013. Proposed by R.D. Rawlins, representative, South Devon Division.

14. Dr Sarah Wollaston MP for Totnes – a town twinned with Narnia and Area 51, Nevada.

15. Lawrence Krauss. http://cosmiclog.nbcnews.com/_news/2010/09/20/5144889-how-to-spot-quantum-quackery?lite

16. www.historytoday.com/Stephen-brogan/james-i-royal-touch

17. www.bbk.ac.uk/boyle/workdiadies/WD2Clean.html

18. Carl Sagan in W.H. Reid *et al*, *Unmasking the Psychopath.* New York: Norton & Co. 1986.

19. MS Goldstein, D.T. Jaffe, C. Sunderland. *Physicians at a holistic medical conference: Who and Why?* Health Values, 10:3-13, September/October 1986.

20. Peter H. Canter. *Vitalism and other Pseudoscience in Alternative Medicine* in *Healing, Hype, or Harm.* Ed. Edzard Ernst. Imprint Academic, Exeter. 2008.

21. http://www.gmc-uk.org/guidance/ethical_guidance/personal_beliefs.asp

22. William. T. Jarvis, *Why Health Professionals Become Quacks.* www.quackwatch. com/01QuackeryRelated Topics/quackpro.html. December 11,1998.

23. Example: Dr Michael Dixon of the College of Medicine had business class flights to Japan for himself, wife and three children paid for by the sponsors of research on Johrei healing. http://edzardernst.com/2015/05/johrei-healing-and-the-amazing-dr-dixon-presidential-candidate-for-the-rcgp/. (He was not elected to the RCGP presidency).

24. D. Goleman. *Brain defect tied to utter amorality of the psychopath.* New York Times, July 7, 1987.

25. Stephen Barrett. *Quackery: how should it be defined?* Quackwatch.com, 2001.

353

26. Rose Shapiro. Suckers: *How Alternative Medicine Makes Fools of Us All*. Vintage Books London. 2009.

27. Arabic for 'a student' is *tālib,* pleural *tullāb*. In Pashto, the pleural is *tālibān*. In Afghanistan/Pakistan the term is applied to insurgents of a notably fundamentalist ideology, which they seek to infiltrate and integrate into other cultures...

28. Charles Grafton Page: *Psychomancy: spirit-rappings and table-tippings exposed*: D. Appleton & Co. New York 1853.

Chapter 20

Rational responses to Complementary and Alternative Medicine

Details that could throw doubt on your interpretation must be given, if you know them. You must do the best you can – if you know anything at all wrong – to explain it. If you make a theory and advertise it, then you must also put down all the facts that disagree with it, as well as those that agree with it…The idea is to try to give all the information to help others to judge the value of your contribution; not just the information that leads to judgment in one particular direction or another…It's a kind of scientific integrity, a principle of scientific thought that corresponds to a kind of utter honesty – a kind of leaning over backwards.
Richard Feynman

That which can be asserted without evidence can be dismissed without evidence. Once the hard won principles of reason and science have been discredited, the world will not pass into the hands of credulous herbivores who keep crystals by their sides and swoon over the poems of Khalil Gilbran. The 'vacuum' will be invaded instead by determined fundamentalists of every stripe who already know the truth by means of revelation and who actually seek real and serious power in the here and now. One thinks of the painstaking, cloud-dispelling labour of British scientists from Isaac Newton to Joseph Priestley to Charles Darwin to Ernest Rutherford to Alan Turing and Francis Crick, much of it built on the shoulders of Galileo and Copernicus, only to see it casually slandered by a moral and intellectual weakling from the usurping House of Hanover.
Christopher Hitchens

I could never manage to understand how 'integrating' quackery with science-based medicine would do anything but weaken the scientific foundation of medicine.
David Gorski

Real Secrets of Alternative Medicine is intended to stimulate further enquiry into placebo effects and their value in improving a sense of wellbeing in those experiencing disease or illness. A more general sense of wellness, happiness, contentment, and a stress free existence is much to be desired, but is part of normal life and is not considered here under the rubric of 'medicine'. Four principal groups of readers have been identified and are invited to consider whether to offer unwavering support for the precepts set out herein, or to reject these foolish notions out of hand.

1. The camee, family and friends

You are my principle readership because the aim is to help you make wise choices and avoid being quacked and defrauded. CAMs do work – but not in the way their practitioners and proponents might wish you to think. If camistry seems to give you benefit, I am pleased for you. But why not consider whether a more empathic conventional practitioner might not do as well. Consider whether a placebist might not give you the same benefits without the false claims, and save you spending time and funds on implausible treatments and remedies.

You must be confident that you are not being groomed as vulnerable with a tendency to accept irrational ideologies by those who wish to take advantage of you. Be sure the cloak of confusion has not been thrown over you and the care and attention you need has not been conflated with therapeutic techniques or remedies which have no plausible effects on any specific condition. Ensure the practitioner is distinguished from the practice.

2. The doctor, nurse and other health professional

You are between a rock and a hard place: You will want to please individual patients, many of whom have irrational beliefs which have to go un-challenged. You will want to apply good scientific critical thinking and ensure alternative systems of healthcare are clearly identified as such.

If you are going to maximise the utility of placebo interventions and harness their effects overtly, you must acknowledge that the science behind such intervention is presently of poor quality, and obtain informed consent on that basis. Not to do so would be deceptive and risk damaging the trust between patient and healthcare professional. If patients know a placebo intervention is being used, any beneficial effect is probably weakened, but not entirely – and honesty demands candidness. That is one difference between an ethical practitioner and a quack.

Physician and lawyer Jay Katz explored these issues in *The Silent World of Doctor and Patient*. Even in the 1980s he found doctors too wedded to the maxim that 'doctors know best' – remaining silent about matters patients should have considered:

> For conversation to be meaningful, both parties must be entitled to make decisions and to have their choices treated with respect. Trust, based on blind faith must be distinguished from trust that is earned after having first acknowledged to oneself and then shared with the other what one knows and does not know about the decision

to be made. Although such mutual trust is difficult to embrace and to sustain, it is important to strive for it. The proponents of informed consent and patient self-determination have insufficiently appreciated that trusting oneself and others to become aware of the certainties and uncertainties that surround the practice of medicine and integrate them with one's hopes, fears and realistic expectations, are inordinately difficult tasks. They are among the tasks, however, that fidelity to disclosure and consent requires physicians and patients to undertake. The opponents of informed consent, on the other hand, have insufficiently appreciated that disclosure and consent do not abolish trust. Disclosure and consent only banish unilateral blind trust; they make mutual trust possible for the first time.

For millennia, patients were expected to do as their magi, priests and physicians told them – now the days of medical paternalism have passed. Today patients expect to understand what is proposed for them and to be involved in decision making. 'The doctrine of informed consent' was first formalised by Justice Bray in the California Court of Appeals in 1957. Taking the term from a brief submitted by the American College of Surgeons, he opined: 'A physician violates his duty to his patient and subjects himself to liability if he withholds any facts which are necessary to form the basis of an intelligent consent by the patient to the proposed treatment....In discussing the elements of risk a certain amount of discretion must be employed consistent with the full disclosure of facts necessary to an informed consent.'

Some registered medical practitioners actually endorse camistry, often disguised as part of 'integrated' care. The previous chapter on *Quacks* will point to their responsibilities and may prick their consciences. They will need to be able to answer patients, with a clear conscience and due professional integrity: 'What is the added value of the intervention you propose, above the care I should expect anyway? What is the evidence that the treatment you propose results in outcomes better than that achieved by use of placebos? What evidence do you have for the existence in reality of *chakras, quantum entanglements, pathways of 'vital energy', zones,* or other esoteric elements you propound? What evidence do you have that the treatment or remedy you propose has any effect on a specific disease or illness? Are you sure you are not just offloading awkward patients, seeking to appease them, to ease your conscience and make your life easier? Can you be trusted to explain the alternative nature and implications of any proposed CAM? With health commissioners now all too keen to obtain services from commercial providers based on 'patient choice', what reassurances can you give you are not conspiring in a racket?'

The GMC requires that doctors must respect patients' beliefs and avoid confrontation. This may present difficulties in dealing with individual patients but should not preclude patients being fully informed nor doctors' engagement in the political process, healthcare commissioning – and the writing of books! Other conventional healthcare professions should exhibit comparable ethical considerations.

Even today, GPs offer placebos – a recent web-based survey showed that 97% have prescribed a placebo at some time in their careers. Examples include: nutritional

357

supplements for conditions unlikely to benefit from them, such as glucosamine (which is not necessary to 'support healthy joints'); antibiotics (for suspected viral infections) and peppermint pills (for pharyngitis). 'Pure' placebos comprising sugar pills that have no active ingredient were prescribed regularly by 1% of GPs.[1]

3. Non-medical camists

You have to consider whether you are in the right profession and whether you should undertake further training to qualify in one of the conventional professions and avoid the irrationality of quackery. Above all please ensure you do not take pecuniary advantage of the gullible and ill-informed. That would be fraud. You will have to consider how patients are to distinguish between a sincere and ethical camist and a quack. And consider how you are to ensure your patients give consent to treatment with full information as to the true nature of the CAM you propose – including placebo effects. And look to your conscience closely to identify why you wanted to be a camist. For example, why a chiropractor and not an osteopath, physiotherapist or a manipulator of un-identified flying energies? Are you sure you are not a quack?

Do you seriously suggest that if the pseudo-science of camistry is not 'integrated' with scientific medicine, patients will suffer? Do you think it reasonable and acceptable that public funds should be provided so you can hallucinate and satisfy your whims?

4. Politicians, healthcare managers and those who support camistry

You have to ensure you can distinguish between the mess of science with its organised scepticism, and ideological belief systems.[2] Your own abilities to think critically, to avoid logical fallacies and to demonstrate integrity are put to the test. Denial is not a big river in Egypt.

BMA policy is that homeopathic remedies should not be funded by the NHS unless and until there is plausible evidence of their effectiveness. That is a standard applied across medicine, and it is surprising that the government has not acceded to the request that the National Institute of Clinical and Healthcare Effectiveness (NICE) should prepare a report on the cost effectiveness of homeopathic remedies and their use in the NHS. In Scotland, Lothian Health Board consulted in 2012 and withdrew funding in 2013. Other politicians must answer as to why they are dilatory is this regard. The US is the Land of the Free and allows the sale of many remedies. Medicines are regulated, but given homeopathic remedies contain no therapeutically active atoms and are not medicines, regulation is difficult. In China, Mao Zedong at first wanted to set Traditional Chinese Medicine and acupuncture aside – but the cost of providing orthodox medicine was simply too great, and barefoot doctors and TCM became the norm in most rural areas.

Macro-economics have a part to play. Until the 1760s and the advent of the industrial revolution, all the world's cultures were based on agriculture. A hundred years later and service industries became the dominant sector. Another hundred years and information technology has brought about a worldwide revolution. We are simply running out of work for us all to do. The healthcare sector is attracting ever more attention, encouraged by some universities which, for a fee, offer a degree in science for the study of pseudo-science. Should this be accepted? Patients and the students themselves might be misled. Likewise the tax payers who are expected to provide funding.

It is hardly in the best interest of politicians to limit the activities of alternative medicine practitioners, nor to deny the desires of voters who ascribe benefit to their systems. That way lies censorship and a nanny state. Fortunately CAM generally avoids serious complications by virtue of the fact that most procedures and remedies do nothing beyond the placebo, and placebos are pleasing. As Jeremy Hunt, UK Secretary of State for Health remarked in a letter to a constituent: 'Homeopathic care is enormously valued by thousands of people.' But so what? He has no evidence that homeopathic remedies effect any specific disease. BMA policy does not oppose 'homeopathic care', just expenditure on homeopathic 'remedies' – unless and until NICE reports.

A problem arises with closer critical analysis of such policies. If a politician, healthcare manager, insurer, celebrity, or even registered doctor allows or encourages un-critical provision of alternative systems of medicine, if they are prepared to be associated with systems for which there is no plausible objective evidence of benefit, if they vicariously support those systems by endorsement and encouraging the interest of others, then we are bound to ask – where will it end? Is there no limit to the time, trouble and funds which might reasonably be expended on these hedonistic systems? On what basis will such treatments and procedures be rationed?

If the transmission of non-existent forces by hand waving, needling of non-existent channels, manipulating non-existent subluxations, prescribing pills with non-existent active ingredients, and herbs with non-existent vital forces is to be funded, then why not angelic healing, crystal ball gazing, tarot card reading? Why not anything which gives pleasure to a sufferer such as free tickets to entertainments or visits to the gardens of Highgrove House? On what basis are those who have faith in angels, crystals, cards or stars to be discriminated against? That is for the politicians to decide. You must be the judge of their decisions.

In September 2012 David Cameron appointed as Secretary of State for Health, Jeremy Hunt, who had stated in a letter to a constituent in 2007 that he supported the spending of public money on homeopathy. Ben Goldacre suggests his appointment was akin to appointing someone who believes in perpetual motion as Secretary for Transport.[3] In August 2013 Mr. Hunt changed tack and speaking on BBC radio he made it clear: 'I don't support homeopathy. I need to follow the science and what science says, what the evidence says. I support doing what the scientific evidence says.'[4] Progress.

The House of Commons Science and Technology Committee Report on Homeopathy concluded: 'By providing homeopathy on the NHS and allowing MHRA

(Medicines and Healthcare products Regulatory Agency) licensing of products which subsequently appear on pharmacy shelves, the government runs the risk of endorsing homeopathy as an efficacious system of medicine. To maintain patient trust, choice and safety, the government should not endorse the use of placebo treatments, including homeopathy. Homeopathy should not be funded on the NHS and the MHRA should stop licensing homoeopathic products.'

The Government Response demurred: 'We note the committee's view ... however we do not believe that this risk amounts to a risk to patient trust, choice or safety, nor do we believe that the risk is significant enough for the Department to remove the (healthcare commissioners') flexibility to make their own decisions.' Fair enough, but all patients must be properly informed that they are on their own to make their choices without guidance from NICE. The government's response was patronising and unworthy.

It is just as well that there is regulation of the manufacturing processes. Andy Lewis reports: 'Manufacturers of Bach Flower Remedies and various homeopathic products had their London factory inspected by the American regulators, as they export to the US. The report was damning. They found no control over broken glass entering their medical products, poor production processes resulting in one in six products failing to receive the homeopathic ingredient, poor labelling and lack of quality control on the products. The US authorities have placed the products on their 'red list' which means they will be seized if imported.'[5]

Professor David Colquhoun has set out a detailed account of the twenty or more regulatory authorities which purport to regulate camists – supposedly making sure their claims are honest, decent and truthful – but which in practice seem to promote the CAM, irrespective of its merits. Some regulators seem deep in denial and may be complicit in fraud. Politicians are implicated by default and by failure to act. Colquhoun opines: 'The regulation of alternative medicine in the UK is a farce. It is utterly ineffective in preventing deception of patients...None of the official regulators seem to be able to grasp the obvious fact that it is impossible to have any sensible regulation of people who promote nonsensical untruths.'[6]

Do politicians support CAM because it seems to be a cheaper alternative for assuaging patients concerns? Cheaper than allowing conventional practitioners the time to properly care for patients, to counsel and support them and offer the hope and consolation they need? You must be the judge.

Real Secrets of Alternative Medicine

This book considers how placebo effects can be harnessed to help sufferers better come to terms with their dis-ease, illness, disability, and achieve to the greatest extent possible a sense of satisfaction, health and well-being. At all times, the advice of qualified conventional health practitioners should be sought. The central concern has been to consider how modern evidence and science-based medicine developed, leaving behind a range of other practices as alternatives and how these alternatives give camees the benefits they desire. These desires are located in the cerebrum, along with hopes, aspirations, emotions, expectations, feelings of transcendence, senses of spiritual experience, and the dynamics of the *ego* and *id.*

All of us interested in the application of placebo effects, do care and try to offer consolation, hope and love. At all times clinical care and therapy is the responsibility of professional clinicians. Placebists offer condimentary care, providing pleasure but without substantial effect on disease processes. Such care will not provide completion of any conventional medicine and cannot be regarded as 'complementary'. Non-scientific medical systems cannot be integrated with conventional medicine without contaminating and corrupting modern scientific healthcare.

It is essential that anyone suffering significantly from emotional distress, or who is 'feeling on the edge' seeks professional help immediately. An excellent guide with this title is provided by the Royal College of Psychiatrists and should be consulted forthwith if indicated.[7]

For patients whose suffering requires professional attention, approaches formalised as 'talking therapies' may have a place. This term describes a distinct evidence based therapeutic approach taken by trained counsellors and psychotherapists. As newer approaches are shown to be more efficacious, outmoded ideas are left behind. That is a different approach from that of camists who remain faithfully wedded to their belief systems. 'Talking therapies' may benefit patients who have conditions which need evidence based treatments.[8] Camees are patients who have decided they want alternatives.

Cognitive Behaviour Therapy (CBT) is becoming a standard treatment for anxiety and depression when troublesome enough for professional attention. The Department of Health started its Improved Access to Psychological Treatments (IAPT) program in 2007 and in the first three years over a million people were helped.[8]

Whether camees seek professional medical attention or not, they do need consolation, hope and love. This is why many turn to camists. Many professionals regard CBT as a self-help therapy, very much dependent upon the patient's own engagement. This is not surprising given that it is within the patient that the suffering is felt.

Not every patient with a problem will need professional medical attention. Many patients feel they do not have an illness in any case. Medical attention can be expensive and hard to obtain – particularly in the developing world. Lay counselling has not only been shown to work, but represents a democratisation of medical knowledge and is empowering for patients. As Vickram Patel has put it: 'If there is to be health for all – all must be involved.'[9] Dr Patel has particular experience of introducing such a system in Goa where community workers are trained to intervene in cases of anxiety and depression. The principles of offering consolation, hope and love can be applied to all in need. Patients who might turn away from regular

361

medicine and seek solace in camistry can have useful support from placebists.

In the West, Eastern practices developed to assist meditation, particularly within the Buddhist tradition, have been adapted as *Mindfulness:* 'the intentional, accepting and non-judgmental focus of one's attention on the emotions, thoughts and sensations occurring in the present moment.' Having studied Buddhism and Zen, in 1979 Professor Jon Kabat-Zinn founded the University of Massachusetts' Mindfulness-Based Stress Reduction (MBSR) program to treat the chronically ill. This led to mindfulness ideas and practices being used for the treatment of a variety of conditions in both healthy and unhealthy people. Mindfulness practice is being used by psychologists to treat obsessive-compulsive disorder, anxiety and to prevent relapse in depression and drug addiction, but has also gained worldwide popularity as a distinctive method and starting point to handle emotions and stress in people with no identifiable psychological illness. As such it is not an 'alternative therapy' and not a CAM.

Complementary, Condimentary and Alternative medical systems do have their attractions. Their proponents cite 'customised lifestyle management', 'person-oriented care', 'dietary advice', 'detailed evaluation not being dependant on time', 'engagement with the healing power of nature', as being important elements of the therapies they offer. Well and good – but this is no more than conventional doctors and healthcare professionals should and will be doing subject to the pressures of time and funding. So what is the added value of camistry? Not a lot, except a nicely branded package of care, consolation and concern. As Edzard Ernst has advised: 'Nothing wrong with that, as long as you don't fall for the hype of those who promote it.'[10]

We have moved on from the days of myth, superstition and the supernatural. We now have alternatives. There should be no need to resort to the occult, thaumaturgic and hermetic. Beliefs in nothingness may not merit much esteem, but patients who nevertheless desire, want and claim a need for nothingness must themselves be respected and supported as they travel the path they have chosen – the path of nothingness, *wudo,* the way of *wu.*

Camees will find attraction in a variety of CAM systems for a variety of reasons – most of which are psychologically repressed and cannot be well articulated. Few camees get beyond 'it seems to me...' or 'it worked for me'. Most are unable to distinguish type I placebo effects from type II effects on disease, or identify what it was that 'worked' for them. The ethical placebist can support patients with consolation, hope and love – but should never suggest or imply that conventional advice is set aside. And should not attempt to explain something until sure there is something to explain (Hyman's Maxim).[11] Placebos are no substitute for conventional care, but camistry may provide patients with the benefits of being condimentary. And that may provide the consolation, hope and solace patients seek.

Endnotes to Chapter 20

1.http://www.plosone.org/article/info:doi/10.1371/journal.

2. 'Manager': from Latin *manus,* hand – hence, 'one who handles'. In a discussion on the deity, the surgeon suggested 'God is clearly a surgeon, for did he not make Eve from Adam's rib?' 'I think not,' replied the manager. 'He is a manager, given that he brought order out of chaos.'. 'No,' countered the politician, 'He is a politician – who do you think created the chaos in the first place?'

3. http://blogs.telegraph.co.uk/news/tomchiversscience/100179258/jeremy_hunt.

4.http://www.dcscience.net/BBC%20Radio%205%20Live%20DC%20Eames.mp3
Also discussion on video at http://www.dcscience.net/?page_id=6105#060813

5.http://www.quackometer.net/blog/2012/08/boots-unconcerned-about-nelsons-products.

6. David Colquhoun (2012). *Regulation of Alternative Medicine – why it doesn't work.* sumj.dundee.ac.uk/data/uploads/epub-article/016-sumj.epub.pdf

7. http://www.rcpsych.ac.uk/mentalhealthinfo/problems/feelingontheedge.aspx

8.www.dh.gov.uk/prod_consum_dh/groups/dh_digitalassets/documents/digitalasset/dh_123 985

9. Vikram Patel. www.TED.com. 12th June 2012.

10. http://edzardernst.com/2014/12/aromatherapy-not-much-more-than-a-bit-of-pampering

11. Ray Hyman, quoted by James Alcock in Joe Nickell, *Psychic Sleuths.* Prometheus Books, Buffalo, 1994.

Bonus Chapter.

Wudo

Those kind friends who suggest a person suffering from a tedious complaint, that he "had better try alternatives to orthodox medicine", are apt to enforce their suggestion by adding, that "at any rate it can do no harm."
This may or may not be true as regards the individual. But it always does very great harm to the community to encourage ignorance, error, or deception in a profession which deals with the life and health of our fellow creatures.
Oliver Wendell Holmes Snr

The universe is full of magical things patiently waiting for our wits to grow sharper.
Eden Phillpots[1]

It seems a depressing reality that while desperate people exist to exploit, scientific reality will often be ignored and dubious fictions substituted in its stead.
David Robert Grimes[2]

Science is founded on the conviction that experience, effort and reason are valid; magic on the belief that hope cannot fail nor desire deceive.
Branislaw Malinowski

Hello clouds, hello sky.
Basil Fotherington-Thomas[3]

The compound word *Wudo* has been conjured to capture the approach to healthcare and well-being chosen by camees and camists who favour an esoteric flavour to healthcare. Wudo is a more arcane lifestyle path and philosophy. Formed by combining *wú* (Chinese: nothing, nothingness, without – as in *wú lì*, non-sense) together with *dō* (Japanese: 'the way or path' – Chinese, *tao*). As in *judo,* the way of gentleness; *shinto,* the way of the spirit, *chadō,* the way of powdered green tea and preparation of its magical properties. Just as practitioners of judo are *judoka,* so followers of *wudo* are *wudoka* (Japanese: *ka,* practitioner). Additionally, *wu* without the inflection means 'spirit medium; shaman; magician; witch doctor'.[4] Either use and both meanings are apposite here.

Wudoka who engage with more paranormal and supernatural aspects of healthcare, may have been disappointed with orthodox medicine, need more time and trouble spent on them, or simply be disenchanted with a scientific approach to healthcare. They may not fully appreciate the background, history, and context of their chosen 'way'. It is for them this book will have particular resonance, as they seek to make wise choices and avoid being misled, taken advantage of, exploited, gulled, hoaxed, given false hope, duped and defrauded.

Wudo requires suspension of belief in rationality and a willingness to accept the authoritarian premises of wise gurus, teachers or founders of alternative healthcare and medical systems. There are many systems to choose from and choices must be made wisely. There may be some anecdotal evidence to support the beliefs held, but this does not meet the standards of science. Evidence of the effectiveness of CAM is based on ideas of innate intelligence, vital forces, the imagination and intuitive experience of perhaps one person, a guru, a relative, or even a personal revelation. Anecdotes abound (French: secret or private stories). Research is carried out to prove camistry does work, not to determine whether it does. Controls are inadequately used. Meaningful statistics are sparse.

Wudo is not itself an established faith, but rather an approach to dealing with belief. In the case of healthcare, a belief in pseudo, non, or even anti-scientific principles. That is, in nothingness, without reason. Therefore – a matter of faith and wishful thinking.

Wudoka also need to consider *Ka Ching* (Japanese: *ka,* practitioner; Chinese, *ching,* great book). The Chinese *I Ching* is a divination system originating five thousand years ago. Hexagrams set down in the *Great Book of Changes* enable the developing balance of opposites to be predicted. This is reflected as the principles of *yin* and *yang* and concepts of harmony. *Ka Ching* will appeal to practitioners who seek harmony in the human spirit – a concept which is dear to the hearts of Wudoka. Of course, *ka-ching* could also represent the onomatopoeic sound of cash registers as quacks rack up further profits from the unsuspecting and gullible. You must be the judge.

The terms *wú* or *wu* can also be applied to all other fields of human endeavour, wherever there is absence of critical thinking and faith in an amorphous transcendent nothingness. It has been intimated that important economic and political decisions have been made on no substantial basis whatsoever and financial crises have resulted.

Suggestions that 'at least CAM does no harm' should be set aside. The most important and real issue is not whether camistry can cause harm, but whether it can have any plausible reproducible beneficial effects beyond placebo. It can be a red herring to claim no harm is caused - a logical fallacy, and misleading. However, by creating and endorsing mind sets susceptible to *wu* and encouraging wudo, CAM can have a most malign and harmful influence. An individual patient may well benefit from camistry. If that is what they believe, let us hope so – but the mind-set of a body politic which accepts wudo can have unintended consequences. The corrosive effect of pseudo-science makes it all the harder to identify what does and does not have a genuine beneficial effect on patients and their pathologies. All the harder to support the carers and counsellors who are genuinely helping patients. All the harder for patients to find caring professionals who practice with integrity. The negative influence of nonsense harms us all.

Can Camistry and Wudo do harm?

All medical practice can harm – but camists generally fail to properly inform patients as to risks of their systems. Camees seem not to fully understand or comprehend the issues. Dishonest camists may convince uncritical thinkers that camistry is a rational and effective approach.

Camees may be lulled into a false sense of security, even to the extent of shunning conventional medical practitioners and ceasing to take conventional medicines they need. They may be given false hope, and charges may be high and unjustified. Patients may be attracted to the world of the supernatural, esoteric and hermetic and lured to wudo. Lack of critical thinking and irrationality undermines the steady progress being made by medicine, affecting the mindset of whole communities and society beyond healthcare.

Illness behaviour may be encouraged – a motivational state which may further entrench chronicity. Gordon Waddell referred to this state as being 'actions and conduct which express and communicate the individual's own perception of disturbed health.' This may be out of proportion to the underlying physical disease and part of a cognitive and affective disturbance. This does not imply malingering (a conscious attempt to mislead), but does suggest that the biomedical model of health, may not be adequate to account for all a patient's experience.[5] At present, science is unable to shine a light on the more occult corners of human imagination.

If 'remedies' in homeopathic pillules really can beneficially affect disease, just think of the 'memories' of toxins and poisons also present which might cause harm. If freeing blood flow, 'innate intelligence', 'subluxation', 'vital forces', *ch'i*, 'healing energy' has any beneficial effect, just think of how a manipulation, a needle, a transmitted 'energy' might be just a fraction misplaced – and cause harm. Does your camist discuss this? Have you all the information on the risks? Does the camist? Have health and safety checks on these novel treatments been carried out? Or perhaps the proposed treatments are harmless, offering only *wu*. You must be the judge.

A particular problem arises if patients suffering from the most serious problems are unduly attracted to camistry. The US National Institutes of Health, National Center for Complementary and Alternative Medicine counsels:

> Beware of Cancer Treatment Frauds: The U.S. Food and Drug Administration (FDA) and the Federal Trade Commission (FTC) have warned the public to be aware of fraudulent cancer treatments. Cancer treatment frauds are not new, but in recent years it has become easier for the people who market them to reach the public using the Internet. Some fraudulent cancer treatments are harmful by themselves and others can be indirectly harmful because people may delay seeking medical care while they try them, or because the fraudulent product interferes with the effectiveness of proven cancer treatments. The people who sell fraudulent cancer treatments often market them with claims such as 'scientific breakthrough,' 'miraculous cure,' 'secret ingredient,' 'ancient remedy,' 'treats all forms of cancer,' or even 'shrinks malignant tumors.' The advertisements may include personal stories from people who have taken the product but such stories and 'testimonials' – whether or not they're real – aren't reliable evidence that a product is effective. Also, a money-back guarantee is not proof that a product works.[6]

Statistics suggest that Apple's founder Steve Jobs, whose neuro-endocrine pancreatic tumour was treatable by radiotherapy and who had a liver transplant late in the day, might still be alive had he not initially decided to treat his cancer by diets.

Every penny and minute spent on alternative treatments could have been spent on conventional medicine, counselling and care. Harriet Hall has commented 'It is irresponsible to recommend that rheumatoid arthritis patients try treatments like bee-sting therapy, feverfew, and homeopathy while avoiding mention of the proven benefits of disease-modifying anti-rheumatic Drugs.'[7]

Spending time with camistry represents the opportunity foregone to have done something else – the 'opportunity costs'. The time and trouble taken by an attentive empathetic practitioner in a constructive therapeutic encounter will provide benefit through placebo effects. That is what all conventional practitioners do and would like to do more if time allowed. But practices prescribing ineffective remedies, waving hands, releasing innate energies and influencing vital forces take time, trouble and funding which can scarcely be afforded by tax payers on behalf of society, let alone enthusiastic individuals.

Today's CAM systems are founded on outmoded precepts and philosophies. Medicine and healthcare has moved on. Not in opposition to outdated concepts but simply by taking the most effective ideas and progressing. Science can never prove anything to the ultimate extent, but we now have alternatives to ancient ideas based on plausible, reproducible evidence. King James I declared 'The age of miracles is past' in 1603.

This book describes ways of utilising placebo effects. It is a given that patients are fully informed that is the intention and that the science behind it remains of poor quality. *Real Secrets* offers no opposition to CAM, but the hope is that understanding will widen and enable patients to be fully informed when making healthcare choices. One of the most comprehensive lists of academic articles on the harmful effects of CAM can be found on a veterinary website.[8] As Scott Replogle points out – any therapy which has any actual influence on the body's processes will also have the potential for unintended effects, some of which may do harm.

The adverse effects of homeopathy have recently been reported in a systematic review of thirty eight primary studies.[9] Of these, thirty adverse effects were direct and due to the homeopathic remedies themselves (some of which seemed to have contained heavy metals), eight were indirect effects. These were potentially more serious as they were caused by standard conventional medicine being ignored and substituted with homeopathic. 11% of patients at Bristol Homeopathic Hospital reported adverse effects of headaches, lethargy or vomiting. Homeopaths recognise these effects and refer to them as 'homeopathic aggravations'. Any preference for homeopathy over conventional medicine is clearly fraught with risk. The more serious the condition, the greater the risk. Certainly any clinician knowing a patient is partial to homeopathy, or any other CAM, must discuss the risks with them.[10]

Some insightful homeopaths do recognise the harm their practice may cause. Luc De Schepper of the Institute of Homeopathic Medicine has commented:

At this point the greatest threat to homeopathy comes not from allopathic practitioners or pharmaceutical companies but from self-professed homeopaths who do not follow the immortal laws and principles laid down by Hahnemann. These pseudo-homeopaths violate the most basic principle of homeopathy: to give a single remedy which covers the totality of the symptom picture. I know of practitioners who are trying to create for themselves the prestige and status of allopathic physicians, imitating the lab coats and stethoscopes as well as the polypharmacy of allopathy. Typically these patients suffer aggravations lasting weeks or months while the homeopath offers no succour. But polypharmacy (giving many prescriptions at once) is harmful in homeopathy as well as in allopathy. Remember that the remedies bear a powerful force.[11]

The basic premise of CAM is that conventional medicine is in error, and that the CAM provides an entirely different, superior way to cure disease. Many patients recognise the implausibility of the camists' claims and take them with a metaphorical pinch of salt along with their regular medicine as may be required. But some patients do not have appropriate insight and the path of *wu* might be dangerous for them. Some camists now prefer to style their systems not as 'alternative' but 'complementary', thereby hoping to imply they complete regular orthodox treatment in some mysterious way. Still others use the term 'integrated', not simply to imply that conventional care should be integrated with social, economic, environmental determinants of health – agreed – but that CAM should actually be incorporated into orthodox care. That is a matter of marketing of metaphysics and belief systems, not practicing medicine. Healthcare conference programmes, college prospectuses, and policy statements need careful scrutiny to spot whether CAM is being smuggled onto the agenda. Camists are often coy about their real intentions of insurgency. Bait and switch as some have suggested. Buyer beware.

Additionally, commissioners, regulators and politicians have the challenge of protecting the public from abuse, fraud and ineffective health care. Rationing must be rational. Quackademic research and outcomes reporting must be approached with scepticism.

The greatest harm of camistry and wudo is *malacephaly:* cerebral softening as a result of fudge, fallacies, fantasy and fraud (*malakos,* soft; *cephale,* head). The very words used by camists points to an attempt to deceive and mislead. Why else would they refer to 'integrative medicine', said by some to represent a 'synthesis of the best ideas and practices of conventional and alternative medicine.' But as said by others – if it works it will be medicine. Why refer to 'complementary approaches' – when they do not complete anything? Why not be honest and declare that for those who like that approach, CAM is alternative *to* rational medicine?

Beware the standards accepted in some countries where practitioners are allowed to claim their CAM remedies can cure serious conditions such as cancer and Aids or render vaccination unnecessary. The UK's Cancer Act (1939) prohibits public advertisements offering to treat cancer, but conferences are still held to consider 'what practitioners have said about certain matters', disclaiming this constitutes illegal 'offers to treat'.[12] Vast sums are spent; lives are lost. In the long run, the promulgation of false beliefs, lack of critical thinking and a weakening of commitment to scientific medicine can benefit no one. Giving patients false hope is simply unethical.[12] The aim of revealing the *Real Secrets* is to enlighten readers, not to save the world from quacks, con-artists, scamists and fraudsters.[14] There, readers must accept their own responsibility – and must be the judge. May the *wu* be with you.

Endnotes to Bonus Chapter

1. *A Shadow Passes* (1919). Often misattributed to WB Yates and even Bertrand Russell (sometimes with one or two words changed). The best-known works by Phillpotts were part of a series set on Dartmoor. Phillpotts was suggesting that there are many other 'magical things' that will be revealed as our knowledge and capabilities grow.

2. http://www.theguardian.com/science/blog/2015/jul/15/autism-how-unorthodox-treatments-can-exploit-the-vulnerable.

3. Geoffrey Willans in *Down with Skool!*

4. Gary Zukav, *The Dancing Wu Li Masters.* 1979. New York. William Morrow and Co.

5. Gordon Waddell et al. *Chronic low-back pain, psychological distress, and illness behaviour.* Spine 9 (2), 1984. G. Waddell et al, *Symptoms and signs: physical disease or illness behaviour?* BMJ (Clin Res Ed). 1984 September 22;289 (6447).
Waddell's papers emphasise the importance of distinguishing illness behaviour from physical disease. This has been a major component of my analysis of claimants for personal injury compensation in my role as an expert medical witness to the courts.

6. http://nccam.nih.gov/health/cancer/camcancer.htm?nav=upd

7. Harriet Hall www.sciencebasedmedicine.org/index.php/anderew-weilaafp-article.

8. Scott L. Replogle MD: www.skeptvet.com/index.php?p=1_21_What-s-The-Harm.

9. P. Posadzki, A. Alotaibi, E. Ernst. *Adverse effects of homeopathy: a systematic review of published reports and case series.* International Journal of Clinical Practice. Blackwell Publishing. 66:   doi: 9.1111/ijcp.12026. December 2012.

10. Edzard Ernst, M.H. Pittler, B. Wider, K. Boddy. *The Desktop Guide to Complementary and Alternative Medicine*, Edinburgh, Elsevier Mosby, 2006.

11. Luc De Schepper. *The Real Danger to Homeopathy: Pseudo-Homeopathy.* http://instituteforhomoeopathicmedicine.wordpress.com/2014/05/17/the-real-danger-to-homeopathy-pseudo-homeopathy

12. http://www.telegraph.co.uk/news/uknews/11624590/cancer-patients-offered-bogus-cures-by-alternative-medicine-practitioners.html

13. Kevin Smith. *The Ethics of Homeopathy.* Bioethics, October 2012. http://onlinelibrary.wiley.com/doi/10.1111/j.1467-8519.2010.01876.x/abstract.

14. In my initial draft I inadvertently typed 'fraudstars'. That might be apposite.

A final conservation with Mrs. Smith

'Well Mrs. Smith, I've done as you suggested and my book is before you. In order to answer your question as to whether alternative medicine might help you I had to review the whole scope of human evolution from the creation until now. I have had to try and understand why it is that some people want to use alternatives to scientific evidence based medical systems and why some people are prepared to practice alternatives and endorse non-scientific approaches. We are alive, we dream, we imagine. Medicine, represented by conventional, orthodox, mainstream practices has changed and, under the revelation of scientific methods – always will. Old ideas will be discarded; the new will follow.

It seems some people prefer alternatives to such medical systems. They feel more comfortable with the occult, supernatural and the magic of thaumaturgic medicine. Their right to hold such beliefs should be respected. There are a plethora of practices originating with the heightened imaginations of their founders and many continuing to be practiced by enthusiastic believers today. There is no plausible rationale for these CAM systems. If there was, they would be conventional. I suggest they are *condimentary*. Their use provides flavour and pleasurable feelings but has no substantial effect on any pathological or physical process.

This book is about trust and truth, which the Oxford English Dictionary has as: 'that which is true or in accordance with fact or reality.' That requires doctors, nurses and health professionals to practice with integrity, be honest about the basis of their beliefs and obtain fully informed consent from patients. Many practitioners try to avoid the term 'alternative', preferring instead 'complementary' and suggest their practice can be 'integrated'. You must judge how honest they are, whether they are seeking to mislead you and whether they are quacks or even frauds.

CAM works – by magic and sex. The same neuro-chemicals released by a mysterious performance and by intimate human relationships engage deep seated neurological pathways and create pleasure. Camistry can provide pleasurable effects as the result of a constructive therapeutic relationship with an empathic practitioner. Manipulation may benefit the local part, but that is a technique not used exclusively by camists. The hand waving, needling and release of occult intelligences, vital forces or energies do nothing. Engagement with spirits may help the soul but there are no effects on disease. The camist engages your imagination, creates a climate of heightened hope, raises your expectations and helps you focus on your own pleasurable feelings as the patterns of your mind are realigned. Whether this is a form of hypnosis or the manifestation of placebo effects is immaterial and a matter of semantics, not science – but camists prefer to keep these secrets from you.

Placebos and hypnosis both work. In practice, I see no difference except in details of the methods used. As a magician I create an illusion just as I said I would. As a hypnotist I suggest that your imagination will be focussed against a background of heightened expectation. As a placebist I must honestly tell you I am engaging placebo effects. As a clinician I need your permission to do so and I must avoid any lack of intellectual honesty and deceit – for that would make me a quack and fraud. How can you tell if a camist is honest and sincere or a fraudulent quack? I cannot advise you further – but I hope the revelations of the *Real Secrets of Alternative Medicine* will provide a basis for your healthcare choices and that you will be a wise judge.

Please bear in mind that all doctors are expected to offer consolation, hope and be compassionate – 'With head and heart and hand' as the motto of the British Medical Association has it. The duties of a doctor require that we do the best for our patients. It is hardly of the best to engage you in outmoded superstition, metaphysical philosophy and non-evidence based practices. Patients may well need more time, care and attention. They will certainly want consolation, hope and love. If a doctor cannot make provision personally, they should develop services which can – without resorting to the occult. Placebists are ideally placed to help doctors and nurses with this task.

That is why I campaign for doctors and members of the regular health professions to support further research into the neurosciences and the ethics of placebo practice, to investigate placebo effects scientifically, and to be honest and open about their use.[1] I share with Professor Michael Baum the hope that 'Hospitals such as the Royal London Homeopathic Hospital should be turned into centres for evidence-based, supportive care for people with life threatening or terminal illnesses. A centre with psychologists; masseurs; counsellors; art and music therapists. Unlike homeopathy, these therapies have been critically evaluated: they have been proven to enhance well-being. And add a research centre so we can further this area of healthcare. This will make a real difference to the quality of people's lives.'[2]

We all know that conventional medicine is not faultless but most conventional practitioners are doing all they can to see their treatments are offered on the basis of properly established clinical and cost-effectiveness. Please avoid the 'red-herring' and 'you too' fallacies which say that because conventional treatment is not perfect, it is acceptable for CAM not to be. Do not be diverted from the actual issue – the lack of effectiveness of CAM. And avoid the 'straw-man' fallacy of misrepresenting the position of orthodox practitioners, none of whom would claim medicine is perfect. All practitioners should act with intellectual integrity, strive to be honest and do all they can to use methods for which there is plausible evidence of clinical effectiveness.

Bear in mind that CAM can also do harm, directly or indirectly. Time and money may be wasted on ineffective treatments. Patients may delay or even avoid treatment from which they could benefit. Grooming by unscrupulous camists may encourage them become dependent and develop 'illness behaviour' with inappropriate attachment to diseases, real or imagined. Children are not able to give their own informed consent. Remedies may contain toxic molecules, most have not been tested, and none reach the standard of regulated medicines. Some manipulations can damage arteries and affect blood flow to the brain. Even if the treatment is gentle, or non-contact, there are issues. Doctors, nurses and healthcare practitioners should be doing their best for patients. Pandering to philosophical fancies and the whims of those who follow *wu* is patronising, paternalistic and unworthy.

Patients who choose to do so should have the right of access to alternatives to medicine and the pleasures of condimentary medicine. But tax payers and funders should have the right to say they do not want the resources they provide spent on treatments with no plausible reproducible scientific evidence of useful clinical effect. Above all, camists should demonstrate intellectual integrity. The practices of camistry can undermine efforts to educate and train healthcare practitioners on a basis of honesty and science. Attempts to integrate camist metaphysics into conventional health systems can only undermine the progress made over the centuries to establish healthcare and wellbeing on a sound scientific, rational and intellectually honest basis.

Cancer researcher David Grimes puts it well: 'By clinging to delusion, belief in alternative medicine denigrates the very wonder of science and medicine and the massive strides we as a species have made over the last century or so in understanding the world around us, and how our bodies work.'[3]

I hope all doctors, nurses, and all other regular healthcare practitioners, whether active or retired, will find some time to study the effects of placebos, act with integrity as placebists, and offer the support of consolation, hope and love to those who might otherwise turn to camistry.[4]

Conventional practitioners care more than you may think. That is the real secret. Thank you.'

Endnotes

1. The Campaign for Alternative Remedy Evaluation (CARE) has been founded to that end.

2. Michael Baum, quoted by Rose Shapiro: *Suckers. How Alternative Medicine Makes Fools of Us All.* Vintage, Random House. 2009.

3.http://www.irishtimes.com/opinion/homeopathy-does-not-work-beyond-a-placebo-effect-1.534500

4. Rev. Dr John Wesley's *On Visiting the Sick* does not impart information by a lecture, but wisdom by a sermon. Wesley admonished that empathy was lacking in eighteenth century England. His call for compassion to be effected by providing practical assistance to the sick, whether in mind, body or spirit, has not been bettered:

> Too many persons of large substance pass over on the other side. How contrary to this is both the spirit and behaviour of even people of the highest rank in a neighbouring nation! In Paris, ladies of the first quality, yea, Princesses of the blood, of the Royal Family, constantly visit the sick, particularly the patients in the Grand Hospital. And they not only take care to relieve their wants (if they need anything more than is provided for them) but attend on their sick beds, dress their sores, and perform the meanest offices for them. Here is a fashion that does honour to human nature. It began in France; but God forbid it should end there!

For further information about styles and titles
used in conventional orthodox medicine, bibliography, further guidance,
frequently asked questions and a glossary, refer to:

www.placedo.co.uk.

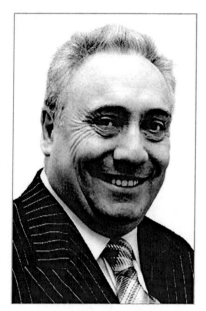

Richard Rawlins

Acknowledgements.

My patients have been most helpful in revealing the *Real Secrets of Alternative Medicine*. They have all given me priceless insights into their concerns and how they have come to terms with them. Audiences at my talks and lectures have asked particularly stimulating questions. My professional colleagues have offered significant support for my clinical practice. I am most grateful.

Colleagues in the British Medical Association, Royal College of Surgeons of England, British Orthopaedic Association, The Worshipful Society of Apothecaries, The General Medical Council, The Magic Circle and the Riviera Circle of Magic have likewise been influential.

I am grateful to the staff and librarians of those institutions and of the Wellcome Institute, the British Library, the King's Fund and the Royal Society of Medicine in London.

The advice of Nick Ross, Edzard Ernst, Bob Calleja, Rodney Croft, Keith Gould, Alan Henness and John Ransley has been much appreciated.

Jayne has been a major source of encouragement and strength. If I were American, I would wax emotional.

354 plexual for plural

CPSIA information can be obtained
at www.ICGtesting.com
Printed in the USA
LVOW12s2329010816
498612LV00045B/1463/P